Visual Aspects of Dyslexia

Visual Aspects of Dyslexia

Edited by

John Stein

Zoï Kapoula

OXFORD

UNIVERSITY PRESS

OXFORD
UNIVERSITY PRESS

Great Clarendon Street, Oxford, OX2 6DP,
United Kingdom

Oxford University Press is a department of the University of Oxford.
It furthers the University's objective of excellence in research, scholarship,
and education by publishing worldwide. Oxford is a registered trade mark of
Oxford University Press in the UK and in certain other countries

British Library Cataloguing in Publication Data
Data available

Library of Congress Cataloging in Publication Data
Library of Congress Control Number: 2012937859

ISBN 978–0–19–958981–4

Printed and bound by
CPI Group (UK) Ltd, Croydon, CR0 4YY

Contents

List of Figures

List of Abbreviations

AB	attentional blink
AM	attentional masking or amplitude modulation
BOLD	blood oxygen level-dependent
CIE	Commission Internationale de l'Elairage
CNS	central nervous system
CS	contrast sensitivity
DD	developmental dyslexia
DTI	diffusion tensor imaging
EEG	electroencephalogram
ERP	event-related potential
FM	frequency modulation
fMRI	functional magnetic resonance imaging
IPRGC	intrinsically photosensitive retinal ganglion cell
LCPUFA	long-chain polyunsaturated fatty acid
LGMV	local grey matter volume
LGN	lateral geniculate nucleus
LIP	lateral intraparietal area
MEG	magnetoencephalography
MMN	mismatch negativity
MRS	magnetic resonance spectroscopy
MTM	multitrace memory model
MT	middle temporal
NIRS	near infrared spectroscopy
OTC	occipital temporal cortex
PET	positron emission tomography
PPC	posterior parietal cortex
RT	reaction time
SAS	sluggish attentional shifting
SCN	hypothalamic suprachiasmatic nucleus
SFDI	spatial frequency doubling illusion
SLI	specific language impairment
SOA	stimulus onset asynchrony
TMS	transcranial magnetic stimulation
UCS	Uniform Chromaticity Scale
VA	visual attention
VBM	voxel-based morphometry
VWFA	visual word form area

List of Contributors

Elizabeth G. Conlon
School of Psychology and Griffith
Health Institute
Griffith University
Gold Coast, Queensland, Australia

Jean-François Démonet
Leenaards Memory Center
CHUV & University of Lausanne
Lausanne, Switzerland

Andrea Facoetti
Dipartimento di Psicologia Generale
Developmental & Cognitive
Neuroscience Lab
Università di Padova, Padova,
Unità di Neuropsicologia dello Sviluppo
Istituto Scientifico 'E. Medea'
di Bosisio Parini
Lecco, Italy

Burkhart Fischer
Optomotor Laboratory
Freiburg, Germany

Caroline Reilhac
Imagerie Cérébrale et Handicaps
Neurologiques, INSERM, UMRS 825
Université Toulouse III Paul Sabatier
Toulouse, France

Zoï Kapoula
IRIS group, UMR 8194
CNRS & University Paris V
Service d'Ophtalmologie
Hôpital Européen Georges Pompidou
Paris, France

Delphine Lassus-Sangosse
Centre du Langage et des troubles
des apprentissages
CHU Grenoble, France

Muriel Lobier
Laboratoire de Psychologie
et NeuroCognition
UMR CNRS 5105
Université Pierre Mendès France
Grenoble, France

Kristen Pammer
The Department of Psychology
The Australian National University
Canberra, Australia

Chris Singleton
Formerly with the Department
of Psychology
University of Hull
Hull, UK (now retired)

John Stein
Physiology Department
University of Oxford
Oxford, UK

Sylviane Valdois
French National Centre of
Scientific Research (CNRS)
Laboratoire de Psychologie
et NeuroCognition
UMR CNRS 5105
Université Pierre Mendès France
Grenoble, France

Trichur R. Vidyasagar
Department of Optometry &
Vision Sciences
The University of Melbourne,
Parkville, Victoria, Australia

Arnold Wilkins
University of Essex
Colchester, UK

Chapter 1

A Neurological Account of Dyslexia

Jean-François Démonet and Caroline Reilhac

Introduction

The neurological conceptualization of developmental dyslexia (DD), also termed specific reading disability, originates from the seminal work of Galaburda and co-workers who discovered microscopic abnormalities in the cytoarchitectonic structure of neocortical regions in the postmortem brains of a few subjects who were known to have received the diagnosis of dyslexia in life (Galaburda et al., 1985). Abnormalities such as ectopias were mainly located in cortical sites strategical for language processing; the authors suggested that dyslexic subjects might have suffered from disorders of cortical ontogenesis and especially impaired neuron migration from the germinal zone to the six-layered cerebral cortex.

While conjectures about the brain correlates of dyslexia had long been based only on the model of acquired dyslexia in adults, recent advances in brain imaging have allowed researchers to acquire considerable evidence about abnormalities of brain structure and function in subjects with DD (both children and adults) compared to standard readers. However, one should note that the neuropathological findings of Galaburda have still not been replicated, and neuroimaging results cannot yet be directly correlated with them because the spatial resolution of brain imaging in humans is not yet high enough. However, alongside neuroimaging, genetic studies have lent increasing support to the biological bases of DD, as they suggest links between a number of chromosomal loci and the typical cognitive deficits in DD. Furthermore, recent work has identified genes such as *DCDC2* and *KIAA0319* whose mutations induce abnormal neural migration during cortical ontogenesis, possibly hampering learning plasticity in the neural networks which support language processes (see, for instance, Meng et al., 2005; Paracchini et al., 2006; Rosen et al., 2007; for a review, Gabel et al., 2010).

This chapter covers some of the main results of brain imaging studies that can help us to understand the structural and functional brain abnormalities in adults and children with dyslexia.

Pathological findings and structural brain imaging

Pathology studies, as well as, more recently, morphological brain imaging mainly in adult subjects, concur to show structural brain abnormalities especially in the neocortex in dyslexics. At a microscopic level, from postmortem histopathology observations in the brain of some dyslexic adults, neural ectopias in the molecular outermost layer of the neocortex as well as dysplasias and microgyrification have been described, especially in perisylvian areas and the left hemisphere (Galaburda et al., 1985); cell abnormalities were also found in the lateral geniculate nuclei of the thalamus, particularly a diminished cell size in the magnocellular layers (Livingstone et al., 1991). More recent results in animal models from Galaburda's group now present evidence of cortical abnormalities resembling those described in the very few human pathology cases. In a mouse model, Jenner et al. (2000) showed that abnormal cortical connectivity is a possible consequence of cortical ectopias. This research line has clearly stimulated a neuroscience approach to DD, a condition that has too often been considered a purely functional learning impairment. The diversity of the language symptoms of dyslexia might be accounted for by the distribution of the microlesions throughout crucial cortical territories. These lesions seem to encompass different brain regions and the diverse localization of such cortical abnormalities would impede appropriate functional specialization in one or more key regions that make fluent reading possible, from visual analysis through phonological encoding, to automatized lexical access. Morphometric magnetic resonance imaging (MRI) studies in adult dyslexic subjects have shown clear brain structural abnormalities compared to standard readers (Habib, 2000; Leonard et al., 2001; Rae et al., 2002; Eckert et al., 2003). However, results have been highly inconsistent; this is probably explained by the small sample sizes, phenotypic heterogeneity, comorbidity, and a priori analyses limited to only a few regions of interest. The advent of statistically sounder methods for analysing structural brain signals in the whole encephalon from relatively large subject samples has yielded more consistent results.

Recent advances in image analyses such as voxel-based morphometry (VBM) have suggested abnormalities of local grey matter volumes (LGMVs) in the temporal cortex, especially in the left inferior temporal regions (e.g. Brown et al., 2001; Kronbichler et al., 2008). However, simple comparisons between impaired and control groups using this method may not be straightforward; results may be more consistent when corroborated by other evidence using different imaging modalities (e.g. positron emission tomography, PET: see Silani et al., 2005) and from the results of cognitive tests. For the latter, studies of correlations between cognitive performance and brain image signals across subjects have been especially revealing of the role of certain key regions, such as the inferior temporal cortex for reading, and the left superior temporal cortex for phonological processing. A recent VBM study using this correlational approach (Pernet et al., 2009) performed in relatively large samples of adult dyslexic and standard readers showed the following results.

First, no significant differences in LGMVs were found between the two groups, matched for non-verbal IQ,; this is at variance with what was claimed in earlier studies involving smaller groups and/or analyses limited to only regions of interest chosen a priori. Secondly, significant differences were obtained between the two groups by correlating LGMV with behavioural variables, namely time taken to read pseudowords aloud, accuracy of phoneme deletion, and for spelling irregular words. For each task, significant correlations were found in each subject group or between them in the following regions: the left superior temporal cortex, the ventral visual cortex, the lateral cerebellar cortex. It is worth noting that each of these results are congruent with one or the other of the main theories that have been put forward to account for the system-level dysfunctions in dyslexia, namely phonological processing (Ramus, 2004), visual decoding of orthography (Vidyasagar & Pammer, 2010), and learning-related cerebellar dysfunction (Nicolson & Fawcett, 2007). The effects found in this study in the cerebellum are particularly noteworthy as they provide one of the few pieces of evidence in favour of Nicolson and Fawcett's 'cerebellar' hypothesis that was not generated by their own group, which has been a source of scepticism. Overall, these results also highlight the phenotypic heterogeneity of dyslexia and show that, far from being mutually exclusive, the main pathophysiological theories of dyslexia probably each relate to one component of the causal mechanisms. Third, despite the negative results of the first anatomical comparison, a more detailed statistical study (Pernet et al., 2009), including subgroups of subjects defined by their cognitive performance, showed that the size of two very small areas in the right cerebellar hemisphere and the right neostriatum achieved very high discrimination between dyslexics compared with non-dyslexics. The right cerebellar site is the region which Stoodley and Schmahmann (2009) showed to activate consistently during language tasks.

Another recent technique introduced in neuroimaging is diffusion tensor imaging (DTI); the analysis of the 'anisotropy' of water diffusion in the brain. In simple terms, this involves measuring the uneven nature of the signal in various directions; anisotropy is especially important for signals associated with large bundles of white matter which generate highly-oriented signals in one direction across adjacent voxels, thus giving the direction of the tracts in a given anatomical location. Compared to normal readers, a decrease in white matter anisotropy has been found in dyslexics in several studies (Klingberg et al., 2000; Beaulieu et al., 2005; Deutsch et al., 2005). This lower anisotropy may reflect a poorer anatomical organization of the fascicles involved. These white matter microstructure disturbances mostly underlie the left temporoparietal junction, an area which is essential for the phonological mediation of reading. Importantly these abnormalities were often correlated with reading scores; lower anisotropy tended to be associated with poorer reading skills.

A number of studies have focused on specific white matter structures especially the corpus callosum and longitudinal fascicles (Frye et al., 2008; Keller & Just, 2009; Rimrodt et al., 2010). In a review paper, Ben-Shachar et al. (2007) reported a positive correlation between phonological performance and the diffusion signal perpendicular to the callosal fibres (and not along the major fibre axis); thus best-performing subjects had larger (though fewer) connection fibres between the two hemispheres, for a constant volume of the corpus callosum.

Functional brain imaging studies

Functional imaging provides indices of brain activity capturing either spontaneous or experimentally-induced variations; correlations are then sought between brain activity changes and experimental conditions (e.g. stimulus presentation against no stimulus; subject response against no response). Historically, the first techniques of this type used the electroencephalographic (EEG) signal, very often through the method of event-related potentials (ERPs), averaged over a time window of several hundred milliseconds during which time-locked effects could be related to the experimental conditions. More recent and costly, magnetoencephalography (MEG) provides more accurate anatomical information than EEG. The key feature of these two techniques is their ability to reveal changes in the neural assemblies supporting cognitive processes in real time. But more fine-grained anatomical resolution requires local electrical recordings that can only be performed during surgical procedures. As reading and writing are dynamic processes that develop over a few hundred milliseconds across neural networks distributed over the whole brain, real-time resolved EEG and MEG bring out crucial information. Many results have been obtained with these techniques in studies on DD. For a detailed review, see Salmelin and Kujala (2006).

Newborns at genetic risk of developing dyslexia present with abnormal auditory-evoked potentials (Guttorm et al., 2010) suggesting very early impairment of cortical processing. However, great phenotypic heterogeneity is seen on recording evoked potentials in adult-hood (Giraud et al. 2005, 2008). Only rarely have follow-up measurements been made as children grow older. Maurer et al. (2007) compared children at risk of dyslexia with control subjects without this risk; all underwent cognitive assessment and ERP measurements before and after initial reading teaching at school. The dyslexic children, unlike the controls, did not show normal development of a neural marker of the perceptual integration of letters (difference in the amplitude of the 'N1' component between perception of letter and symbol strings); there was a correlation between the amplitude of this marker and reading performance assessed at second grade.

Two methods for tomographic brain imaging can be used in a functional mode: PET and functional magnetic resonance imaging (fMRI). These techniques are used to measure indices of brain activity in the entire volume of the brain with good enough resolution to reconstruct images in millimetre slices or volumes; each image unit (or 'voxel') yields an activity rate. This activity is variable in time, spontaneously and under various experimental conditions, such as reading or phonological language tasks. These variations, although very weak, are subject to statistical calculations and estimation of the correlation between activity fluctuations in brain structures and cognitive processes manipulated in the experimental paradigm (for a review, see Démonet et al. 2005).

Functional imaging studies have revealed which brain areas involved in reading and cognitive processes are dysfunctional in dyslexia. Some limitations and methodological difficulties with these techniques must first be highlighted. PET is based on the use of water labelled with oxygen-15. This technique is very sensitive, but less used because of its high cost. In addition, it can not be used on children without clinical indications because of the use of radioactive tracers, even though the radiation dose is low. FMRI, however, is suitable for all subjects including children and has become the standard technique for functional neuroimaging, even though the blood oxygen level-dependent fMRI signal has a relatively low signal/noise ratio and poor time resolution. Brain correlates of language functions consist of low amplitude, transient events and are widely distributed throughout the brain. Variables such as the age of the subjects, handedness, their familiarity with the stimuli or experimental procedures, duration of stimulus presentation, and frequency of presentation can all affect the data collected and must be controlled for in any study (Démonet et al. 2005). Functional neuroimaging studies of language impairments are especially difficult as the task patients are required to complete must be carried out in spite of the language disorder whilst at the same time it should bring out effects relevant to the issue at stake. In the case of dyslexia, specific difficulties exist such as the phenotype diversity of deficits in qualitative and quantitative terms and the effects of compensatory mechanisms over childhood and adolescence.

Main results of functional neuroimaging studies

Georgiewa et al. (1999, 2002) were the first to report the results first only of fMRI studies and then combined with ERPs, comparing dyslexics with controls. Differences between the two groups were found using visual language tasks in the left inferior frontal cortex, between 250 and 600 ms (Georgiewa et al., 2002). Using a line or word detection task, Helenius et al. (1999) showed that dyslexic subjects had a deficit in prelexical processing usually involving the left inferior temporo-occipital cortex. However, the presence of a normal N100 suggested that early visual processing was normal. This conclusion is uncertain, however, since the same team reported early components that were abnormal, but in the auditory domain (Helenius et al., 2002).

In normal adult readers, the brain regions involved in isolated word reading are widely distributed but dominated by a left-hemispheric network with two posterior circuits and one anterior circuit (Pugh et al., 2000). The ventral or temporo-occipital circuit focuses on the fusiform gyrus (visual word form area or VWFA; Cohen et al., 2002) and seems to underlie letter string matching with their phonological equivalents; the dorsal or temporoparietal circuit includes the angular gyrus and supramarginal gyrus (Price et al., 1998); the precise interplay between these structures and circuits remains to be clarified. Recent work in effective connectivity describes the existence of an occipitoparietal link which would be involved in a global addressing and attentional system while a 'detour' between the parietal and occipital cortex via the fusiform VWFA would be necessary for the detailed assembly process (Levy et al., 2009).

The anterior circuit is mainly focused on the left inferior frontal gyrus and is connected to both posterior circuits (Price et al., 2001); it seems to be involved in phonological and articulatory processes in preparing oral production.

In adult dyslexics compared with non-impaired readers, a reduction in the activity of the posterior part of the reading system (occipital-temporal cortex and lateral parietal cortex) has been shown. Activation of the key region in the dorsal circuit, the angular gyrus, shows a positive correlation with reading scores in normal readers and a negative correlation in dyslexic subjects (Rumsey et al., 1999). A PET study (Paulesu et al., 2001) in well-compensated adult dyslexics and controls, from three different nationalities

(English, Italian, and French) described a lack of activation in the ventral circuit in dys-lexics whatever their mother tongue. These results match those reported in studies with MEG (Helenius et al., 1999).

Although the left inferior frontal region and right hemispheric regions seem less active in dyslexics in some studies (Paulesu et al., 1996; Rumsey et al., 1997), in others, on the contrary, the authors found an increase in activity suggesting mechanisms in premotor cortex that compensate for the disruption in posterior regions; this was shown in the left frontal cortex (Shaywitz et al., 1998; Brunswick et al., 1999; Georgiewa et al., 2002) and over right perisylvian regions (Simos et al., 2002).

Results obtained in children and adolescents complement and help interpret some of the discordant results from studies in adults. Shaywitz's group have made major contri-butions to this subject (see, e.g. Shaywitz & Shaywitz, 2008). Shaywitz et al. (2002) stud-ied 144 dyslexic and non-impaired children and showed that during a rhyme judgement task activity increases with age in the left and right inferior frontal regions only in chil-dren with dyslexia. These results support the compensatory hypothesis: increases in activation in frontal regions and/or right hemispheric regions reflect the way alternative brain circuits help to overcome the disruption in left posterior regions. Shaywitz et al. (2002) also showed that the decrease in brain activity in the ventral reading circuit observed in adults with dyslexia is not the result of continuing difficulties in reading since they found a positive correlation between the activity of this area and the level of reading in children with dyslexia. However, Simos et al. (2000) described in MEG stud-ies that this region had a level of activity in children with dyslexia comparable to con-trols and that the difference was located primarily in the time course of involvement of these brain areas: the neural activity from 250–1200 ms after stimulus presentation 'jumped' to the right temporal cortex in children with dyslexia (Simos et al., 2000) whereas in normal-readers it spread to the left temporal and parietal regions. Finally, van der Mark et al. (2009) studied the specialization of the occipital-temporal cortex in children with dyslexia, varying letter familiarity and lexicality. Unlike in control sub-jects, gradual specialization of the posteroanterior cortical response was not observed in the dyslexics.

In summary, these results suggest abnormal connectivity within temporal-parietal-frontal circuits involving language, perhaps particularly affecting the circuit underlying the working memory phonological loop. In addition, dyslexia affects the interaction between the 'dorsal and ventral circuits of reading' (as conceptualized by Pugh et al., 2000), which concur with the findings of other studies such as those by Horwitz et al. (1998) and Klingberg et al. (2000). Blomert's group has carried out two major studies in normal and dyslexic readers using a letter-to-sound matching task. First, they empha-sized the importance of the left superior temporal cortex in multisensory integration of speech sounds and written letters (a crucial step for reading acquisition) in skilled read-ers. This process was found to be impaired in adult dyslexics, and the superior temporal cortex, the neural structure mediating this processing, was underactivated compared to skilled readers (Blau et al., 2009). Secondly, they obtained similar results in normal early reading development with reduced neural integration of letter and speech sounds in the left superior temporal lobe (the planum temporale/Heschl sulcus and superior temporal sulcus) in dyslexic children compared to fluent readers (Blau et al., 2010).

All these results have been obtained in alphabetical languages. One intriguing issue is whether dyslexia would affect the underlying brain circuits in non-alphabetical, ideographic languages in a different way, as suggested by (Siok et al., 2004). A recent study (Hu et al., 2010) investigated how differences in the patterns of reading activation in dyslexic and skilled readers depend on the language spoken and its orthography (writing system). These authors showed, in a direct comparison of Chinese and English reading in monolingual subjects, that reduced brain activation for Chinese and English dyslexics is remarkably similar during semantic word matching. Furthermore, these similarities contrast with the activation differences between Chinese and English normal readers that they localized to the left inferior frontal sulcus (Chinese >English) and left posterior superior temporal sulcus (English >Chinese). This pattern of similarities and differences strongly suggests a common neural basis for dyslexia regardless of the language spoken and its orthography. Dyslexics from both cultures activated both the left inferior frontal and the superior temporal cortex; this suggests that culturally independent strategies are used when reading is less efficient. This result also illustrates that the neural underpinnings of reading are determined by the interaction of cognitive abilities and the learning environment.

An important issue to consider is the influence of reading performance on brain functional activation; very often dyslexic subjects are less proficient than controls when matched for chronological age and this must be controlled for by choosing younger reading age-matched controls. Hoeft et al. (2007), using fMRI and a visual word rhyming task, compared adolescent dyslexic with both chronological-age and reading-age matched control subjects. While hyperactivation was observed in the frontal regions in the dyslexic group relative to the chronological-age control group (as did Shaywitz's group), this difference was not seen when compared to the reading-age control group, suggesting that this hyperactivation reflected mainly reading performance and not the influence of dyslexia. By contrast, hypoactivation in left temporal and parietal cortex was consistently observed in the dyslexic group when compared with either of the control groups, suggesting that hypoactivation in these regions definitely reflects defective information processing for reading. Most interestingly, this study also involved a morphometric VBM study and revealed that the hypoactivated left parietal cortex also showed lower grey matter volume in the dyslexic subjects than in the chronological-age control subjects.

Pathophysiological hypotheses on dyslexia tested by neuroimaging

The numerous pathophysiological hypotheses about the origin of dyslexia have all received empirical support from neuroimaging studies confirming the existence of differential effects predicted. (Much greater progress would have been made if these empirical data had clearly spoken against one or other of the hypotheses!) These theories as to the aetiology of dyslexia can be classified into two types. The first postulates a deficit affecting processing of phonological or lexical representations stored in long-term memory. Second, a number of theories imply abnormalities affecting real-time sensorimotor processing; the deficits would hamper rapid processing of information in the magnocellular systems as well as the engagement and resources of attention (Stein & Walsh, 1997; Vidyasagar & Pammer, 2010) together with sensorimotor learning abilities that might especially rely on the cerebellum (Nicolson & Fawcett, 2007). Only some aspects of this abundant literature will be considered.

Because a phonological deficit is thought to be a predominant aetiological factor in dyslexia, the majority of functional imaging studies have evaluated these processes using rhyming tasks (Rumsey et al., 1997; Simos et al., 2000), verbal working memory tasks (Paulesu et al., 1996), or during the auditory presentation of verbal stimuli (Rumsey et al., 1992; Simos et al., 2000). Most studies have found a hypofunction of perisylvian regions particularly in the left hemisphere. Paulesu et al. (1996) suggested that the pattern found in individuals with dyslexia may be related to a disconnection in the left perisylvian circuit.

Our team has studied categorical perception of phonemes using PET and fMRI. Adult dyslexic subjects were found to have decreased activity in the left supramarginal gyrus (Ruff et al., 2002), a key region for phonological awareness (Demonet et al., 1996). Another recent study has focused on disorders of phonological categorization and the tendency of some dyslexics to discriminate incorrectly between acoustic variants of the same stop consonant; in these subjects Broca's region was overactive compared to other dyslexic subjects who did not show erroneous within-category discrimination. Among normal readers those showing increased activation in the same cluster in Broca's area were those who showed the best between-category discriminations; so we proposed that motor coding of speech supported this optimal phoneme discrimination. We therefore speculated that the subgroup of dyslexics we identified lack language based motor coding of acoustic variants of phonemes (Dufor et al., 2009). These findings are in line with the 'allophonic' theory of speech perception deficit in dyslexia proposed by W. Serniclaes (Serniclaes et al., 2001).

Temple et al. (2000) studied fMRI responses to rapid changes of the acoustic speech signal in fMRI and showed, in normal readers, an increased activation in the left inferior frontal region and the right cerebellar hemisphere during rapid as compared to slower changes of the acoustic signal. In dyslexic subjects, the authors noted an increase in activation in these regions for slow variations. Similarly, Nagarajan et al. (1999) found a decrease in subjects with dyslexia in the M100 obtained in MEG recordings in response to acoustic stimuli with rapid changes, whereas they had a larger M100 amplitudes than the controls for slower stimuli.

These effects were also studied with natural syllables (ma/na), sometimes modified by stretching the formant transitions (Ruff et al., 2002). Brain regions sensitive to acoustic changes were identified in the left frontal region; and the slowing of the transitions resulted in increased activation in this region for the dyslexic subjects. However, activation in the left supramarginal gyrus was not influenced by these acoustic variations, whereas this region is consistently shown to be hypoactive in adults with dyslexia. Two important effects involved in the basic mechanisms of dyslexia were thus identified by this study: first neuronal activity is enhanced by slowing of speech transitions in certain brain regions; and secondly absence of neuronal activity in the supramarginal gyrus is the likely 'signature' of the phonological awareness deficit so often seen in subjects with dyslexia. This dependence of different brain regions on speech rate could account for some of the discrepancies in the literature.

Measuring MMN (mismatch negativity) has proved especially relevant to the perceptual deficit hypothesis. This neurophysiological component is obtained by introducing in a repeating stimulus series an unexpected change. The MMN is independent of the subject's attentional engagement in the experiment (Kujala & Näätänen, 2001); this independence from attention suggests that it reflects an automatic process in the cortical neural populations responsible. Initial studies in children with a learning disorder showed a decrease in the amplitude of the MMN, but the specificity of this effect seems uncertain. Schulte-Körne et al. (1998) proposed that the MMN decrease relates to an impaired processing of language-specific features; Kraus et al. (1996) described the importance of a phonetic factor, the voice onset time (a temporal speech cue which allows speakers to discriminate the between 'ga' and 'ka', for example). By contrast, Baldeweg et al. (1999) described impaired MMNs in dyslexic subjects in a non-language experiment involving pitch changes in tones. These results represent neurophysiological correlates of the speech discrimination disorders seen in dyslexic subjects, although there is a large phenotype heterogeneity. Note that Giraud et al. (2005) have confirmed the existence of a disorder of temporal processing of the speech signal (lack of a characteristic electrophysiological component reflecting the specific processing of the pre-voicing sound of the phoneme 'b' which characterizes this phoneme in French) but only in a subgroup of dyslexics with severe disabilities, while another also markedly deficient subgroup showed an electrophysiological profile characterized not by the absence of this component but by multiple components. Further, an unpublished part of this study showed a *normal* electrophysiological profile in a third subgroup involving less severely impaired patients. Similar paradigms have allowed Leppänen et al. (1999) to compare children at genetic risk or not at risk of developing dyslexia: the results of these studies suggest that from the age of 6 months subjects with a family history of dyslexia process auditory stimuli differently.

In several studies, concordant arguments for a visual magnocellular system dysfunction have been reported. For example, Eden et al. (1996) found a lack of activation of area MT/ V5 during a task of motion detection and highlighted a correlation between the level of activation in area V5 and reading speed in dyslexic subjects and normal readers. However, other studies have not confirmed these results (Johannes, 1996; Vanni, 1997; Amitay, 2002). The effects of the magnocellular system seem in fact subtle and highlighted only under certain experimental constraints (Bednarek & Grabowska, 2002).

In collaboration with the group of Valdois, we have used fMRI to explore the hypothesis that dyslexic children have a deficient visual attention span. We used a variant of a visual letter discrimination task originally designed by Pernet et al. (2004, 2006) involving both a centrally presented letter and a parafoveal letter (either in the right- or left-visual hemifield); subjects were required to detect the (rare) trials in which the two letters differed. Visual attention load was differentially taxed according to whether the parafoveal stimulus was flanked or not by distracter letters. The dyslexic children performed the task as well as control readers, but more slowly. FMRI results involved only (no response) trials with matched letters; compared with control children, the dyslexics showed an activation deficit in parietal and temporal cortices in the flanked condition, but no difference was seen in the isolated condition. A statistically robust, specific effect was observed in a cluster in the left superior parietal lobule showing higher activation in the flanked condition in the control readers (regardless of the lateralization of the parafoveal stimulus), which was not seen in the dyslexic subjects, who showed reduced brain activity in this brain region. This very recent study strongly supports the idea that these 5th grade dyslexic children have a deficit in the magnocellular dominated, dorsal visual pathway. Importantly these children, while showing the typical reading deficit, had *normal* phoneme awareness performance.

Despite a very large amount of work in recent years results have been very variable. It is unlikely that a single unified theory will emerge from this phenotypic diversity. Psychological concepts from the fields of memory and perception and their applications to the corresponding neuropsychological domains may offer useful frameworks that could help clarify the neuropsychology of dyslexia. For instance, Nicolson and Fawcett (2007) rightly point out the importance of procedural memory; furthermore, the concept of categorical perception seems relevant to account for phonology-related speech perception; likewise, the framework of working memory with limitations of attention-driven buffers could probably help reconcile a number of research lines relating to perturbations of the dorsal visual pathway (see, for instance, Lallier, 2010). In any case acknowledging this phenotypic diversity seems the most sensible standpoint, as the genetic origin of dyslexia is highly likely to be diverse too. As already proposed (Ramus, 2004), dyslexia, conceived as a clinical syndrome, may result from diverse abnormalities of cortical ontogenesis that would involve disordered neuron migration in many different cortical regions. Depending on the location of these neuronal ectopias in a given subject different dyslexia phenotype may result, for instance a preponderance of phoneme awareness deficits might be associated with ectopias in the superior temporal cortex, while preponderance of microlesions in the parietal cortex would generate 'magno cell'-like dysfunctions.

References

Amitay, S., Ben-Yehudah, G., Banai, K., & Ahissar, M. (2002). Disabled readers suffer from visual and auditory impairments but not from a specific magnocellular deficit. *Brain*, 125, 2272–85.

Baldeweg, T., Richardson, A., Watkins, S., Foale, C., & Gruzelier, J. (1999). Impaired auditory frequency discrimination in dyslexia detected with mismatch evoked potentials. *Annals of Neurology*, 45, 495–503.

Beaulieu, C., Plewes, C., Paulson, L.A., Roy, D., Snook, L., Concha, L., & Phillips, L. (2005). Imaging brain connectivity in children with diverse reading ability. *NeuroImage*, 25, 1266–71.

Bednarek, D.B., & Grabowska, A. (2002). Luminance and chromatic contrast sensitivity in dyslexia: the magnocellular deficit hypothesis revisited. *NeuroReport*, 13, 2521–5.

Ben-Shachar, M., Dougherty, R.F., & Wandell, B.A. (2007). White matter pathways in reading. *Current Opinion in Neurobiology*, 17, 258–70.

Blau, V., van Atteveldt, N., Ekkebus, M., Goebel, R., & Blomert, L. (2009). Reduced neural integration of letters and speech sounds links phonological and reading deficits in adult dyslexia. *Current Biology*, 19, 503–8.

Blau, V., Reithler, J., van Atteveldt, N., Seitz, J., Gerretsen, P., Goebel, R., *et al.* (2010). Deviant processing of letters and speech sounds as proximate cause of reading failure: a functional magnetic resonance imaging study of dyslexic children. *Brain*, 133, 868–79.

Brown, W.E., Eliez, S., Menon, V., Rumsey, J.M., White, C.D., & Reiss, A.L. (2001). Preliminary evidence of widespread morphological variations of the brain in dyslexia. *Neurology*, 56, 781–3.

Brunswick, N., McCrory, E., Price, C.J., Frith, C.D., & Frith, U. (1999). Explicit and implicit processing of words and pseudowords by adult developmental dyslexics: A search for Wernicke's Wortschatz? *Brain*, 122, 1901–17.

Cohen, L., Lehéricy, S., Chochon, F., Lemer, C., Rivaud, S., & Dehaene, S. (2002). Language-specific tuning of visual cortex? Functional properties of the visual word form area. *Brain: A Journal of Neurology*, 125, 1054–69.

Demonet, J.-F., Fiez, J.A., Paulesu, E., Petersen, S.E., & Zatorre, R.J. (1996). PET Studies of Phonological Processing: A Critical Reply to Poeppel. *Brain and Language*, 55, 352–79.

Démonet, J.-F., Thierry, G., & Cardebat, D. (2005). Renewal of the neurophysiology of language: functional neuroimaging. *Physiological Reviews*, 85, 49–95.

Deutsch, G.K., Dougherty, R.F., Bammer, R., Siok, W.T., Gabrieli, J.D.E., & Wandell, B. (2005). Children's reading performance is correlated with white matter structure measured by diffusion tensor imaging. *Cortex*, 41, 354–63.

Dufor, O., Serniclaes, W., Sprenger-Charolles, L., & Démonet, J.F. (2009). Left premotor cortex and allophonic speech perception in dyslexia: a PET study. *NeuroImage*, 46, 241–8.

Eckert, M.A., Leonard, C.M., Richards, T.L., Aylward, E.H., Thomson, J., & Berninger, V.W. (2003). Anatomical correlates of dyslexia: frontal and cerebellar findings. *Brain*, 126, 482–94.

Eden, G.F., VanMeter, J.W., JRumsey, J.M., Maisog, J.M., Woods, R.P., & Zeffiro, T.A. (1996). Abnormal processing of visual motion in dyslexia revealed by functional brain imaging. *Nature*, 382, 66–9.

Frye, R.E., Hasan, K., Xue, L., Strickland, D., Malmberg, B., Liederman, J., *et al.* (2008). Splenium microstructure is related to two dimensions of reading skill. *NeuroReport*, 19, 1627–31.

Gabel, L.A., Gibson, C.J., Gruen, J.R., & LoTurco, J.L. (2010). Progress towards a cellular neurobiology of reading disability. *Neurobiology of Disease*, 38, 173–80.

Galaburda, A.M., Sherman, G.F., Rosen, G.D., Aboitiz, F., & Geschwind, N. (1985). Developmental dyslexia: four consecutive patients with cortical anomalies. *Annals of Neurology*, 18, 222–33.

Georgiewa, P., Rzanny, R., Hopf, J.M., Knab, R., Glauche, V., Kaiser, W.A., *et al.* (1999). fMRI during word processing in dyslexic and normal reading children. *NeuroReport*, 10, 3459–65.

Georgiewa, P., Rzanny, R., Gaser, C., Gerhard, U.J., Vieweg, U., Freesmeyer, D., *et al.* (2002). Phonological processing in dyslexic children: a study combining functional imaging and event related potentials. *Neuroscience Letters*, 318, 5–8.

Giraud, K., Démonet, J.F., Habib, M., Marquis, P., Chauvel, P., & Liégeois-Chauvel, C. (2005). Auditory evoked potential patterns to voiced and voiceless speech sounds in adult developmental dyslexics with persistent deficits. *Cerebral Cortex*, 15, 1524–34.

Giraud, K., Trébuchon-DaFonseca, A., Démonet, J.F., Habib, M., & Liégeois-Chauvel, C. (2008). Asymmetry of voice onset time-processing in adult developmental dyslexics. *Clinical Neurophysiology*, 119, 1652–63.

Guttorm, T.K., Leppänen, P.H.T., Hämäläinen, J.A., Eklund, K.M., & Lyytinen, H.J. (2010). Newborn event-related potentials predict poorer pre-reading skills in children at risk for dyslexia. *Journal of Learning Disabilities*, 43, 391–401.

Habib, M. (2000). The neurological basis of developmental dyslexia: an overview and working hypothesis. *Brain*, 123, 2373–99.

Helenius, P., Tarkiainen, A., Cornelissen, P., Hansen, P.C., & Salmelin, R. (1999). Dissociation of normal feature analysis and deficient processing of letter-strings in dyslexic adults. *Cerebral Cortex*, 9, 476–83.

Helenius, P., Salmelin, R., Richardson, L., Leinonen, S., & Lyytinen, H. (2002). Abnormal auditory cortical activation in dyslexia 100 msec after speech onset. *Journal of Cognitive Neuroscience*, 14, 603–17.

Hoeft, F., Meyler, A., Hernandez, A., Juel, C., Taylor-Hill, H., Martindale, J.L., *et al.* (2007). Functional and morphometric brain dissociation between dyslexia and reading ability. *Proceedings of the National Academy of Sciences of the United States of America*, 104, 4234–9.

Horwitz, B., Rumsey, J.M., & Donohue, B.C. (1998). Functional connectivity of the angular gyrus in normal reading and dyslexia. *Proceedings of the National Academy of Sciences of the United States of America*, 95, 8939–44.

Hu, W., Lee, H.L., Zhang, Q., Liu, T., Geng, L.B., Seghier, M.L., *et al.* (2010). Developmental dyslexia in Chinese and English populations: dissociating the effect of dyslexia from language differences. *Brain*, 133, 1694–706.

Jenner, A.R., Galaburda, A.M., & Sherman, G.F. (2000). Connectivity of ectopic neurons in the molecular layer of the somatosensory cortex in autoimmune mice. *Cerebral Cortex*, 10, 1005–13.

Johannes, S., Kussmaul, C.L., Münte, T.F., & Mangun, G.R. (1996). Developmental dyslexia: passive visual stimulation provides no evidence for a magnocellular processing defect. *Neuropsychologia*, 34, 1123–7.

Keller, T.A., & Just, M.A. (2009). Altering cortical connectivity: remediation-induced changes in the white matter of poor readers. *Neuron*, 64, 624–31.

Klingberg, T., Hedehus, M., Temple, E., Salz, T., Gabrieli, J.D., Moseley, M.E., *et al.* (2000). Microstructure of temporo-parietal white matter as a basis for reading ability: evidence from diffusion tensor magnetic resonance imaging. *Neuron*, 25, 493–500.

Kraus, N., McGee, T.J., Carrell, T.D., Zecker, S.G., Nicol, T.G., & Koch, D.B. (1996). Auditory neurophysiologic responses and discrimination deficits in children with learning problems. *Science*, 273, 971–3.

Kronbichler, M., Wimmer, H., Staffen, W., Hutzler, F., Mair, A., & Ladurner, G. (2008). Developmental dyslexia: gray matter abnormalities in the occipitotemporal cortex. *Human Brain Mapping*, 29, 613–25.

Kujala, T., & Näätänen, R. (2001). The mismatch negativity in evaluating central auditory dysfunction in dyslexia. *Neuroscience and Biobehavioral Reviews*, 25, 535–43.

Lallier, M., Tainturier, M.J., Dering, B., Donnadieu, S., Valdois, S., & Thierry, G. (2010). Behavioral and ERP evidence for amodal sluggish attentional shifting in developmental dyslexia. *Neuropsychologia*, 48, 4125–35.

Leonard, C.M., Eckert, M.A., Lombardino, L.J., Oakland, T., Kranzler, J., Mohr, C.M., *et al.* (2001). Anatomical risk factors for phonological dyslexia. *Cerebral Cortex*, 11, 148–57.

Leppänen, P.H., Pihko, E., Eklund, K.M., & Lyytinen, H. (1999). Cortical responses of infants with and without a genetic risk for dyslexia: II. Group effects. *NeuroReport*, 10, 969–73.

Levy, J., Pernet, C., Treserras, S., Boulanouar, K., Aubry, F., Démonet, J.F., *et al.* (2009). Testing for the dual-route cascade reading model in the brain: an fMRI effective connectivity account of an efficient reading style. *PloS One*, 4, e6675.

Livingstone, M.S., Rosen, G.D., Drislane, F.W., & Galaburda, A.M. (1991). Physiological and anatomical evidence for a magnocellular defect in developmental dyslexia. *Proceedings of the National Academy of Sciences of the United States of America*, 88, 7943–7.

Maurer, U., Brem, S., Bucher, K., Kranz, F., Benz, R., Steinhausen, H.C., *et al.* (2007). Impaired tuning of a fast occipito-temporal response for print in dyslexic children learning to read. *Brain*, 130, 3200–10.

Meng, H., Smith, S.D., Hager, K., Held, M., Liu, J., Olson, R.K., *et al.* (2005). DCDC2 is associated with reading disability and modulates neuronal development in the brain. *Proceedings of the National Academy of Sciences of the United States of America*, 102, 17053–8.

Nagarajan, S., Mahncke, H., Salz, T., Tallal, P., Roberts, T., & Merzenich, M.M. (1999). Cortical auditory signal processing in poor readers. *Proceedings of the National Academy of Sciences of the United States of America*, 96, 6483–8.

Nicolson, R.I., & Fawcett, A.J. (2007). Procedural learning difficulties: reuniting the developmental disorders? *Trends in Neurosciences*, 30, 135–41.

Paracchini, S., Thomas, A., Castro, S., Lai, C., Paramasivam, M., Wang, Y., *et al.* (2006). The chromosome 6p. 22 haplotype associated with dyslexia reduces the expression of KIAA0319, a novel gene involved in neuronal migration. *Human Molecular Genetics*, 15, 1659–66.

Paulesu, E., Démonet, J.F., Fazio, F., McCrory, E., Chanoine, V., Brunswick, N., *et al.* (2001). Dyslexia: cultural diversity and biological unity. *Science*, 291, 2165–7.

Paulesu, E., Frith, U., Snowling, M., Gallagher, A., Morton, J., Frackowiak, R.S., & Frith, C.D. (1996). Is developmental dyslexia a disconnection syndrome? Evidence from PET scanning. *Brain*, 119, 143–57.

Pernet, C., Franceries, X., Basan, S., Cassol, E., Démonet, J.F., & Celsis, P. (2004). Anatomy and time course of discrimination and categorization processes in vision: an fMRI study. *NeuroImage*, 22, 1563–77.

Pernet, C., Valdois, S., Celsis, P., & Démonet, J.F. (2006). Lateral masking, levels of processing and stimulus category: a comparative study between normal and dyslexic readers. *Neuropsychologia*, 44, 2374–85.

Pernet, C., Andersson, J., Paulesu, E., & Demonet, J.F. (2009). When all hypotheses are right: a multifocal account of dyslexia. *Human Brain Mapping*, 30, 2278–92.

Pernet, C.R., Poline, J.B., Demonet, J.F., & Rousselet, G.A. (2009). Brain classification reveals the right cerebellum as the best biomarker of dyslexia. *BMC Neuroscience*, 10, 67.

Price, C.J., Howard, D., Patterson, K., Warburton, E.A., Friston, K.J., & S.J. Frackowiak. (1998). A functional neuroimaging description of two deep dyslexic patients. *Journal of Cognitive Neuroscience*, 10, 303–15.

Price, C.J., Warburton, E.A., Moore, C.J., Frackowiak, R.S., & Friston, K.J. (2001). Dynamic diaschisis: anatomically remote and context-sensitive human brain lesions. *Journal of Cognitive Neuroscience*, 13, 419–29.

Pugh, K.R., Mencl, W.E., Jenner, A.R., Katz, L., Frost, S.J., Lee, J.R., *et al.* (2000). Functional neuroimaging studies of reading and reading disability (developmental dyslexia). *Mental Retardation and Developmental Disabilities Research Reviews*, 6, 207–13.

Rae, C., Harasty, J.A., Dzendrowskyj, T.E., Talcott, J.B., Simpson, J.M., Blamire, A.M., *et al.* (2002). Cerebellar morphology in developmental dyslexia. *Neuropsychologia*, 40, 1285–92.

Ramus, F. (2004). Neurobiology of dyslexia: a reinterpretation of the data. *Trends in Neurosciences*, 27, 720–6.

Rimrodt, S.L., Peterson, D.J. Denckla, M.B., Kaufmann, W.E., & Cutting, L.E. (2010). White matter microstructural differences linked to left perisylvian language network in children with dyslexia. *Cortex*, 46, 739–49.

Rosen, G.D., Bai, J., Wang, Y., Fiondella, C.G., Threlkeld, S.W., LoTurco, J.J., *et al.* (2007). Disruption of neuronal migration by RNAi of Dyx1c1 results in neocortical and hippocampal malformations. *Cerebral Cortex*, 17, 2562–72.

Ruff, S., Cardebat, D., Marie, N., & Démonet, J.F. (2002). Enhanced response of the left frontal cortex to slowed down speech in dyslexia: an fMRI study. *NeuroReport*, 13, 1285–9.

Rumsey, J.M., Andreason, P., Zametkin, A.J., Aquino, T., King, A.C., Hamburger, S.D., *et al.* (1992). Failure to activate the left temporoparietal cortex in dyslexia. An oxygen 15 positron emission tomographic study. *Archives of Neurology*, 49, 527–34.

Rumsey, J.M., Donohue, B.C., Brady, D.R., Nace, K., Giedd, J.N., & Andreason, P. (1997). A magnetic resonance imaging study of planum temporale asymmetry in men with developmental dyslexia. *Archives of Neurology*, 54, 1481–9.

Rumsey, J.M., Horwitz, B., Donohue, B.C., Nace, K.L., Maisog, J.M., & Andreason, P. (1999). A functional lesion in developmental dyslexia: left angular gyral blood flow predicts severity. *Brain and Language*, 70, 187–204.

Salmelin, R., & Kujala, J. (2006). Neural representation of language: activation versus long-range connectivity. *Trends in Cognitive Sciences*, 10, 519–525.

Schulte-Körne, G., Deimel, W., Bartling, J., & Remschmidt, H. (1998). Auditory processing and dyslexia: evidence for a specific speech processing deficit. *NeuroReport*, 9, 337–40.

Serniclaes, W., Sprenger-Charolles, L., Carré, R., & Demonet, J.F. (2001). Perceptual discrimination of speech sounds in developmental dyslexia. *Journal of Speech, Language, and Hearing Research*, 44, 384–99.

Shaywitz, B.A., Shaywitz, S.E., Pugh, K.R., Mencl, W.E., Fulbright, R.K., Skudlarski, P., *et al.* (2002). Disruption of posterior brain systems for reading in children with developmental dyslexia. *Biological Psychiatry*, 52, 101–10.

Shaywitz, S.E., & Shaywitz, B.A. (2008). Paying attention to reading: the neurobiology of reading and dyslexia. *Development and Psychopathology*, 20, 1329–49.

Shaywitz, S.E., Shaywitz, B.A., Pugh, K.R., Fulbright, R.K., Constable, R.T., Mencl, W.E., *et al.* (1998). Functional disruption in the organization of the brain for reading in dyslexia. *Proceedings of the National Academy of Sciences of the United States of America*, 95, 2636–41.

Silani, G., Frith, U., Demonet, J.-F., Fazio, F., Perani, D., Price, C., *et al.* (2005). Brain abnormalities underlying altered activation in dyslexia: a voxel based morphometry study. *Brain*, 128, 2453–61.

Simos, P.G., J.I.Breier, Fletcher, J.M., Bergman, E., & Papanicolaou, A.C. (2000). Cerebral mechanisms involved in word reading in dyslexic children: a magnetic source imaging approach. *Cerebral Cortex*, 10, 809–16.

Simos, P.G., Breier, J.I., Fletcher, J.M., Foorman, B.R., Bergman, E., Fishbeck, K., *et al.* (2000). Brain activation profiles in dyslexic children during non-word reading: a magnetic source imaging study. *Neuroscience Letters*, 290, 61–5.

Simos, P.G., Breier, J.I., Wheless, J.W., Maggio, W.W., Fletcher, J.M., Castillo, E.M., *et al.* (2000). Brain mechanisms for reading: the role of the superior temporal gyrus in word and pseudoword naming. *NeuroReport*, 11, 2443–7.

Simos, P.G., Fletcher, J.M., Foorman, B.R., Francis, D.J., Castillo, E.M., Davis, R.N., *et al.* (2002). Brain activation profiles during the early stages of reading acquisition. *Journal of Child Neurology*, 17, 159–63.

Siok, W.T., Perfetti, C.A., Jin, Z., & Tan, L.H. (2004). Biological abnormality of impaired reading is constrained by culture. *Nature*, 431, 71–6.

Stein, J., & Walsh, V. (1997). To see but not to read; the magnocellular theory of dyslexia. *Trends in Neuroscience*, 20, 147–52.

Stoodley, C.J., & Schmahmann, J.D. (2009). The cerebellum and language: evidence from patients with cerebellar degeneration. *Brain and Language*, 110, 149–53.

Temple, E., Poldrack, R.A., Protopapas, A., Nagarajan, S., Salz, T., Tallal, P., *et al.* (2000). Disruption of the neural response to rapid acoustic stimuli in dyslexia: evidence from functional MRI. *Proceedings of the National Academy of Sciences of the United States of America*, 97, 13907–12.

van der Mark, S., Bucher, K., Maurer, U., Schulz, E., Brem, S., Buckelmüller, I., *et al.* (2009). Children with dyslexia lack multiple specializations along the visual word-form (VWF) system. *NeuroImage*, 47, 1940–9.

Vanni, S., Uusitalo, M.A., Kiesilä, P., & Hari, R. (1997). Visual motion activates V5 in dyslexics. *NeuroReport*, 8, 1939–42.

Vidyasagar, T.R., & Pammer, K. (2010). Dyslexia: a deficit in visuo-spatial attention, not in phonological processing. *Trends in Cognitive Sciences*, 14, 57–63.

Chapter 2

Subitizing, Dynamic Vision, Saccade and Fixation Control in Dyslexia

Burkhart Fischer

General introduction

About 2 million years ago the evolution of human beings from other primates began. Pretty early on, human beings were able to communicate with each other by an articulated language. Written language, by contrast, developed only very recently. Five thousand years ago human beings were still using pictures to communicate. This was relatively easy, because the human brain was already able to recognize abstract pictures of things seen. Today, picture language has been re-established in the interactions between computers and their users. For example, Windows shows small pictures (pictograms, icons) on your desktop, which are used via mouse clicks to tell the computer what the user wants to do next. Similarly today pictograms are used in public life to direct and inform people, e.g. to find their way around an airport. The advantage of pictograms is that they can be used in any country around the world regardless of the language.

The use of a written language and its obligatory learning at school started in Europe only 250 years ago. Before schools were established, only a minority of the population were able to read and write at all. This means that on a 1-year scale of overall human development, written language for everybody was introduced only 1 hour ago.

That some people have particular difficulties acquiring literacy was recognized by the end of the nineteenth century. The problem was called word blindness, implying that it has to do with a disorder of vision, but not of the eyes. Because of the extremely late introduction of written language it does not come as a surprise that we do not find a literacy centre in our brains, nor a reading or spelling centre. But we have a language centre (Broca's), responsible for spoken language. Most of us learn to speak our language all by ourselves by imitation within the first few years of our lives, without the need for any special teaching.

In contrast, we do not acquire literacy by ourselves. Beginning at the age of 6 years, we need many years of instruction at school and hundreds of hours of daily practice at home to acquire it. In other words, our brains have not been prepared for reading and writing. Letters are useless, biologically speaking. They do not smell, one cannot eat or drink them. To be able to use them was never a criterion for survival. Even today it is not crucial for survival. In Asian countries a large percentage of the population is still illiterate. After catastrophes like the Haiti earthquake in 2010, what people needed most urgently were water, food, clothes, and medical care, not schools. It is only our modern culture over the last few hundred years that has made reading and writing so important.

But to learn to read and write is a huge challenge for our brains. The learning process leads to an establishment of complex neural networks with many different functions. Perhaps the most important is vision, a highly complex system. It is therefore clear from the beginning that several different aspects of vision must be investigated when it comes to the question of whether or not dyslexics suffer from visual deficits. One needs specific tasks to test the different functions and one needs to assess quantitative performance in these tasks by control subjects at different ages in order to compare this with that of dyslexics. These tasks should not require any language processing in order to be sure that they are purely visual.

The sensory organs for vision, the eyes, will not be covered at all in this chapter, since we do not see with our eyes but rather with our brains. We will, however, discuss the control of eye movements and fixation, because these are integral parts of vision in general, and especially of the reading process. There have been several studies of the role of saccadic eye movements in dyslexia, but most of them have failed to use adequate tasks.

First of all, measuring eye movements during reading does not make much sense, because the chaotic patterns of saccades seen may simply be the result of poor reading skills, rather than the result of poor saccadic control. One should use non-reading eye movement tasks and compare the results with those obtained from normally reading control subjects of the same age. If one finds deficits in saccade control of dyslexics performing non-reading tasks, this suggests that defective eye control could contribute to their reading problems.

Then one wants to know what happens to the reading process if the optomotor deficits are reduced by daily practice. Of course, one expects improvement in reading, but it could be that it was only the learning process of reading which improves due to the training, because proper reading needs more than correct saccade and fixation control.

Therefore this chapter deals with the following 4 subfunctions of vision:

1. Subitizing and visual number counting. This is the basic capacity of our visual system to estimate the number of up to four or five items without counting them, when they have been seen for only a very short period of time (say, 100 ms). One can actually count up to nine items displayed for a very short time, but this needs more time and the percentage of correct responses decreases. This capacity for subitizing contributes to reading, because it allows us to know how many letters are in a word or how many letters are still to be visited within a fixation, without having to count them.

2. Dynamic vision. Since vision requires a series of saccadic eye movements, one must be able to correctly store a certain number of pictures within a limited period of time. Vision takes place in time and the speed of vision must be as fast as required by the sequence of saccades. These temporal aspects of vision have been almost completely neglected in classical ophthalmology.

3. Saccade control must be synchronized with the ongoing process of reading. It is not enough to have intact eyes; the control of their movements is what counts in reading.

4. Fixation control. In between saccades the eyes are supposed to stay in one place, i.e. saccades as well as slow converging or diverging eye movements must be suppressed.

This book demonstrates clearly that dyslexics do indeed suffer from visual deficits. These are not necessarily the only problems they may have. The fact that only a proportion of dyslexics suffer from visual and/or optomotor deficits already suggests that other problems must play an important role. For example, the auditory system must be taken into account. The role of low-level auditory differentiation will be discussed at the end. Comparison of auditory and optomotor data shows that one cannot clearly separate a group of visual or auditory dyslexics from others. In the case of acquired dyslexia the patient has learned a written language successfully before the accident or disease causing the brain damage. The symptoms are different from those in developmental dyslexia, which seems to be a congenital deficit in learning to read that did not affect the acquisition of spoken language. Since most of the visual and optomotor deficits can be improved by training, we are dealing with a neurodevelopmental condition, which is probably a consequence of genetic vulnerability.

Subitizing and number counting

Introduction

Cycles of saccades and fixation form the optomotor basis for natural vision; so our brain receives different 'pictures' in a fast sequence. Visual processing must be correspondingly fast in order to keep these pictures in the correct temporal order while constructing a stable perception of the visual scene. Short words and parts of longer words are scanned by saccades. Losing the temporal order of these scans and misidentifications of the letters seen results in more or less chaotic reading. During reading, we see more than one letter during one period of fixation. Due to the size of the 'window' around the fovea one sees only four to six letters at a time (O'Regan, 1990). The next saccade must be programmed to jump across these letters in order to analyse the content of the next 'window'.

Whether or not the special visual capacity of subitizing and/or number counting helps in the process of reading is an open question. It is possible that subitizing limits the number of letters analysed during a single fixation. The results of an attempt to answer this question are presented in this chapter. A special task to assess subitizing and number counting quantitatively was designed. Data for control subjects were collected and the development of subitizing was measured (Fischer, 2006) see also (Starkey & Cooper, 1995). Giving the task to dyslexics showed that the development of this specific visual capacity lags behind the development of control subjects doing the same task. To see whether poor task performance could be improved, the task was given in a modified version for daily practice at home for 3 weeks. Clear improvements were observed in most children. The transfer to basic arithmetic of such training was studied in children with dyscalculia (Fischer et al., 2008b). Similar positive effects in dyslexic children were seen.

Methods

Subjects

Control subjects were recruited from German schools. They had normal or high grades in reading, writing, and in basic arithmetic and no history of neurological problems.

Table 2.1 The number of subjects in the different age groups are shown for the controls and the dyslexics

Subitizing	7–8 years	9–10 years	11–13 years	14–17 years	All
Controls	35	36	62	85	218
Dyslexics	227	330	241	20	818
Training	50	63	47	10	170

Dyslexic subjects had below normal grades in reading and spelling but their general intelligence was normal or above. Subjects who did not pass reading or spelling tasks, but were not tested for intelligence, formed another group of poor readers. Results from the latter two groups were compared with respect to their performance in the subitizing task and no significant differences were found. Therefore both groups were combined into one experimental group, labelled 'dyslexic' in this chapter. The subjects were aged 7–17 years old. They were divided into four age groups as shown in Table 2.1.

Design of the task

One to nine items (small circles) were presented simultaneously on a small LCD display (2.5 × 6 cm, outer borders) corresponding to 5.7 × 11.4 degrees of visual angle at a viewing distance of 30 cm. The circles were 2 mm in diameter. They were presented in black against a greenish background. The stimuli were too small, their contrast was too low, and the presentation time too short to give rise to after images. The minimum distance between the stimuli was 8 mm horizontally and 5 mm vertically. The spatial positions of the randomly selected number of items were randomized within a 4 × 4 array. Fig. 2.1 shows examples of the presentation of four, six, and eight items. By chance, some of the presentations looked like the dots on a die, while others looked irregular. A fixation mark was presented in the centre of the display at the beginning of each trial. It was turned off when the items were presented. Thus all items were presented parafoveally. The presentation time was 100 ms which is shorter than the shortest possible saccadic reaction time even for express saccades (Fischer & Ramsperger, 1984). This way the subjects could not possibly count the stimuli by scanning saccades. The limited presentation time did not imply a limited response time (see later). The visual display, the keyboard, and data collection were all implemented on a small hand-held instrument. The data stored in the instrument were down loaded after the training and were analysed for this presentation. Parents were given a written report about the success of the training.

Procedure

The subjects were introduced to the task by presenting each set of items for an unlimited period of time. They were instructed to press the key corresponding to the number of

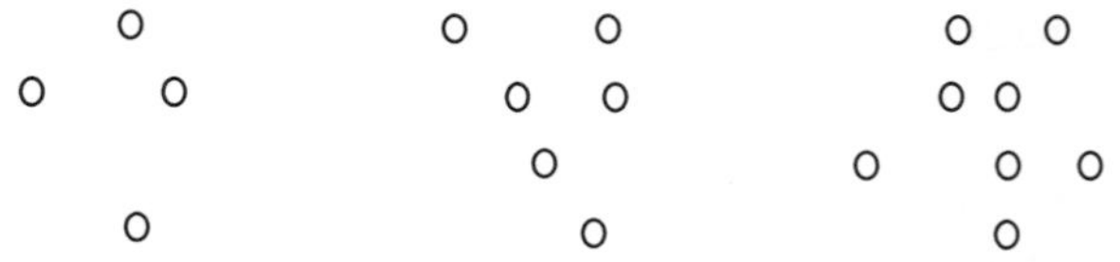

Fig. 2.1 Three examples of stimulus presentation of 4, 6, and 8 items.

items in the display. The spatial arrangement of the digit keys was identical to those on computer keyboards. Subjects were asked to respond as rapidly as possible. Therefore they were also instructed to start with their hand above the centre of the keyboard. At least 12 practice trials were given. After they understood the task subjects were given another five trials of the real task with a presentation time of 100 ms. After 1 s the fixation point disappeared and the test pattern was presented for 100 ms only (shortest saccadic reaction time). The subject reacted by pressing the response key. The next trial was initiated only after another key press by the subject. Even though reaction time was important within a trial the speed of the complete task performance could be controlled by the subject. Each number of items was shown 20 times with the exception of a single item, which occurred only 10 times. The total time for a test session was about 20 min.

Data collection and analysis

The data were recorded by the test instrument and downloaded to a personal computer for later analysis. For each trial the number of items (N) presented and the digit of the pressed response key were recorded together with the response time. For each subject and for each number of items we calculated the percentage of correct responses p(N) and the corresponding mean response time r(N). For N > 3 an almost linear relationship was obtained for r(N) as a function of N (see Fig. 2.2). Therefore we calculated the linear regression between response times and the item number for N = 4 – 8. The slope t of the regression line gives the average extra time t needed for each additional item. The basic reaction time T was calculated as the mean value of r(1). The mean percentage of the correct responses P was calculated for item numbers between 4 and 8. Item number 9 was excluded from this analysis, since most children noticed that 9 was the highest digit on the key board and pressed 9, whenever the item number was 'large'. They hit the correct

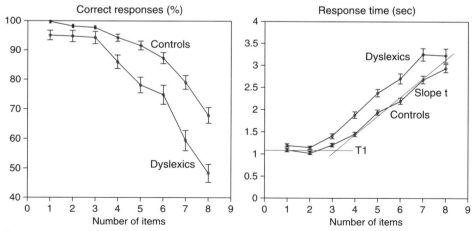

Fig. 2.2 The percentage of correct responses (left panel) and the response times (right panel) were plotted as a function of the number of items. T1 indicates the basic response time. The slope of straight line shows the definition of the time per item. See text for details.

key often by this kind of guessing. To compare the performance of the control and test subjects age curves were plotted for basic response time $T = r(1)$, the time per item (called the effective recognition speed), the correctness P = the mean value of correct responses for item numbers 4 to 8. ANOVAs with age as a covariate were used to determine the significance of the differences between groups and the effects of age. More details have already been published in (Fischer et al., 2008a).

Training

To improve performance in the task, dyslexic subjects were given training at home. The training followed Hebbian principles, attempting to improve the efficacy of relevant synapses. If an impulse in a neuron is successful in eliciting one in the next neuron then the synapse is strengthened so that the chances that the next impulse will also be transferred are increased (Hebb, 1949). The training task was the same as that used for diagnosis, but initially it was made very easy, by setting the maximum number of items at only 3 and the presentation time was increased to 300 ms. As subjects improved, the task was made more difficult by increasing the maximum number of items and by decreasing the presentation time. Before beginning the training the diagnostic task was administered, and again after 20 days of training. This way one could see if any improvements were directly due to the training. The subjects were recruited as described earlier, but only those who failed in at least one of two variables derived from the task performance were included in the study. Table 2.1 shows the age groups.

Results

Subitizing and counting

To see the processes of subitizing and counting, the percentage of correct responses and the response times were plotted as a function of item number for a control group and a group of age matched dyslexics (age 11–13 years). Fig. 2.2 shows the two pairs of curves. For item numbers below 4 almost all the controls' responses were correct and their response times were about the same, indicating the range of subitizing. For item numbers above 4 the percentage of incorrect responses and the response times began to increase almost linearly: for each additional item an almost constant amount of extra time was needed to find the correct response (right panel of Fig. 2.2). Comparing the two groups one sees that in the subitizing range almost all responses were correct, with the dyslexics showing a slight tendency to lower values. Note, that the dyslexics reached mean values of 95%. Thus response accuracy does not different the two groups. A clearer difference between the groups, however, can be seen in the time domain: response times were much longer for the dyslexics. With increasing item numbers above 4 both groups exhibit a linear increase in response time, but the slope of the regression line is lower for the controls compared with the dyslexics.

Development of subitizing and counting

Plotting the basic response time and the effective recognition speed as a function of age gives Fig. 2.3. Both groups show improvement lasting right through to adulthood. The left panel shows that the controls were faster in finding the correct response, even

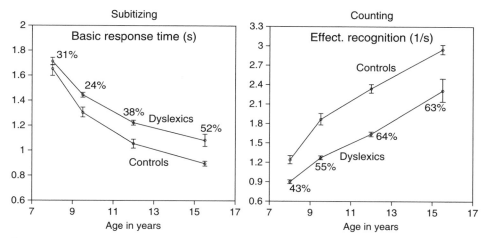

Fig. 2.3 Basic response time (left panel) and effective recognition (right panel) vs. age. Numbers indicate the proportion of dyslexics below the 16th percentile.

when there was only 1 item. (Of course, if there had been always only 1 item, the response times would have been much shorter and probably the dyslexics would have been as fast as the controls. But this task required a decision as to the number of items.) The percentage of dyslexics failing to reach the 16th percentile achieved by the controls is given by the numbers on the curves.

The controls did much better than the dyslexics at all ages. The percentage of dyslexics falling below the control 16th percentile increased with age from 43% to 63%. The effective recognition speed is composed of two variables: the time per item and the percentage of correct responses. Both variables are plotted as a function of age in Fig. 2.4. With increasing age the time per item differs more and more between the two groups. The difference between the groups' proportion of correct responses is large, but stays about the same over the age range considered. Since the time per item decreases with age and the percentage of correct responses increases, the effective recognition is a sensitive index of the differences between the groups.

Training in subitizing and counting

Fig. 2.5 shows the effects of daily practice on two variables (basic response time and effective recognition) before and after the training as a function of age, with the proportion who reached the 16th percentile after training. So far we do not know whether successful training of subitizing alone transfers to improved reading skills. We do know, however, that as a consequence of the training, basic arithmetic skills improve in children with dyscalculia; such children also show deficits in subitizing and number counting (Fischer et al., 2008b).

Discussion

It could be argued that subitizing and number counting should not be regarded as visual functions, because higher cognitive functions are needed to do the task. Yet, it certainly is

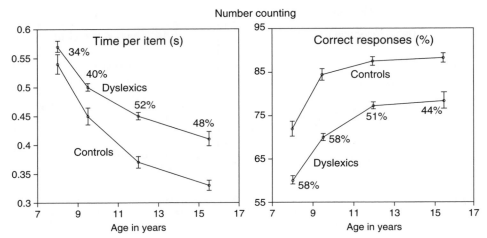

Fig. 2.4 Time per item (left panel) and percent correct (right panel) vs. age for item numbers 4 to 8.

a function which needs fast and correct visual processing up to the primary visual cortex and beyond. Most probably, the inferior temporal cortex is involved, because receptive fields of single cells there are large (Desimone et al., 1980) and cover both foveal and parafoveal vision. Therefore, defects in subitizing and number counting, as tested in this study, should be included in the list of possible visual deficits in dyslexics. While it is not clear at the outset, why subitizing should play a role in reading one can easily imagine that this parafoveal visual achievement facilitates the optomotor component of the reading process, because it allows us to 'see' how many letters there are to the right of the present fixation. It will also indicate how far away the next space in the text is. Perhaps the deficit

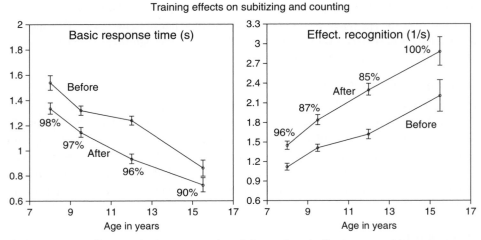

Fig. 2.5 Training effects on basic response time (left panel) and effective recognition (right panel).

is only in fast parafoveal vision, which is needed for the performance of the task as well as for fluent reading.

Irrespective of these considerations, we have to accept that subitizing and number counting differentiates dyslexics from controls at all ages between 7–17 years. The important point is that subitizing may still be regarded as dependent on low-level visual processing, because it does not require any language processing. However, since there are more visual and optomotor deficits encountered in dyslexia, one cannot expect improvements in reading unless these other deficits are also addressed. Nevertheless in cases where the deficit in subitizing and number counting is definitely the only deficit the child has, we can hope to see improvements in reading by this training alone.

Dynamic vision

Introduction

Visual processing in the brain takes place in time, therefore some measure of the speed of vision is needed. This is most evident, when talking about the perception of movement. It has been found, that two subsystems of visual processing exist: the parvocellular and the magnocellular system. The first works on object identification to answer the question of *what* it is that we see; the second works on the question *where* things are in space. The magno system is sensitive to stimuli changing in time, e.g. movement. Originating in the retina, the two systems follow the same anatomical pathway up to the primary visual cortex (Tootell et al., 1988). From there the magno system projects dorsally to the parietal cortex and the parvo system projects ventrally to the inferior temporal cortex. This kind of dichotomy must be kept in mind from the beginning, whenever we talk about vision. Surprisingly, in classical ophthalmology time does not play any role at all. Static vision is what is diagnosed by tests of visual acuity. Dynamic vision has been neglected in the investigation of the quality of vision, despite the fact that under natural viewing conditions we 'see' by fast sequences of saccades. Many studies have suggested that it is the magno system which exhibits visual deficits in dyslexia. Here we describe a simple test to obtain a measure of the speed of vision in adults as well as in children. It will be applied to control and dyslexic subjects.

Methods

Subjects

Participants for this study were recruited in a similar way to those in the previous study. Table 2.2 gives the numbers of the participants in each age group. Fig. 2.6 shows the stimuli.

Table 2.2 Number of controls and dyslexics in each age group participating in the study of dynamic vision

Dyn. vision	7–8 years	9–10 years	11–13 years	14–17 years	All
Controls	33	37	43	27	140
Dyslexics	79	214	168	43	504

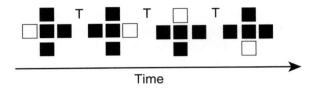

Fig. 2.6 Stimuli used in the task of dynamic vision. T means the time of the presentation of each stimulus in the sequence.

Time

The size of stimulus was large enough to be identified 100% correctly, when it was presented as a stationary stimulus. Its orientation was changed every 170 ms for a random duration. When the trial series ended, the subject's task was to press the arrow key corresponding to the last orientation. After 100 trials the percentage of correct responses was calculated in relation to random guessing (25% correct). Physically the test instrument was identical to the one used in the previous study.

Fixation-task

To test foveal dynamic vision a small stimulus consisting of the capital letter T was presented in one of its four possible orientations: right, left, up, down.

Jump-task

In another version of the fixation task the centrally presented stimulus jumped to the right or left at some unpredictable time in the trial. The best strategy to detect the last orientation was a prosaccade to the new position of the stimulus. The visual task remained the same, but the subject most probably made a saccade just before the end of the trial. In 20% of the 100 trials—randomly interspersed—the stimulus jump did not take place. This required the subject to maintain fixation in the middle until the jump.

Anti-task

Another version of the task was to present a strong distractor at one side while the stimulus was presented on the opposite side. The best strategy to detect the orientation was an antisaccade with respect to the distractor. In order to prevent a prosaccade to the distractor followed by a second saccade to the stimulus, the stimulus occurred only once in one of the four orientations. A sequence of two saccades would take too much time and the subject would reach the correct side only when the stimulus had already disappeared. Again, in 20% of the trials the distractor was not presented and the series of orientations ended with the stimulus still in the centre. These methods have been described in detail (Fischer & Hartnegg, 2000; Fischer et al., 2000). Altogether, the test of dynamic vision had three conditions from which five variables could be obtained: fixation trials, jump centre trials, jump trials, anti-centre trials, anti-trials.

Results

All three tasks were given to control subjects and students with dyslexia. The percentage of correct responses was the dependent variable in each of the five conditions. Fig. 2.7 shows the age curves for both groups. The three panels on the left correspond to the conditions with the stimulus in the centre. In principle these conditions should be the same, because the stimulus whose orientation has to be detected falls on the fovea. One sees,

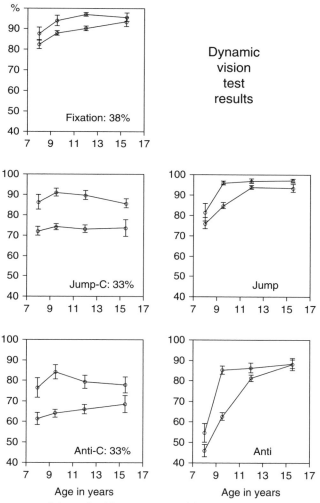

Fig. 2.7 The age curves of dynamic vision as measured by the percentage of correct responses. The lower curves in each panel represent the data from the dyslexics.

however, that the results in the jump centre and anti-centre condition are clearly different from the fixation condition.

It seems that the subjects had expected the stimulus to appear on the right or left, they defocused their attention, hence they missed the correct orientation in the centre. The important point is that the dyslexics performed worse than the controls. The two panels on the right give the results of the jump and anti tasks. Here also there was a difference between the two groups. In the three left panels one sees little or no change with age. Therefore, the four age groups were collapsed into one in order to estimate the percentage of subjects failing to achieve the 16th percentile criterion. The numbers in the lower right corner of the panels give these percentages: about one-third of the dyslexics failed the test of dynamic vision. Thus by no means all dyslexics exhibited deficits that were detected by these tasks.

Training and transfer

As in the study on subitizing we attempted to improve the deficits in dynamic vision by daily practice. This question will be postponed to later sections, where the training of saccade and fixation control will be described. The three tasks of dynamic vision were used for training purposes in the optomotor domain. Thereby dynamic vision was improved at the same time. Most of the dyslexic children learned to do the task 100% correctly, even when the series of stimuli became faster (down to 90 ms presentation time).

Discussion

The tasks described in this section are tasks which challenge dynamic vision. Other tasks may be designed that serve the same goal. The crucial point is to introduce temporal changes into the visual pattern to be perceived by the subject. One task of this kind is the detection of a small random dot pattern within a larger random dot pattern. The small one will remain invisible unless the dots begin to move coherently within the surrounding larger dot pattern. Using this task the development of dynamic vision and its early decline in the age range of 35–40 years has been described (Schrauf et al., 2000). The age curve is almost identical to the one obtained by applying the fixation version of the tasks described here to participants above the age of 17 years (Fischer & Hartnegg, 2002).

Evidence of deficits in the magno system of dyslexics has been reported by several authors in this book. The significance of these deficits for dyslexia becomes clear, however, only if one knows the percentage of dyslexics who do not reach a criterion, e.g. the 16th percentile reached by age matched controls; 33–38% failed this. The change from the original task to the jump and to the anti-version had a strong effect for both groups, but the effect for the dyslexics was much stronger than for the controls.

Saccade control

Introduction

Saccades are obligatory under natural viewing conditions. We do not notice these fast movements of the eyes nor can we see them by watching our eyes in a mirror. One way of becoming aware of their significance in natural vision is to look at geometrical illusions that disappear when we stop making saccades (Fischer et al., 2003). This also emphasizes how difficult it is not to make saccades. When reading, saccade control must be highly accurate because the coordination of language processing and a saccade control is key to accurate fluent reading.

Quite a number of studies on the role of eye movements in reading have been published with contradictory results. One problem is that poor saccade control during reading could be either a consequence of poor reading or a cause. Therefore, saccade tasks have been used, that did not require reading. Pavlidis (1981) showed that in dyslexics, generation of a series of sequential saccades, similar to reading eye movements, but to non-alphabetic targets was interrupted by more regressive saccade than in controls. However this result could not be replicated (Olson et al., 1991).

The EZ-reader model of the reading process (Reichle et al., 2003) postulates that coordination of saccade control and reading needs control by the frontal lobe. Therefore, since automatic saccade generation does not involve the frontal component of saccade control, it should not be affected in dyslexia. However, successful antisaccade performance does rely on intact frontal function (Guitton et al., 1985); hence antisaccade control should be affected in children with reading problems. In contrast prosaccade control, especially express saccades, can be made without the frontal eye fields using the superior colliculus (tectum; Schiller et al., 1979, 1987).

In addition, steady fixation between saccades needs to be close to perfect for fluent reading. Fixation can be destabilized by intrusive saccades (simple instability) and/or by slow drifts of one or the other or both eyes (binocular instability). The optomotor cycle is shown in Fig. 2.8. It illustrates the coordination of fixation, reflexive saccades, and voluntary control by the frontal lobe. It allows us to understand how deficits in saccade and/or in fixation control may contribute to poor reading. Here I will describe diagnostic eye movement tasks and the results of using them in control subjects and in students with dyslexia. Training and its transfer to reading is also explained. Finally I will concentrate on the stability of fixation.

Methods

Subjects

The participants in both control (N = 182) and dyslexic (N = 624) groups were recruited the same way as for the studies previously described. Most of the dyslexics were tested for intelligence and performed at a normal or higher level. We did not have the IQ values for another group of poor readers, but all of them had normal grades in maths. The two groups of poor readers did not show any significant differences and therefore both groups were combined (N = 3782).

Children with a diagnosis of attention deficit (ADHD) were excluded. All participants were aged 7–22 years old. The groups were classified into five age groups as shown in Table 2.3.

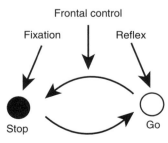

Frontal control

Fixation   Reflex

Stop   Go

Fig. 2.8 The optomotor cycle shows schematically the basic organization of saccade and fixation control. For details see text.

Table 2.3 Number of subjects in the study of saccade control

Saccade Control	7–8 years	9–10 years	11–13 years	14–17 years	17–22 years	All
Controls	31	47	43	32	29	182
Dyslexics	961	1517	983	252	69	3782
Training	50	87	57	14	0	208

Eye movement recording

The movements of both eyes were recorded in the horizontal direction using infrared light corneal reflection (Iris Scalar or ExpressEye; Hartnegg & Fischer, 2002). The resolution was 1 ms in time and 12 min of arc in space. Saccades were identified automatically by a computer program under trial-by-trial visual control (Fischer et al., 1997).

Optomotor saccade tasks

Two tasks were used to analyse saccade control. The temporal aspects are shown in Fig. 2.9. In the prosaccade task a fixation point was shown in the centre of the screen and after one second another stimulus was presented randomly 4 degrees to the right or left. This task condition is called 'overlap', because the stimulus and the fixation point overlap in time during the second part of each trial. The subject was instructed to look at this new stimulus (prosaccade) as quickly as possible. In the antisaccade task the fixation point was also shown, but it was extinguished after a second. 200 ms later (the gap) a new stimulus was presented randomly 4 degrees to the right or left. This task condition is called 'gap', because of the temporal gap between fixation target offset and stimulus onset. The subject was instructed to look to the side opposite to where the stimulus had appeared (antisaccade).

Variables

The variables are defined as shown in the upper and lower parts of Fig. 2.9. The full set of variables included reaction time (SRT) of pro- and antisaccades, the percent number of express saccades in the overlap condition, and the percent number of erratic saccades (% errors) in the antisaccade gap task. The percentage of corrective saccades

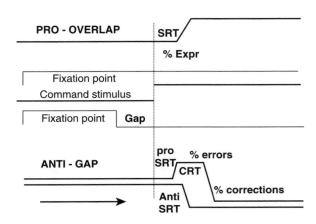

Fig. 2.9 Time course of the visual stimuli in the overlap prosaccade task and the gap antisaccade task.

(% corrections) after errors bringing the eyes to the opposite side of the stimulus and the corresponding correction time (CRT) were also determined. All variables were calculated separately for left and right stimulation. A complete description of the tasks and the definition of the variables have been given earlier (Fischer et al., 1997).

Training

The subjects were grouped into four age groups (7–17 years). In addition to the classification of the experimental group described earlier these subjects exhibited deficits in saccade control by scoring below the 16th percentile in two or more variables describing antisaccade performance (see later). Their post-training data were compared with their pre-training data as well as with corresponding data of an age-matched control group. The number of participants was N = 208 (see Table 2.3).

Corresponding to the three components of saccadic control the training consisted of up to three versions of a visual orientation detection task, which was used to investigate dynamic vision (see preceding section) i.e. to probe the magnocellular subsystem of vision. A full description has been published (Fischer & Hartnegg, 2000). The training was scheduled individually for each child depending on the individual diagnostic results obtained from the analysis of the eye movement records. Daily training required 200 repetitions and lasted 8–13 min depending on subject progress. The training instrument controlled the difficulty of the tasks adaptively by controlling the speed by which the stimulus changed its orientation. As the subjects increased their correct responses the difficulty was increased by using faster rates of orientation change from 210 ms at the beginning to 90 ms.

Transfer to reading

Transfer of the training to reading was studied in two groups: the experimental group (n = 11) was given the training required by the diagnosis, the control group (n = 10) had to wait until the training group finished training. For this study only small groups were available, because all subjects were being treated for dyslexia. The children chosen had a common teacher, who would provide identical help for both groups. After the training, both groups received the same lessons in reading for 6 weeks. During this study nine children were lost (21 remained), because not all variables could be collected from each child. There was no placebo group, because the training by itself specifically affects the components of saccade and fixation control depending on the task version. Reading competence was tested by counting the reading errors in a special reading task before and after the reading lessons. The reading test was specially designed for this study of children of different ages from 7–13 years.

Results

Fig. 2.10 shows the age development of pro- and antisaccade reaction times in dyslexics and controls. Both groups showed significant changes with age. Prosaccade reaction times were slower for the dyslexics only in the youngest and the oldest age groups, where the proportion of subjects failing the 16th percentile criterion was 31% and 32%, respectively. Since 16% is by definition the percentage of the control group that fail, the

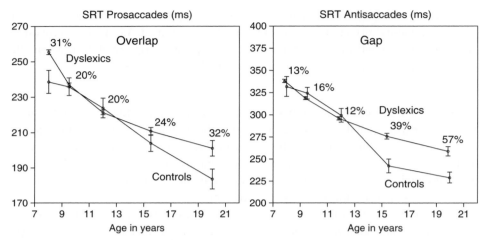

Fig. 2.10 Comparison of age curves of the reaction times of the prosaccade with overlap conditions (left panel) and antisaccade with gap condition (right panel).

numbers of 20–24% indicate that reaction times were significantly different only in some of the age groups. While for theoretical reasons this might indicate that in this age range the dyslexics are not different from the controls, in practice one has to test every child to make sure that the reaction times are within or outside the limits of the controls. Reaction times for the antisaccades (right panel Fig. 2.10) indicate that the three youngest groups did not differ and the percentages of off-limit dyslexics were even smaller than the 16th percentile. However, the two oldest groups differed significantly with off-limit percentages of 39% and 57%, respectively.

Errors

When looking at the errors occurring in the antisaccade task (Fig. 2.11) one sees also a strong development with age in both groups. However, here the differences between the two groups are very clear for all age groups except the youngest. At age 7 or 8 years both groups reached mean error rates of just below 80%, i.e. neither group was able to perform the antisaccade task without glancing at the stimulus. As they become older both groups decreased their error rate significantly, but the differences between the groups became larger. The percentage of off-limit responses increased from 18% to almost 60%. Unlike the reaction times, the error rate did differentiate between the groups at all ages except the youngest. It seems that with the beginning of school both groups start the development of a new capacity, namely the ability of their frontal cortex to control their saccades.

Error correction in the antisaccade task: most studies on antisaccade performance count the errors, but they ignore the question of whether or not the subjects correct their errors. In our analysis of the eye movement traces we also analysed the second corrective saccades after stimulus onset in cases where the first saccade was an error. Only those secondary saccades that reached the opposite side (as was required by the antisaccade instructions) were considered as corrective saccades. For each subject the percentage of

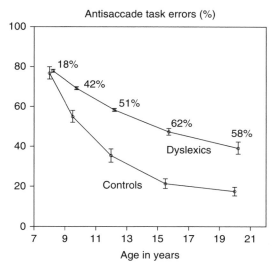

Fig. 2.11 Comparison of error rates in the antisaccade task with gap conditions.

uncorrected saccades was calculated and served as another index describing the performance in the antisaccade task. Fig. 2.12 shows that indeed quite a large percentage of errors remained uncorrected.

The children not only followed their reflexes but they were also unable to generate a saccade to the opposite side on command, thereby leaving the errors uncorrected. The numbers beside the curves indicate the percentage of dyslexic subjects failing the 16th percentile criterion.

As can be seen in Fig. 2.13, the correction times decrease with age similar to the reaction times. The proportion of subjects failing the 16th percentile criterion increase from 21%

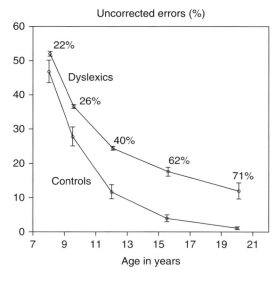

Fig. 2.12 The number of uncorrected errors is larger in dyslexics in the age-matched controls. Only the controls reach the ideal value of almost zero.

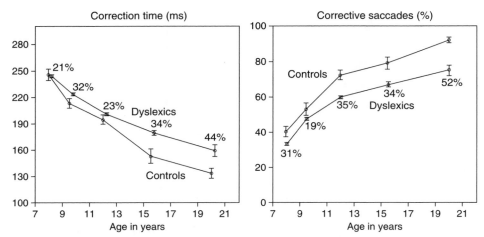

Fig. 2.13 Comparison of age curves of the correction times (left panel) and the percentage of corrective saccades.

to 44%. The rate of corrective saccades was 31% in the youngest group and increased to 52% in the oldest group.

Altogether, we analysed five variables derived from the pro- and antisaccade tasks: the reaction times (2), the error rate (1), the rate of corrective saccades (1), and the correction times (1). If one requires that all variables have to meet the 16th percentile criterion, before one states that a subject's performance on the saccade tasks is different from controls, one needs to determine the percentage of dyslexics that fail the 16th percentile criterion in at least one out of the five variables. With this stringent requirement the percentage of dyslexic subjects ranged from 63% in the youngest group to 90% in the oldest (see 'General discussion' section).

Saccadic control training

To improve the control of saccades one has to remember, that there are three components: the reflexive saccade, the frontal component, and the stop component, which prevents the occurrence of too many express saccades. Depending on the results of the diagnostic tests the schedule for each child must contain one, two, or all three components. We decided to use three versions of the dynamic vision task: Fixation, Jump, and Anti. On the basis of earlier training experience (Fischer & Ramsperger, 1986) a minimum of 7 days of daily practice were planned for each component. Longer durations were given in periods of 7 days. Thus the total training durations varied between 3–8 weeks.

Fig. 2.14 shows the effects of training on reaction times for the pro- and antisaccades. While the prosaccade reaction times remained about the same, the antisaccade reaction times decreased considerably. Thus the prosaccade reaction times did not allow differentiation between the two groups, before or after training. Before training, the antisaccade reaction time differentiated the two groups only in the older children. The antisaccade reaction times became faster in all age groups.

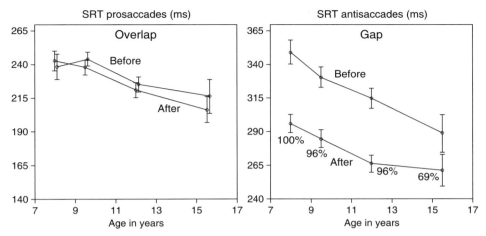

Fig. 2.14 Pre- and post-training age curves of the reaction times of prosaccades with overlap conditions (left panel) and antisaccades with gap conditions (right panel). The numbers at the lower curve indicate the percentage of dyslexics who reached the range of the age-matched controls (p16 criterion).

Fig. 2.15 shows the effect of the training on the percentage of uncorrected errors. Roughly, performance in the antisaccade task improved by a factor of two. The proportion of dyslexics, who reached the 16th percentile criterion depends on age as can be seen in Fig. 2.15. Almost all members of the younger groups were successful.

Training specificity

The training study did not include a placebo group, because it is quite unlikely that such a basic brain function as saccadic control would be influenced by psychological factors.

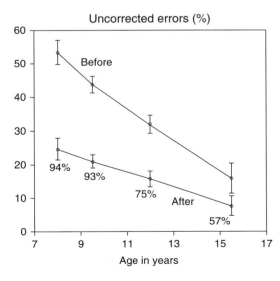

Fig. 2.15 Trainings effects on the percentage of uncorrected errors. The numbers at the lower curve indicate the percentage of dyslexics who reached the p16 criterion of the controls.

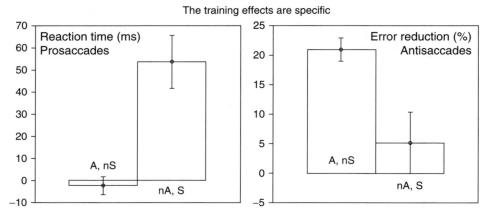

Fig. 2.16 The specificity of saccade training is shown by the change of prosaccadic reaction times in two groups and by the change of antisaccade errors in the same two groups. A, the antitask and the fixation task were trained, or not, nA. S, the saccade task was trained, or not, nS.

Analysis of the effects of training with different schedules confirmed this view. Two groups with different training schedules were compared. If the anti- and fixation tasks were trained, but not the saccade task, the training did not reduce the reaction times for prosaccades, but reduced errors in the antisaccade task. If the saccade task was trained but not the anti-task, the reaction times of the prosaccades were reduced but the error rate remained about the same. Fig. 2.16 shows these results graphically. This implies that placebo effects did not affect the training. The effects of training saccade control have been confirmed (Dyckman & McDowell, 2005).

Transfer to reading

Transfer of saccade training to reading was studied separately. Reduction in reading errors due to the saccade training are compared between the trained and control (waiting) groups. Fig. 2.17 shows the significant differences in the percentage of reading error reduction between the trained and control groups. Reading speed was also assessed, but did not differ significantly before and after the training. The assessment of reading was repeated after 6 weeks of reading instruction for both groups recombined into one. While further reductions in errors were seen, the strength of the effect was greatest right after the training. A common effect of the training was a clear improvement of handwriting as reported by the parents and teachers. So far, long-term studies have not been carried out, but relapses are rare, because most subjects improved their reading and went on reading from then on.

Discussion

After the introduction of the antisaccade task to detect deficits in saccade control (for review, see Everling & Fischer, 1998; Munoz & Everling, 2004) there is no question any more, that in dyslexia brainstem and muscle control of eye movements is quite normal.

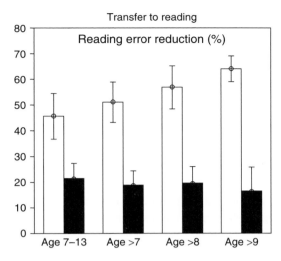

Fig. 2.17 The transfer of the saccade training to reading. White columns: experimental group; black columns: waiting group.

It is the frontal control of saccades, which exhibits increasing developmental deficits in poor readers and dyslexics. Because the antisaccade task does not rely on language processing it is also clear, that the chaotic patterns of saccades that occur during reading are not a consequence of poor language processing. Just the opposite: poor reading is often a consequence of poor saccade control by the frontal lobe. This experimental result was predicted by one of the most complete models of eye movement control during reading (Reichle et al., 2003). Yet, this does not imply, that no other deficits play an important role in dyslexia, such as auditory impairments (see 'Stability of fixation' and 'General discussion' sections).

Stability of fixation

Introduction

An important function of the optomotor control system is to achieve stable fixation. Fixation may be interrupted or destabilized in two different ways: conjunctive saccades (simple instability) or by small slow drifts of one or both eyes (binocular instability). In the case of simple instability the angle of convergence remains the same, in binocular instability the angle of convergences changes in a dynamic way and temporary double vision may be the consequence. The stability of fixation has been neglected to a great extent, because oculomotor research has been mainly interested in the movements of the eyes not in the 'resting' eyes. Only when it was discovered that neurons in the frontal eye fields (Goldberg et al., 1986), in the parietal cortex (Robinson et al., 1978), in the tectum (Munoz & Wurtz 1992, 1993), and in the substantia nigra (Hikosaka & Wurtz 1983) are active during periods of active fixation, oculomotor research reacted and began to contribute to the concept of the optomotor cycle.

The prosaccade task with overlap provides a fixation stimulus throughout a trial. We therefore analysed eye movement traces during the last 400 ms before stimulus onset and during the 700 ms after stimulus onset. Thus the short period during the saccade was excluded. A full account of this study on fixation instability in dyslexia was published recently (Fischer & Hartnegg, 2009). Note that here we deal with a dynamic deficit. By contrast, squint or heterophoria are static deficits and may be corrected by static means, e.g. cylindrical correction. The existence of visual and optomotor deficits and their relations to reading are well documented by optometry (Kulp & Schmidt, 2010).

Methods

The diagnostic saccade task is the prosaccade task with overlap.

Simple instability

To quantify simple instability, we counted the number of unwanted saccades occurring during the 400 ms while waiting for the target to move (intrusive saccades). At the end of the diagnostic session the mean value of unwanted saccades per trial was calculated.

Binocular instability

The relative velocity of the two eyes was calculated during each eye movement. A binocular index (bindex) was then calculated, i.e. the total duration that these velocities exceeded a minimum of 2 degrees/s expressed as a percentage of the total duration of each trial. The proportion of trials in which each subject's bindex exceeded 15% provided an index of his binocular instability. This threshold of 15% was chosen because shorter periods within a trial of 1100 ms duration can hardly be considered as a functionally significant disturbance of binocular vision. Table 2.4 shows the number of participants in both studies of fixation control.

Results

Simple instability

This is readily defined as the mean number of intrusive saccades detected during periods of attempted fixation when no saccade should be made at all. Almost all of these saccades were small (<2 degrees) and most were followed by a second corrective saccade back to the fixation point. In addition, these saccades occurred mostly during the time before the stimulus was presented. Fig. 2.18 shows the age curves. While the two younger age groups did not exhibit significant differences, the two older groups contain 31% and 48% of participants, respectively, who failed the 16th percentile criterion of the controls.

Table 2.4 Number of subjects in the study of fixation control

Simple Instab	7–8 years	9–10 years	11–13 years	14–17 years	All
Controls	35	59	42	34	170
Dyslexics	635	973	653	167	2428
Binoc. Instab.	7–8 years	9–10 years	11–13 years	14–17 years	All
Controls	26	45	41	17	129
Dyslexics	587	912	615	153	2267

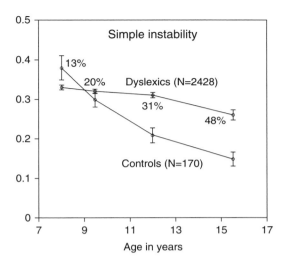

Fig. 2.18 The number of intrusive saccades per trial are used as a measure of simple instability of fixation. The numbers at the curves indicate the percentage of dyslexics who failed the p16 criterion.

Note that even at the age of 13–17 years the number of unwanted saccades did not reach the ideal value of zero.

Binocular instability

Fig. 2.19 shows the age curves of the controls and dyslexics. Interestingly the controls also exhibit quite strong instability—between 25–36%. However, the mean instabilities of the dyslexics exceeded the values of the controls in all age groups. Because of the large inter-individual scatter those of dyslexics failing the 16th percentile criterion is of the order of 25% independent of age.

Eye dominance

In principle, only one of the two eyes could dominate binocular instability by its slow movements, while the other eye could maintain its direction. To test this, the original

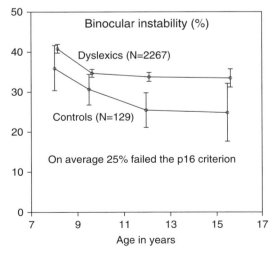

Fig. 2.19 The age curves of the binocular instability show only small decreases with age.

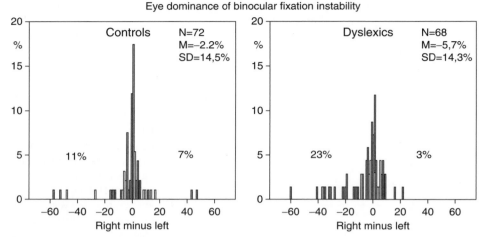

Fig. 2.20 The distribution of the differences between the right and the left eye. Bindex are not significantly different. Only in a limited number of single cases (11% and 23%) the left eye was responsible for the binocular instability.

records of two smaller groups (72 controls, 68 dyslexics) were analysed by assigning a bindex to each eye. Fig. 2.20 shows the distributions of the mean values of the differences of the bindex assigned to the right and left eyes. The mean values of the distributions were not significantly different from zero, but in a few cases (11% among the controls, and 23% among the dyslexics) the left eye was causing the instability more than the right eye. In other words, stable eye dominance was rarely encountered in either group.

Independence of the two types of instability

There was no significant correlation between the simple and binocular instabilities in any of the age groups indicating that the two phenomena are independent of each other. This does not come as a surprise, because the saccade control system is different from the binocular control system.

Fixation training

To improve fixation, we adopted the idea of Stein and Fowler (1985), to cover one eye in dyslexics with binocular problems (failing the Dunlop test). In our case, the training of saccade and fixation control was performed with one eye covered only for the duration of the daily training sessions, i.e. 7–15 min. Improvements in simple and binocular stability were measured by the per cent difference between pre- and post-training values.

Fig. 2.21 shows the results. While binocular instability was significantly ($p < 0.01$) improved by a factor of about 2, simple instability was only reduced by 20%, hardly reaching significance ($p < 0.05$). This difference in improvement supports the notion that the two types of instability are independent of each other.

Discussion

Instability of fixation must be considered an important problem during reading. Even though the fixation periods between two saccades are relatively short, the optomotor

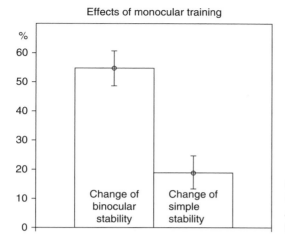

Fig. 2.21 Per cent improvement of binocular and simple stability of fixation by monocular training.

system has to maintain the direction of the line of sight for both the eyes. If this changes as a consequence of involuntary movement the correct sequence of words or of parts of words may be lost. Slow movements of one eye or both may result in a perception of temporarily 'blurred' images. The effort needed to keep the eyes from moving may add considerably to the effort required to master the oculomotor demands of reading. As a consequence the subject may fail to comprehend the text. Reading may sound almost perfect, but the subject cannot tell, what the text means.

General discussion

In conclusion, there may be quite a number of different sensory deficits (including visual and/or auditory deficits) even in a single dyslexic person. One needs to identify as many of these as possible in order to help each child to learn how to read, write and to do basic arithmetic. This chapter concentrated on visual and optomotor deficits.

The significance of visual and optomotor deficits in dyslexia

To estimate the significance of visual and optomotor deficits in dyslexia we calculated the percentage of dyslexics failing the 16th percentile criterion, using only the results of the nine variables from the optomotor and the subitizing tasks or only the seven variables from the optomotor tasks. Table 2.5 gives the number of subjects that could be included in this analysis.

Of the 753 dyslexics, 675 (89.6%) failed the tests on one or more of the nine variables. If only the optomotor variables were used 1796/2293 dyslexics (78.3%) failed in one or

Table 2.5 Number of subjects in each age group for which 9/7 variables were available to estimate the percentage of affected dyslexics. For details see text

All Group	7–8 years	9–10 years	11–13 years	14–17 years	17–22 years	All
9 variables	206	289	194	45	19	753
7 variables	585	900	612	153	43	2293

more of the seven. This result shows that it is valuable to look for visual and optomotor deficits using non-linguistic tests. These optomotor and the visual deficits class as causal factors in dyslexia, because improvements in these deficits improve reading. The high incidence of optomotor and visual deficits in dyslexia does not imply that other low level deficits will not be found in children with dyslexia, e. g. in the auditory domain. Neither does it imply that there are not language-related problems in dyslexia. The wide spectrum of deficits in dyslexia is shown by the size of a recent book; it has 300 pages of text and a reference list of 61 pages containing about 1830 citations (Beaton, 2004).

Gender differences

When analysing the variables separately for females and males few differences were found. But—as in other studies—the percentage of males was clearly higher. The youngest age group contained 60% males and 40% females. With increasing age this relationship changes to 80% males and 20% females in the adults (17–22 years).

Low-level auditory deficits

The first non-visual domain to be considered in dyslexia should be low-level auditory processing. We have developed four different tests of auditory discrimination (Fischer & Hartnegg, 2004): (1) intensity discrimination, (2) frequency discrimination, (3) gap detection, (4) time order. All of these were two-alternative forced-choice tasks that depend on low-level central processing, but do not involve language. They were given to 2329 dyslexic children and the results were compared with those of 282 control children, all in the age range of 7–17 years. The four subdomains of auditory processing are independent from each other and do not depend on general intelligence (Fischer & Hartnegg, 2004). Ninety-nine to 99.9% of dyslexics, depending on age, have either visual or auditory deficits. In other words, the chance of finding at least one visual, optomotor or auditory deficit in a single dyslexic person is close to 100%. This high incidence shows that low-level processing of sensory functions is an important factor causing dyslexic problems. If one can decrease these low-level deficits, e. g. by daily practice, we can help most dyslexics (Schäffler et al., 2004).

These results show that perceptual deficits are causal to reading and spelling problems. Therefore, even though it is clear that genetic factors play a large part, this does not imply that remediation is impossible. If genetic factors lead to deficits in a sensory domain or to a slow development in this domain, nevertheless one can often improve this sensory function, and thereby improving reading and spelling. Thus the question of whether or not dyslexia can be cured or persists throughout life becomes irrelevant for individual dyslexics. It may be regarded as purely theoretical concerning the nature of dyslexia.

Is 'visual dyslexia' a subgroup of dyslexia? From what we have discussed so far it is not very likely that a subclass of dyslexics can be separated as suffering from 'visual dyslexia' alone. From the large numbers of dyslexic subjects, in whom we have all three of visual, optomotor, and auditory measures we can estimate that: (1) only between 3–7% (depending on age) suffer from visual or optomotor deficits alone, without auditory deficits. Therefore a pure 'visual' subgroup of dyslexics would be very small. (2) On the other hand, between 80–92% (depending on age) suffer from visual, optomotor, and also auditory deficits. Thus to separate out a pure visual/optomotor subgroup does not make much sense. This means that one has to look for the deficits in each individual dyslexic person and try to reduce the identified problem as has been pointed out in a recent report (Fischer, 2010).

The magnocellular or temporal hypothesis of dyslexia

The idea that abnormality of a certain group of nerve cells within the visual system accounts for the deficits encountered in dyslexics goes back to observations made in the brains of dyslexic adults after death (Galaburda & Aboitiz, 1986). Specifically, it was found, that the density of large cell bodies in layers 1 and 2 of the lateral geniculate body was lower as compared with normal adults (Livingstone et al., 1991). This cell type is already present in the population of ganglion cells in the retina. The system of these cells, called the magnocellular system, projects from the layers in the lateral geniculate body to the primary visual cortex, where the magno system is still kept separate from the parvo system (Tootell et al., 1988). It projects dorsally to the prestriate cortex and further on to the parietal and to the frontal brain, whereas the parvo system projects ventrally to the inferior-temporal cortex. The frontal cortex is involved in controlling the voluntary component of saccade generation, which is the one which exhibits most of the optomotor deficits observed in dyslexia. From this point of view one may argue, that both the visual and optomotor deficits support the magnocellular hypothesis of dyslexia (Stein & Walsh, 1997). The cells of the magnocellular system respond differently to those in the parvocellular system to prolonged visual stimuli. While the magno cells respond by a transient burst of nerve impulses, the parvo cells respond by a sustained increase in impulse frequency. This physiological difference means that the magno cells respond preferentially to movement and to other visual stimuli that contain fast changes in the time. The magnocellular hypothesis of dyslexia was therefore generalized to a temporal hypothesis which includes also the auditory system (Witton et al., 1998; Stein & Talcott, 1999; Talcott et al., 2002).

Our own data support this generalized hypothesis to the extent, that dyslexics exhibit deficits in dynamic vision (Fischer et al., 2000) as well as in the optomotor domain. In addition, dyslexics exhibit also deficits in subitizing and number counting. Simon et al. (1998) suggested that this visual function also uses the magnocellular system. Within the auditory domain the strongest and most common deficits are found in time-order tasks, in which the subjects have to tell the order of two short stimuli of quite different frequencies (Fischer & Hartnegg, 2004). The time interval between the two stimuli was decreased until the threshold was reached. Dyslexic subjects failed in up to 70% of the cases to reach the range of age-matched controls (Fischer & Hartnegg, 2004). From these observations one may conclude that indeed the time factor plays an important role in reading and spelling as well as in the list of non-reading deficits encountered in dyslexics. Therefore, the data reported here are in agreement with a temporal theory of dyslexia (Stein & Walsh, 1997), but they do not prove that other problems of different nature do not play an important role in dyslexia. If the deficits of dyslexics are due to poor functioning of the magnocellular system one may expect to see deficits everywhere in brain structures, which receive their input directly or indirectly through the magnocellular system.

References

Beaton, A.B. (2004). *Dyslexia, Reading, and the Brain*. New York: Psychology Press.

Desimone, R., Albright, T.D., Gross, C.G., & Bruce, C. (1980). Responses of inferior temporal neurons to complex visual stimuli. *Neuroscience Abstracts*, 6, 194.13, 581.

Dyckman, K.A., & McDowell, J.E. (2005). Behavioural plasticity of antisaccade performance following daily practice. *Experimental Brain Research*, 162, 63–9.

Everling, S., & Fischer, B. (1998). The antisaccade: a review of basic research and clinicalstudies. *Neuropsychologia*, 36, 885–99.

Fischer, B. (2006). Subitizing and counting by visual memory in dyslexia and dyscalculia: Development, deficits, training, transfer. In: C.B. Hayes (Ed.) *Dyslexia in children: New research*, pp. 93–102. New York: Nova Publishers.

Fischer, B. (2010). A sensory fix for problems in school. *Scientific American Mind* 21, 32–7.

Fischer, B., & Hartnegg, K. (2000). Effects of visual training on saccade control in dyslexia. *Perception*, 29, 531–42.

Fischer, B., & Hartnegg, K. (2002). Age effects in dynamic vision based on orientation identification. *Experimental Brain Research*, 143, 120–5.

Fischer, B., & Hartnegg, K. (2004). On the development of low-level auditory discrimination and deficits in dyslexia. *Dyslexia* 10, 105–18.

Fischer, B., & Hartnegg, K. (2009). Instability of fixation in dyslexia: development—deficits- training. *Optometry and Vision Development*, 40, 221–8.

Fischer, B., & Ramsperger, E. (1984). Human express saccades: extremely short reaction times of goal directed eye movements. *Experimental Brain Research*, 57, 191–5.

Fischer, B., & Ramsperger, E. (1986). Human express saccades: effects of randomization and daily practice. *Experimental Brain Research*, 64, 569–78.

Fischer, B., Gezeck, S., & Hartnegg, K. (1997). The analysis of saccadic eye movements from gap and overlap paradigms. *Brain Research Protocols* 2, 47–52.

Fischer, B., Hartnegg, K., & Mokler, A. (2000). Dynamic visual perception of dyslexic children. *Perception*, 29, 523–30.

Fischer, B., daPos, O., & Stürzel, F. (2003). Illusory illusions: The significance of fixation on the perception of geometrical illusions. *Perception*, 32, 1001–8.

Fischer, B., Gebhardt, C., & Hartnegg, K. (2008a). Subitizing and visual counting in children with problems acquiring basic arithmetic skills. *Optometry and Vision Development*, 39, 24–9.

Fischer, B., Köngeter, A., & Hartnegg, K. (2008b). Effects of daily practice on subitizing, visual counting, and basic arithmetic skills. *Optometry and Vision Development*, 39, 30–4.

Galaburda, A.M., & Aboitiz, F. (1986). Biological foundations of dyslexia. A review. *Archivos de Biología y Medicina Experimentales (Santiago)*, 19, 57–65.

Goldberg, M.E., Bushnell, M.C., & Bruce, C.J. (1986). The effect of attentive fixation on eye movements evoked by electrical stimulation of the frontal eye fields. *Experimental Brain Research*, 61, 579–84.

Guitton, D., Buchtel, H.A., & Douglas, R.M. (1985). Frontal lobe lesions in man cause difficulties in suppressing reflexive glances and in generating goal-directed saccades. *Experimental Brain Research*, 58, 455–72.

Hartnegg, K., & Fischer, B. (2002). A turn-key transportable eye-tracking instrument forclinical assessment. *Behavior, Research Methods, Instruments, & Computers*, 34, 625–9.

Hebb, D. (1949). *The organization of behaviour: A neuropsychological theory*. New York: Wiley.

Hikosaka, O., & Wurtz, R.H. (1983). Visual and oculomotor functions of monkey substantia nigra pars reticulata. II. Visual responses related to fixation of gaze. *Journal of Neurophysiology*, 49, 1254–67.

Kulp, M.T., & Schmidt, P.P. (2010). Effect of oculomotor and other visual skills on reading performance: A literature review. *Optometry and Vision Science*, 73, 283–92.

Livingstone, M.S., Rosen, G.D., Drislane, F.W., & Galaburda, A.M. (1991). Physiological and anatomical evidence for a magnocellular defect in developmental dyslexia. *Proceedings of the National Academy of Sciences of the United States of America*, 88, 7943–47.

Munoz, D.P., & Wurtz, R.H. (1992). Role of the rostral superior colliculus in active visual fixation and execution of express saccades. *Journal of Neurophysiology*, 67, 1000–2.

Munoz, D., & Wurtz, R. (1993). Interactions between fixation and saccade neurons in primate superior colliculus. *Society of Neuroscience Abstracts*, 19, 787, 321.

Munoz, D.P., & Everling, S. (2004). Look away: the anti-saccade task and the voluntary control of eye movement. *Nature Reviews/Neuroscience*, 5, 218–28.

O'Regan, J.K. (1990). Eye movements and reading. [Review]. *Reviews of Oculomotor Research*, 4, 395–453.

Olson, R.K., Conners, F.C., & Rack, J.P. (1991). *Eye movements in dyslexic and normal readers*. In: J.F. tein (Ed.) *Vision and Visual Dysfunction, Vol 13, Vision and Vision Dyslexia*, pp. 243–250. London: Macmillan.

Pavlidis, G.T. (1981). Do eye movements hold the key to dyslexia? *Neuropsychologia*, 9, 57–64.

Reichle, E.D., Rayner, K., & Pollatsek, A. (2003). The E-Z-Reader model of eye-movement control in reading: comparison to other models. *Behavioral and Brain Sciences*, 26, 445–526.

Robinson, D.L., Goldberg, M.E., & Stanton, G.B. (1978). Parietal association cortex in the primate: Sensory mechanisms and behavioral modulations. *Journal of Neurophysiology*, 41, 910–32.

Schäffler, T., Sonntag, J., & Fischer, B. (2004). The effect of daily practice on low-level auditory discrimination, phonological skills, and spelling in dyslexia. *Dyslexia*, 10, 119–30.

Schiller, P.H., True, S.D., & Conway, J.L. (1979). Effects of frontal eye field and superior colliculus ablations on eye movements. *Science*, 206, 590–2.

Schiller, P.H., Sandell, J.H., & Maunsell, J.H. (1987). The effect of frontal eye field and superior colliculus lesions on saccadic latencies in the rhesus monkey. *Journal of Neurophysiology*, 57, 1033–49.

Schrauf, M., Wist, E.R., & Ehrenstein, W.H. (2000). Development of dynamic vision based on motion contrast. *Experimental Brain Research*, 124, 469–73.

Simon, T.J., Peterson, S., Patel, G., & Sathian, K. (1998). Do the magnocellular and parvocellular visual pathways contribute differentially to subitizing and counting? *Perception and Psychophysics*, 60, 451–64.

Starkey, P., & Cooper, R.G. (1995). The development of subitizing in young children. *British Journal of Developmental Psychology*, 13, 399–420.

Stein, J., & Fowler, S. (1985). Effect of monocular occlusion on visuomotor perception and reading in dyslexic children. *Lancet*, 2, 69–73.

Stein, J., & Talcott, J. (1999). Impaired neuronal timing in developmental dyslexia—The magnocellular hypothesis. *Dyslexia*, 5, 59–77.

Stein, J., & Walsh, V. (1997). To see but not to read; the magnocellular theory of dyslexia. *Trends in Neuroscience*, 20, 147–51.

Talcott, J.B., Hansen, P.C., Assoku, E.L., & Stein, J.F. (2002). Visual motion sensitivity in dyslexia: evidence for temporal and energy integration deficits. *Neuropsychologia*, 38(7), 935–43.

Tootell, R.B., Hamilton, S.L., & Switkes, E. (1988). Functional anatomy of macaque striate cortex. IV. Contrast and magno-parvo streams. *Journal of Neuroscience*, 8, 1594–609.

Witton, C., Talcott, J.B., Hansen, P.C., Richardson, A.J., Griffiths, T.D., Rees, A., *et al.* (1998). Sensitivity to dynamic auditory and visual stimuli predicts nonword reading ability in both dyslexic and normal readers. *Current Biology*, 8, 791–7.

Chapter 3

Movements of the Eyes in Three-Dimensional Space: Deficits of Vergence and Binocular Coordination in Dyslexia

Zoï Kapoula

Introduction

Reading starts with vision. Vision is a highly active process because of saccadic and fixation eye movements. Saccades allow us to bring one word after another onto the fovea where fine visual analysis takes place during the subsequent fixation period. Reading without saccades is unnatural. Bouma and de Voogd (1974) attempted artificial reading without saccades by presenting each word to fixating eyes. Although reading was still possible, it was slower; but comprehension was not evaluated.

Many studies of eye movements during reading have allowed us to pinpoint important regularities present in non-dyslexic readers. For instance, 90% of reading time is devoted to fixations, while saccades take only 10% of the time; the majority of saccades are made from left to right and have a mean length of seven to nine characters, i.e. 2–3°. About 12% of the saccades are in the opposite direction. These regressive saccades allow for the verification of misread words; their typical length being four characters. For rightward saccades, a privileged landing position exists, bringing the eyes just to the left of the centre of each word (O'Regan, 1990, 1992).

Since the 1980s, various models have been proposed as to how these eye movements are controlled during reading. Some claim that their control is automatic, governed by coarse visual analysis in the periphery; others claim that when and where the eyes will fixate next is decided on a moment-to-moment basis in conjunction with language processing (O'Regan & Lévy-Schoen, 1987). Intensive modelling activity continues (Reichle et al., 1998; Engbert et al., 2005); such models integrate lexical information processing, saccade programming, and covert shifts of spatial attention.

Research on eye movements in dyslexia follows two lines. The first deals with abnormalities in the regularities of eye movements during reading relative to non-dyslexic readers. For instance, shorter saccade lengths and longer fixation durations for dyslexics have often been reported (Rayner, 1998; De Luca et al., 1999), as well as more regressive saccades (Pavlidis, 1981). Olson et al. (1991) reported that compared with normal readers such differences do not exist when dyslexics read pseudowords or during a non-lexical string processing task, suggesting that dyslexics' ocular motor abnormalities are caused by their reading difficulties rather than vice versa.

A second line of research focuses on the neurophysiology of eye movements per se, and uses simple tasks to stimulate eye movements, mostly saccades. For instance, the latency of the saccades has been extensively studied with emphasis on the occurrence of express types of latency (very short latencies of 80–120 ms) that could be attributed to deficits in fixation control (Biscaldi et al., 1994). A few, rather qualitative studies, have described fixation instability, including poor vergence and problems with binocular control (Stein et al., 1987).

The studies conducted by our team have focused on the neurophysiology of eye movements in non-reading tasks. Our goal is to provide complete characterization of fixations and eye movements in dyslexics and non-dyslexics independently from reading. We emphasize that reading involves coordinated movements of the two eyes in all three dimensions: in horizontal and vertical directions as well as in the depth plane. In other words, eye movement activity during reading is physiologically similar to that which takes place during the exploration of natural three-dimensional space. When exploring the environment we engage in saccades, be they horizontal, vertical, or oblique (combining the two directions), or vergence. Vergence eye movements allow one to adjust the angle of the visual axes to the depth at which the object of interest is located. At the cortical level, saccades and vergence are both under the control of parietal and frontal areas; at the level of the brainstem each type of eye movement is controlled by a distinct area—the so-called saccade and vergence motor generators, however dynamically organized and interconnected they may be (Leigh & Zee, 2006).

Reading is a proximal activity and involves sustained control in order to maintain an appropriate vergence angle with respect to the distance of the book or screen from the reader. An inappropriate vergence angle may cause a blurring effect or double vision. While making horizontal saccades the vertical position of the eyes should also be controlled carefully so that the eyes do not deviate up or down with respect to the text line in question. At the end of each line a large oblique saccade is made from right to left and from top to bottom in order to replace the eyes at the beginning of the next line.

A further complicating factor involves maintaining the stability of the vergence angle during saccades. To do so, horizontal and oblique saccades should all be well coordinated for the two eyes. Any inequality in the amplitude of the saccades between the two eyes would modify the vergence angle and could interfere with single clear vision of the word. During the fixation following each saccade, it is important to maintain the stability of the eyes and to avoid conjugate drifts in the horizontal or vertical direction. It is also important to avoid disconjugate (different for the two eyes) drifts, as such drifts producing both retinal slip and changes in the vergence angle. Recall that visual acuity degrades if retinal slip exceeds 2°/s (Westheimer & McKee, 1975).

In the next section we will present a hypothesis on how fine binocular coordination of saccades is learned during development. Then we will present studies on the quality of the binocular coordination of saccades in dyslexics and non-dyslexics and on fixation instability. These studies reveal a link between binocular coordination and vergence.

In the final part we will review studies dealing with the initiation of saccades and vergence.

Binocular coordination—Hering–Helmholtz controversy: a reconciling hypothesis

Fine binocular coordination of saccades is essential for clear binocular vision. What mechanisms the central nervous system (CNS) uses to achieve such coordination has been a controversial issue ever since the early debates between Hering (1868) and Helmholtz (1856–1866). According to Hering, binocular coordination is based on neuro-anatomical connections, allowing the same innervation to be sent to conjugate muscles so that the two eyes move as a single organ. According to Helmholtz, neuroanatomical connections are separate for each eye and thus binocular coordination of movements can only be achieved by training and binocular visual experience.

Hering's thinking has dominated both basic and clinical research. Electrophysiological evidence in favour of Hering's law of equal innervation has been found in monkeys: burst saccade neurons project to motor neurons innervating the lateral, external rectus of one eye and also project to interneurons that relay to the motor neurons innervating the contralateral medial rectus (Leigh & Zee, 2006).

Hering's law of equal central innervation of the two eyes is not incompatible with learning, however. The control of the extraocular muscles in the two eyes cannot be identical; the relay for innervating the abducting lateral rectus (turning the eye outward) is longer than that for innervating the adducting medial rectus. Learning will therefore be necessary to adjust the central command so that finally the eyes move by the same amount.

Our overall hypothesis is that the CNS uses natural existing mechanisms of saccade–vergence interaction to render saccades equal for the two eyes. To illustrate this, one can consider the case of rightward saccades. Because of the asymmetry of the oculomotor plant (difference in muscles and/or in innervation relays), a central saccade command results in a saccade that is larger in the abducting than in the adducting eye (Fig. 3.1a). We hypothesize that the CNS learns to couple the conjugate saccade command with an appropriate rapid vergence command tailored to reduce the initial inequality of the two eyes' saccades (Fig. 3.1b). Thus the resulting saccade has only a small residual divergent disconjugacy that can be subsequently corrected by convergent postsaccadic drift, as we see frequently in adults (Collewijn et al., 1988; Zee et al., 1992). Convergence has to occur rapidly during the saccade; this is possible as shown by studies on combined movements in direction and in depth (e.g. Enright, 1984). When the eyes are already converging at near distance, the CNS learns to programme an additional convergence command to eliminate the peripheral asymmetry. Perhaps under such circumstances it is more difficult to tailor the size of the rapid intrasaccadic convergence needed to cancel the peripheral asymmetry.

Next we will review studies in dyslexic and non-dyslexic children, supporting the contention that binocular coordination is the result of slow learning during development and depends on the vergence state.

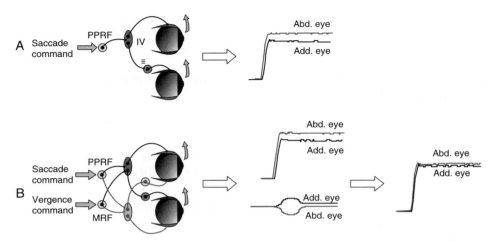

Fig. 3.1 a) Hering's view: the lateral rectus of the abducting eye and the contralateral medial rectus of the adducting eye receive an equal saccadic command. Asymmetry of viscoelastic properties of muscles and/or delay in innervation cause unequal saccades. b) Hypothesis: a small vergence command is sent together with the saccades, compensating for the peripheral asymmetries. III: oculomotor nucleus; IV: abducens nucleus; MRF: mesencephalic reticular formation; PPRF: paramedian pontine reticular formation. Note that the pathway for vergence is hypothetical.

Slow development of binocular coordination in non-dyslexic children—vergence specificity

Fioravanti et al. (1995) reported that in young children binocular coordination of saccades is poor, but improves with age. Yang and Kapoula (2003) reinvestigated this issue, comparing children aged from 4.5–12 years and adults aged from 22–45 years. They recorded binocularly, with an infrared system (Dr Bouis Oculometer). Twenty-degree horizontal saccades were made at near (20 cm) and at far (150 cm) distance; the corresponding convergence angles required were 17° and 2°.

For the far distance the quality of saccadic coordination reached adult levels by the age of 7–8 years but for the near distance coordination remained poor until the age of 10–11 years (Fig. 3.2). Moreover, the small saccadic disconjugacy (the difference in amplitude of the saccade between the two eyes) was found to be mostly divergent in adults. But in children saccade disconjugacy was much more variable and could be divergent or convergent. These results clearly show that the quality of coordination of saccades is based, at least partially, on learning. Learning is complex and involves specific adjustments according to viewing distance and to the vergence angle. The data support the idea that when the eyes are already converging, learning to produce appropriate intrasaccadic convergence is more difficult.

As reading is an activity at near distance, our data imply that learning to read and learning to coordinate movements of the two eyes occur in parallel. Perhaps, reading stimulates further improvement of binocular control.

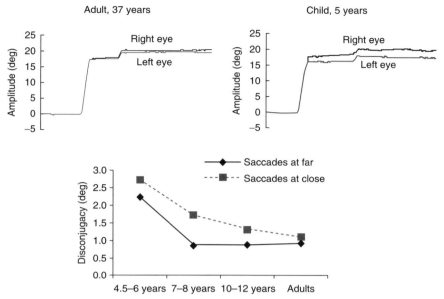

Fig. 3.2 Top: binocular recording of a rightward saccade from an adult and a child. Bottom: saccade disconjugacy for children as a function of age. Saccade disconjugacy in children is worse at close distance.

Before presenting studies on binocular control in dyslexics we will first present a study on vergence using orthoptic testing.

Dyslexia and vergence problems

Stein et al. (1987, 1988) reported that fixation instability and reduced vergence capacity occur frequently in dyslexics. Evans and Drasdo (1990) reported similar observations, e.g. significantly lower convergence and divergence capacities relative to non-dyslexics; but they did not find a correlation between visual deficits and reading disability. Furthermore Ygge et al. (1993a, 1993b) reported that problems of accommodation, stereoacuity, vergence, or strabismus occurred at similar rates in dyslexics and non-dyslexics.

Kapoula et al. (2007) performed exhaustive orthoptic evaluation in 57 dyslexic and 47 non-dyslexic children of comparable age (mean: 11 years). Dyslexics and non-dyslexics were recruited mostly from a college in Paris with classes specialized for dyslexia. Dyslexics were diagnosed before entering the college by a specialized medical centre, using standard criteria. Examination included neurological, psychological, and phonological tests, repeated before oculomotor testing. Reading speed, text comprehension, and word/pseudoword reading were also evaluated using the L2MA battery (Chevrie-Muller et al., 1997). All children included in the study had reading ages more than two standard deviations behind that expected from their age. Wechsler Intelligence Scale for Children-III (WISC III IQ) was measured, and was in the normal range, i.e. between 85 and 115.

Table 3.1 Percentages of dyslexic and non-dyslexic children with stereoacuity (measured with the TNO test) better or equal to 60 seconds of arc and percentages of children with near point of convergence (NPC) below 6 cm

Subjects	TNO (seconds of arc)		NPC (cm) ≤ 6
	<60	60	
Dyslexics (57)	21%	78%	58%
Non-dyslexics (46)	31%	69%	85%

Non-dyslexic children were recruited predominately from the same college and they had normal school performances, most of them superior to the mean scores of their class. Similar criteria and recruitment centres were used for all our studies of dyslexics.

The major orthoptic findings were: normal scores in the TNO stereoacuity test (60 seconds of arc) were slightly more frequent in dyslexics than in non-dyslexics; yet, stereoacuity scores better than normal (< 60 seconds of arc) were slightly more frequent in non-dyslexics (Table 3.1). In contrast, normal values of the near point of convergence (NPC), that is, below 6 cm, occurred in 85% of non-dyslexics while only 58% of dyslexic children reached this value. Many dyslexics (42%) showed NPC greater than 7 cm, 6% of them beyond 10 cm. Divergence amplitude was also measured using a prism bar to test disparity-driven divergence. This test was carried out both at near (40 cm) and at far distances (400 cm). It should be noted that at near distance, divergence response to the prisms could be partially assisted by relaxation of convergence, but this mechanism cannot be involved when the child fixates at far distance. Dyslexics' vergence amplitudes elicited by the prisms were lower both at near and at far distance: dyslexics 10 prism dioptres (pD) at near and 4 pD at far versus non-dyslexics 12 pD at near and 6 pD at far (Fig. 3.3).

Kapoula et al. (2007) argue that reduced divergence capacity at far distance (400 cm) indicates a deficit in divergence per se, occurring independently from convergence and accommodation. Indeed, physiological studies indicate distinct control of convergence and divergence both at cortical and subcortical levels. At the cortical level Gamlin and

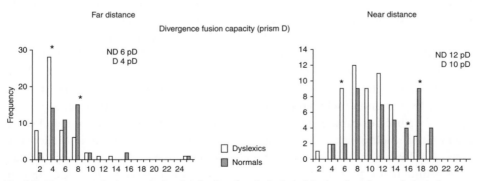

Fig. 3.3 Divergence fusion capacity distribution for dyslexic (white bars) and non-dyslexic (grey bars) children at far and near distance. The median of dyslexic and non-dyslexics is also given. Asterisks indicate a significant difference between dyslexics and non-dyslexics.

Yoon (2000) identified an area close to the saccade area in the frontal eye fields containing separate subgroups of cells that discharge before and during convergence or divergence movements. An electroencephalography study from Tzelepi et al. (2004) indicated that cortical activation prior to divergence movements was located more posteriorly than that prior to convergence. At the subcortical level, Mays (1984) identified distinct groups of cells activated prior and during divergence versus convergence eye movements in the monkey mesencephalic reticular formation. Kapoula et al. (2007) concluded that specific vergence abnormalities assessed by orthoptics occur more frequently among dyslexics. This observation motivated the following studies on the binocular coordination of saccades in dyslexics.

Poor binocular coordination of saccades in dyslexic children

Bucci et al. (2008a) studied the binocular coordination of saccades in 18 dyslexic children (average age 11.4 years) compared with 13 non-dyslexic children of comparable age (11.2 years). They used a simplified single-word reading task (introduced by Vitu, 2004). The task was carried out at a near distance (40 cm). Briefly, each trial started with the presentation of the sign '+' on the left side of the computer screen. After 500 ms the '+' was replaced by a cross and simultaneously a word was presented in the middle of the screen and a '+' on the right side. The child was asked first to fixate the cross on the left side, then to read the word silently, and then to fixate the '+' on the right side. Saccades from this task were compared with another standard saccade task, during which the child had to fixate a LED that jumped randomly from 0° to 10° or 20° to the right or left remaining at each location for 2 s.

The amplitudes of the saccades during the word reading task ranged between 6.5° and 10°, depending on the length of the word and were similar for the two groups of children. The amplitudes of the saccades during the LED task were about 15° and were also similar for dyslexics and non-dyslexics. Thus the binocular coordination of saccades presented next concerns similar saccade amplitudes for dyslexics and non-dyslexics.

Fig. 3.4 shows typical binocular recordings of saccades in a dyslexic and in a non-dyslexic child in the single-word reading task. The dyslexic child's saccades are poorly coordinated and are followed by a large disconjugate drift. Quantitative results from this study showed a statistically significant difference in the disconjugacy of the saccades between the two groups of children: for dyslexics the mean disconjugacy of saccades was 1.17 ± 0.11° for the word reading task and 0.95 ± 0.07° for the LED-target task. In contrast, for non-dyslexics the mean disconjugacy was only 0.41 ± 0.05° for saccades to words, and 0.34 ± 0.02° for saccades to LED targets (Fig. 3.5a).

The disconjugate postsaccadic drift (difference in the drifts of the two eyes), measured in the first period of fixation before the corrective saccade (Fig. 3.5b) was significantly greater in dyslexics (0.45 ± 0.05° for the word reading task and 0.46 ± 0.07°, for the LED-target task). Non-dyslexics showed smaller values (0.25 ± 0.03° and 0.26 ± 0.03° respectively).

For non-dyslexics, the majority of saccades had a divergent disconjugacy (due to a larger amplitude of the saccade in the abducting eye), while the disconjugacy of the postsaccadic drift was predominantly convergent (see positives values on the y axis; Fig. 3.6); the

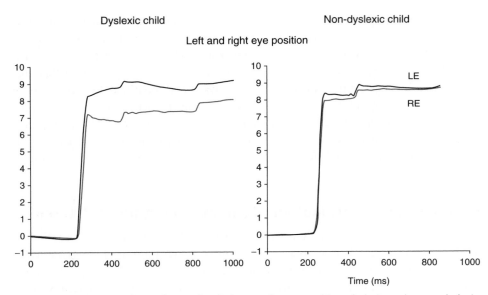

Fig. 3.4 Binocular recordings of saccades during reading a word in a dyslexic and a non-dyslexic. Individual eye positions are shown for the left (dark trace) and the right eyes (grey trace); the word appeared at time zero.

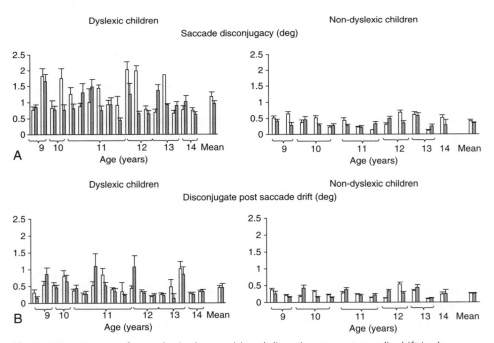

Fig. 3.5 Disconjugacy of saccades in degrees (a) and disconjugate postsaccadic drift in degrees (b) measured during reading of single words and during saccades to the LED.

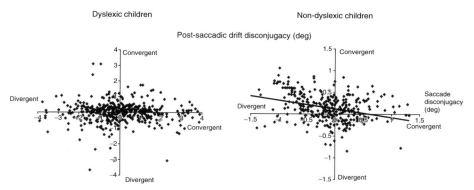

Fig. 3.6 Relationship between saccade and drift disconjugacy. For each saccade in the reading task, the disconjugacy of the saccade is shown in degrees (x-axis) and the disconjugacy of the postsaccadic drift (y-axis). Positive values indicate convergent disconjugacy, negative values divergent disconjugacy. Note the different scales.

correlation between the two was statistically significant (r = 0.35, p <0.05). In contrast, for dyslexics, the disconjugacy was almost randomly convergent or divergent, as was the disconjugacy of the postsaccadic drift, and there was no correlation between the disconjugacy and the postsaccadic drift.

The lack of a stereotyped pattern of saccadic disconjugacy and the lack of correlation imply that dyslexics experience substantial and variable binocular disparity during the fixation period following a reading saccade because their disconjugate postsaccadic drift does not systematically reduce the disparity resulting from their saccadic disconjugacy. Such disparity probably interferes with visual processing of words and needs further investigation. Dyslexics may have to exert their sensory fusional system more, to achieve single vision of the word. Such extra sensory effort during reading could cause visual fatigue. Further investigation with text reading should combine physiological measures of binocular coordination of saccades, of residual fixation disparity and measures of reading performance and of visual fatigue.

Binocular coordination of saccades during free exploration of paintings in dyslexics and non-dyslexics

In order to see if horizontal binocular coordination problems also occur during spontaneous free exploration of paintings, Kapoula et al. (2009) examined the binocular coordination of saccades in dyslexics and non-dyslexics during free exploration of the cubist artwork of Fernand Léger.

The study was conducted with eight non-dyslexic (average age 11.1 years) and 15 dyslexic children (average age 11.2 years). The children were seated in front of a computer screen placed at 30 cm. Initially, they fixated a line target at the bottom-left of the screen; then one of the three paintings (The Alarm Clock, The Contrast of Forms or The Wedding; angular size 18 × 25.4°) was displayed on the screen for a period of 30 s. They explored the painting spontaneously; and were given no specific instructions.

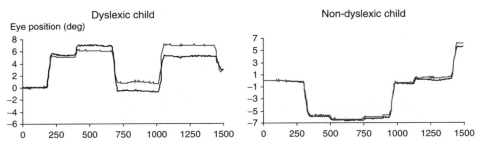

Fig. 3.7 Dyslexic and a non-dyslexic binocular recordings of horizontal saccades looking at a painting. For the dyslexic, the saccade was larger in the right eye, so that at the end of the saccade the eyes converged or diverged relative to their angle at the beginning. During the fixation period following the saccade the eyes were drifting mildly but differently and this modified the vergence angle further. For the non-dyslexic child the disconjugate drift of the eyes was minimal and improved the binocular alignment of the eyes.

Fig. 3.7 shows a sequence of horizontal saccades during free exploration ['of a painting'] (Fig. 3.7a) from a dyslexic and a non-dyslexic child. Clearly, the dyslexic showed larger disconjugacy than the non-dyslexic. The disconjugacy was significantly larger for the whole group of dyslexics than non-dyslexics. Again saccade disconjugacy and post-saccadic drift disconjugacy were uncorrelated in the dyslexics but were correlated in the non-dyslexics. Thus saccade disconjugacy and uncorrelated disconjugate drifts during fixations in dyslexics occur in a non-reading situation; they seem to have an intrinsic physiological problem, leading to poor control of binocular eye alignment.

Poor binocular control in dyslexics could reflect immaturity of the saccade–vergence interaction learning mechanisms that are needed to coordinate saccades, particularly at near distances (i.e. with the eyes converging). One of the theories about the origin of dyslexia proposes a deficit in the magnocellular system, the posterior parietal cortex being a major target of this system (Livingstone et al., 1991; Stein & Walsh, 1997). In other studies carried out with healthy adults, Vernet et al. (2008) used transcranial magnetic stimulation to interfere with the function of the posterior parietal cortex; they demonstrated a deterioration of the binocular coordination of saccades and of the stability of vergence angle during fixation. This area is actively involved in the binocular coordination of saccades and perhaps keeps the brainstem and cerebellar circuits calibrated. Thus, poor binocular coordination in dyslexics could be one of the multiple manifestations of the immaturity of the circuits involving the magnocellular system and the cerebellum. It may not be the sole cause of dyslexia but it could be an aggravating factor, particularly during reading acquisition. An ongoing study tests the persistence of poor binocular coordination in dyslexics up to 17 years; it also examines whether the deficit is specific to near vision.

Latency of saccades and vergence eye movements in dyslexic children

The latency of an eye movement is the period between the appearance of a new stimulus and starting an eye movement to foveate it. During this time interval several processes need to occur, such as the shift of visual attention to the new stimulus, the disengagement of oculomotor fixation, and the computation of the new parameters (Fischer & Ramsperger, 1984; Findlay & Walker, 1999).

Dossetor and Papaioannou (1975) and Pirozzolo and Rayner (1979) showed that the latency of saccades was longer in dyslexics than in non-dyslexics. In contrast, Adler-Grinberg and Stark (1978) and Black et al. (1984) found no such latency difference. Fischer and Weber (1990) reported longer mean latencies and a larger standard deviation for dyslexics. However, Biscaldi et al. (1994) reported shorter mean latencies and more express saccades in dyslexic children and teenagers compared with controls. According to these authors, abnormal function of the fixation system, which is most likely modulated by attention mechanisms, could be responsible for the generation of a large number of express saccades in dyslexics. In other words, the engagement of attention to the fixation point and its inhibitory effect on the saccade system could be deficient in dyslexics. More recently, Bednarek et al. (2006) studied saccades from 10-year-old dyslexic children and age-matched controls. They reported significantly reduced saccade latencies in dyslexics compared to the control group; they did not report express latencies in dyslexics, but a high occurrence of anticipatory latencies. When the attentional shift was facilitated by a cue (Posner et al., 1980), saccade latencies were no different between the two groups of children. These authors also proposed a deficit of the attention system in dyslexics and supported the hypothesis of Facoetti et al. (2003) that dyslexics may have difficulty in narrowing their focus of attention.

Bucci et al. (2008b) examined the latency of saccades at far and at near distance, as well as the latency of convergence and divergence, and of combined saccade–vergence movements. The study was performed with 16 dyslexic children; mean age 11.12 ± 1.08 years, the mean IQ was 104 ± 7 and the mean reading age was 8.4 ± 1.2 years; 14 non-dyslexic children were also tested (mean age: 12.08 ± 0.99 years).

The spatial arrangement used to stimulate eye movements is shown in Fig. 3.8a. Computer-controlled LEDs were placed in two isovergence circles at different distances (at 20 and 150 cm) from the child. Three LEDs were placed on the circle closest to the child, one at the centre and the others at $\pm 20°$. Thus the mean vergence angle required to fixate any of these three LEDs on the near circle was $17°$. Five LEDs were placed on the circle most distant from the child: one at the centre, two at $\pm 10°$, and two at $\pm 20°$; fixation to any of these LEDs required a vergence angle of $2.3°$.

Two paradigms, simultaneous and gap, were used (Fig. 3.8b). In the simultaneous paradigm, after a 2.5-s fixation period, the central LED was switched off and simultaneously the target LED was switched on for 1.5 s. A delay of 0.5 s was introduced before the next trial. In the gap paradigm at the beginning of each trial, a fixation LED was lit up at the centre of one of the circles, and remained lit for 2.5 s. Then it was turned off, and a target LED appeared 200 ms later (gap period). The target LED appeared for 1.5 s. A delay of 0.5 s was introduced before the next trial. This paradigm was used to promote express saccades. Blocks of gap and simultaneous stimuli were randomly interleaved.

For all the eye movements recorded and for both paradigms the mean latencies of dyslexics were longer than those of non-dyslexics (see Fig. 3.9). However, this difference was

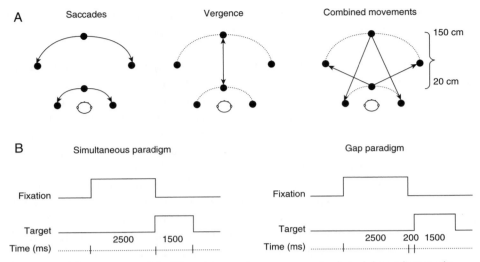

Fig. 3.8 Spatial arrangement (a); different types of eye movements elicited depending on the combination of the central fixation target and the target LEDs: pure saccades at far (150 cm) and at near (20 cm) distance, pure vergence (convergence and divergence) along the median plane and combined saccade—vergence movements. Temporal arrangement (b); schematic diagram of the temporal arrangement used in the two different paradigms (simultaneous and gap).

not always statistically significant. In the simultaneous paradigm the mean latency of dyslexics was significantly longer for saccades at far distance and for the saccadic components of movements combined with convergence and divergence. In the gap paradigm the mean latency was significantly longer for saccades at far distance and for the saccade component of movements combined with convergence.

Previous studies from our group dealing with latency of saccades at different viewing distances in normal children (Yang et al., 2002; Bucci et al., 2005), as well as in children with vertigo (Bucci et al., 2004) and in children with strabismus (Bucci et al., 2006), have shown that saccades at far distance naturally have a longer latency than saccades at near; the same difference occurs for adults and aged subjects (Yang et al. 2002). Multiple mechanisms could explain the longer latency at far distance: sensory, oculomotor, and attentional (Yang et al., 2002). It is likely that initiating a saccade from far distance would require more involvement of parietal–frontal pathways believed to be activated for voluntary saccade triggering (Pierrot-Deseilligny et al., 1995; 2002). The finding of significantly longer latencies for saccades (pure and combined) starting from far distance suggests that dyslexic children may have problems with the initiation of the more voluntary eye movements. Our results allow us to reconcile the contradictory findings reported previously (Dossetor & Papaioannou, 1975; Bednarek et al., 2006) as these two studies used different distances (1 m versus 50 cm).

More express eye movements in dyslexics

As expected, express latencies occur more frequently in the gap than in the overlap paradigm (see Table 3.2). The percentage of express latencies in dyslexics was high for many

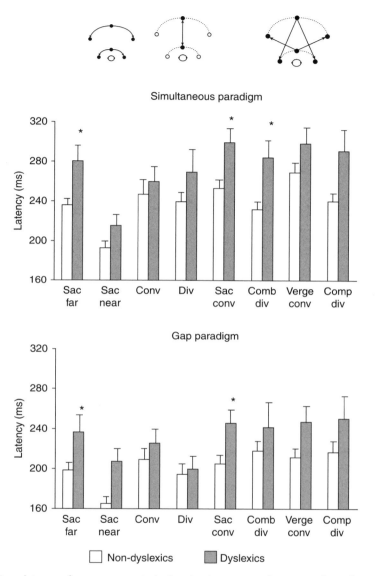

Fig. 3.9 Mean latency of eye movements in the simultaneous and gap paradigms for non-dyslexic (white bars) and dyslexic (grey bars) children. Vertical lines indicate standard error. Significant differences between the two groups shown by an asterisk (Mann–Whitney).

types of eye movements, while for non-dyslexics such latencies occur for fewer subtypes of eye movements (mainly for divergence and saccades at near). Express latencies found in dyslexics could be due to greater disengagement of attention. This idea is in line with Mackeben and Nakayama (1993) who suggested that express latencies use mechanisms involving an unusually rapid shift of attention. Our observations suggest that such an unusually rapid shift of attention is more spatially extended in dyslexics.

Table 3.2 Percentage of express latencies (80–120 ms) for each type of eye movements, in the simultaneous and in the gap paradigm for non-dyslexic and dyslexic children

| | Sacc far | Sacc near | Conv | Combined movements | | | | |
| | | | | Div | Sacc comp | | Vergence comp | |
					Conv	Div	Conv	Div
Gap								
Non-dyslexic	6	34	1	19	10	7	3	10
Dyslexic	12	15	8	23	7	18	8	14
Simultaneous								
Non-dyslexic	0	5	1	4	3	0	2	0
Dyslexic	1	2	3	1	2	0	3	1

To summarize, dyslexic children show longer latencies for saccades starting from a far point but they also show frequent express latencies. While for non-dyslexics express latencies occur mainly for saccades at near distance and diverging, for dyslexics express latencies can also occur frequently for other types of eye movement (saccades at far distance, divergence components of combined movements). Such paradoxical findings can be reconciled; regular latencies and express latencies are believed to involve different initiation mechanisms and perhaps different cortical-subcortical circuits (Pierrot-Deseilligny et al., 1995; Brown et al., 2004; Isa & Kobayashi, 2004). Dyslexics seem to have problems with both types of initiation mechanism.

Normal speed accuracy of saccades and vergence eye movements in dyslexia

Bucci et al. (2009) investigated the velocity and the accuracy of saccades and vergence in dyslexic and non-dyslexic children at mean age 12 ± 1 year for both groups. This study showed that the mean velocity and the accuracy of all eye movements in natural space (saccades, vergence, and combined eye movements) in dyslexics were as good as in non-dyslexic children (see Fig. 3.10).

These findings elucidate the oculomotor capabilities of dyslexics. Studying the latency of eye movements provides information about cortical function: speed/accuracy provides information about premotor and brainstem circuits involved in the generation of eye movements (Leigh & Zee, 2006). Thus, the cortical processes involved in the preparation of eye movements seem to be disturbed in dyslexic children whereas the premotor and brainstem areas responsible for the execution of eye movements seem more normal.

Concluding remarks and future studies

These studies address most eye movement variables involved in reading: binocular coordination, stability of fixation and vergence angle, latency of eye movements, accuracy, and speed. Problems in dyslexic children are specific and only affect some of these—binocular coordination of saccades, fixation instability due to disconjugate drifts,

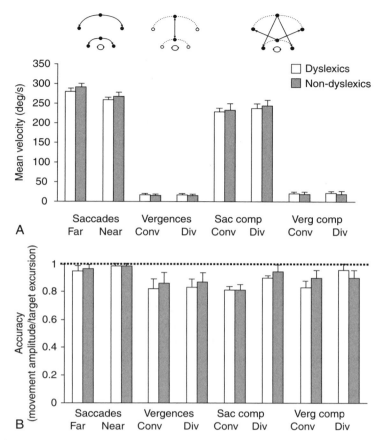

Fig. 3.10 a) Mean velocity (amplitude of the movement/duration) of eye movements in dyslexics and non-dyslexics. Velocities were lower for vergence than for saccades but similar for the two groups. b) Mean accuracy. 1 = perfectly accurate movements. Vergence accuracy is lower than for saccades but there were no differences between dyslexics and non-dyslexics.

and latency. These are eye movement features that develop slowly, achieving adult quality only by the age of 12 years. The saccade and vergence systems are distinct one from the other at least at the level of the brainstem, but need to interact continuously. Deficits in the vergence system may therefore influence the quality of the binocular coordination of saccades. Difficulties in achieving fine binocular coordination in dyslexics, at least at the same age as non-dyslexics, could be seen as a sort of micro-dyspraxia related to magnocellular and cerebellar misfunction.

Precise binocular oculomotor function is a prerequisite for clear vision in general and particularly during reading. Our next step will be to conduct similar studies of binocular control and fixation stability during actual text reading, as such binocular recordings and analysis of vergence and accommodation control are lacking. The consequences of poor binocular saccadic control on reading efficiency have to be evaluated. Inaccurate binocular control results in binocular disparities, which, however small in amplitude, can nevertheless create vergence and accommodation errors when accumulated over time and result in visual fatigue. Visual fatigue and its various consequences on reading performance also need to be measured both subjectively and objectively.

Although much remains to be done, the data reported here allow some clinical conclusions. First, as vergence problems can occur frequently in dyslexics they should be searched for and treated with existing orthoptic training techniques. Indeed, the eye movement control system is a model of cerebral plasticity, and difficulties encountered by dyslexics can be greatly reduced with appropriate training. Vision therapy has been shown to be effective throughout life, even among the elderly or subsequent to brain injury (Ciuffreda et al., 2007, 2008). Development of appropriate new techniques is also needed. This is because the difficulties encountered by dyslexics due to their poor binocular motor control are transient, occurring during saccades, changing from one saccade to the next, and only last a few milliseconds. Exposure to dynamic disparities would be more appropriate.

Another consideration is the importance of reading distance, affecting vergence angles. We are currently investigating the importance of this aspect by measuring eye movements when reading at different distances.

Finally, it is important to emphasize the need for innovative studies examining eye movement behaviour in dyslexics, not only during reading but also during free exploration of visual scenes and paintings. Such studies will help to assess context specificity of motor imperfections and may shed light on general eye scanning strategies in dyslexia.

References

Adler-Grinberg, D., & Stark, L. (1978). Eye movements, scanpaths, and dyslexia. *American Journal of Optometry and Physiological Optics*, 55, 557–70.

Bednarek, D.B., Tarnowski, A., & Grabowska, A. (2006). Latencies of stimulus-driven eye movements are shorter in dyslexic subjects. *Brain and Cognition*, 60, 64–9.

Biscaldi, M., Fischer, B., & Aiple, F. (1994). Saccadic eye movements of dyslexic and normal reading children. *Perception*, 23, 45–64.

Black, J.L., Collins, D.W., De Roach, J.N., & Zubrick, S.R. (1984). Dyslexia: saccadic eye movements. *Perceptual and Motor Skills*, 58, 903–10.

Bouma, H., & de Voogd, A.H. (1974). On the control of eye saccades in reading. *Vision Research*, 14, 273–84.

Brown, J.W., Bullock, D., & Grossberg, S. (2004). How laminar frontal cortex and basal ganglia circuits interact to control planned and reactive saccades. *Neural Networks*, 17, 471–510.

Bucci, M.P., Kapoula, Z., Yang, Q., Wiener-Vacher, S., & Bremond-Gignac, D. (2004). Abnormality of vergence latency in children with vertigo. *Journal of Neurology*, 251, 204–13.

Bucci, M.P., Pouvreau, N., Yang, Q., & Kapoula, Z. (2005). Influence of gap and overlap paradigms on saccade latencies and vergence eye movements in seven-year-old children. *Experimental Brain Research*, 164, 48–57.

Bucci, M.P., Kapoula, Z., Yang, Q., & Bremond-Gignac, D. (2006). Latency of saccades, vergence, and combined movements in children with early onset convergent or divergent strabismus. *Vision Research*, 46, 1384–92.

Bucci, M.P., Bremond-Gignac, D., & Kapoula, Z. (2008a). Poor binocular coordination of saccades in dyslexic children. *Graefe's Archive for Clinical and Experimental Ophthalmology* 246(3), 417–28.

Bucci, M.P., Bremond-Gignac, D., & Kapoula, Z. (2008b). Latency of saccades and vergence eye movements in dyslexic children. *Experimental Brain Research*, 188, 1–12.

Bucci, M.P., Vernet, M., Gerard, C.L., & Kapoula, Z. (2009). Normal speed and accuracy of saccade and vergence eye movements in dyslexic reader children. *Journal of Ophthalmology*, 2009, 325214.

Chevrie-Muller, C., Simon, A.M., & Fournier, S. (1997). *Batterie Langage oral écrit. Mémoire. Attention (L2MA)*. Paris: Editions du Centre de Psychologie Appliquée.

Ciuffreda, K.J., Kapoor, N., Rutner, D., Suchoff, I.B., Han, M.E., & Craig, S. (2007). Occurrence of oculomotor dysfunctions in acquired brain injury: a retrospective analysis. *Optometry*, 78, 155–61.

Ciuffreda, K.J., Rutner, D., Kapoor, N., Suchoff, I.B., Craig, S., & Han, M.E. (2008). Vision therapy for oculomotor dysfunctions in acquired brain injury: a retrospective analysis. *Optometry*, 79, 18–22.

Collewijn, H., Erkelens, C.J., & Steinman, R.M. (1988). Binocular co-ordination of human horizontal saccadic eye movements. *Journal of Physiology*, 404, 157–82.

De Luca, M., Di Pace, E., Judica, A., Spinell, D., & Zoccolotti, P. (1999). Eye movement patterns in linguistic and non-linguistic tasks in developmental surface dyslexia. *Neuropsychologica*, 37, 1407–20.

Dossetor, D.R., & Papaioannou, J. (1975). Dyslexia and eye movements. *Language and Speech*, 18, 312–17.

Engbert, R., Nuthmann, A., Richter, E.M., & Kliegl, R. (2005). SWIFT: a dynamical model of saccade generation during reading. *Psychological Review*, 112, 777–813.

Enright, J.T. (1984). Changes in vergence mediated by saccades. *Journal of Physiology*, 350, 9–31.

Evans, B.J., & Drasdo, N. (1990). Review of ophthalmic factors in dyslexia. *Ophthalmic and Physiological Optics*, 10, 123–32.

Facoetti, A., Lorusso, M.L., Paganoni, P., Umilta, C., & Mascetti, G.G. (2003). The role of visuospatial attention in developmental dyslexia: evidence from a rehabilitation study. *Brain Research. Cognitive Brain Research*, 15, 154–64.

Findlay, J.M., & Walker, R. (1999). A model of saccade generation based on parallel processing and competitive inhibition. *Behavioral and Brain Sciences*, 22, 661–74; discussion 674–721.

Fioravanti, F., Inchingolo, P., Pensiero, S., & Spanio, M. (1995). Saccadic eye movement conjugation in children. *Vision Research*, 35, 3217–28.

Fischer, B., & Ramsperger, E. (1984). Human express saccades: extremely short reaction times of goal directed eye movements. *Experimental Brain Research*, 57, 191–5.

Fischer, B., & Weber, H. (1990). Saccadic reaction times of dyslexic and age-matched normal subjects. *Perception*, 19, 805–18.

Gamlin, P.D., & Yoon, K. (2000). An area for vergence eye movement in primate frontal cortex. *Nature*, 407, 1003–7.

Helmholtz, H. (1856–1866). *Treatise on physiological optics*. Rochester, NY: The Optical Society of America.

Hering, E. (1868). *The theory of binocular vision* (B. Bridgeman, trans.). New York: Plenum Press, (1977).

Isa, T., & Kobayashi, Y. (2004). Switching between cortical and subcortical sensorimotor pathways. *Progress in Brain Research*, 143, 299–305.

Kapoula, Z., Bucci, M.P., Jurion, F., Ayoun, J., Afkhami, F., & Bremond-Gignac, D. (2007). Evidence for frequent divergence impairment in French dyslexic children: deficit of convergence relaxation or of divergence per se? *Graefe's Archive for Clinical and Experimental Ophthalmology*, 245, 931–6.

Kapoula, Z., Ganem, R., Poncet, S., Gintautas, D., Eggert, T., Bremond-Gignac, D., *et al.* (2009). Free exploration of painting uncovers particularly loose yoking of saccades in dyslexics. *Dyslexia*, 15, 243–59.

Leigh, R.J., & Zee, D.S. (2006). *The neurology of eye movements*. New York: Oxford University Press.

Livingstone, M.S., Rosen, G.D., Drislane, F.W., & Galaburda, A.M. (1991). Physiological and anatomical evidence for a magnocellular defect in developmental dyslexia. *Proceedings of the National Academy of Sciences of the United States of America*, 88, 7943–47.

Mackeben, M., & Nakayama, K. (1993). Express attentional shifts. *Vision Research*, 33, 85–90.

Mays L.E. (1984). Neural control of vergence eye movements: convergence and divergence neurons in midbrain. *Journal of Neurophysiology*, 51, 1091–108.

Olson, R.K., Conners, F.C., & Rack, J.P. (1991). Eye movements in dyslexic and normal readers. In: J.F. Stein (Ed.) *Vision and Visual Dysfunction*, pp. 243–250. London: Macmillan.

O'Regan, J.K. (1990). Eye movement and reading. In: E. Kowler (Ed.) *Eye movements and their role in visual and cognitive processes*, pp. 393–453. Amsterdam: Elsevier.

O'Regan, J.K. (1992). Optimal viewing position in words and the strategy-tactics theory of eye movements in reading. In: K. Rayner (Ed.) *Eye movements and visual cognition: Scene Perception and Reading*, pp. 333–54. New York: Springer-Verlag.

O'Regan, J.K., & Lévy-Schoen, A. (1987). Eye movement strategy and tactics in word recognition and reading. In: M. Coltheart (Ed.) *Attention and Performance XII: The psychology of reading*, pp. 363–83. Hillsdale, NJ: Erlbaum.

Pavlidis, G.T. (1981). Do eye movements hold the key to dyslexia? *Neuropsychologica*, 19, 57–64.

Pierrot-Deseilligny, C., Rivaud, S., Gaymard, B., Muri, R., & Vermersch, A.I. (1995). Cortical control of saccades. *Annals of Neurology*, 37, 557–67.

Pierrot-Deseilligny, C., Muri, R.M., Rivaud-Pechoux, S., Gaymard, B., & Ploner, C.J. (2002). Cortical control of spatial memory in humans: the visuooculomotor model. *Annals of Neurology*, 52, 10–19.

Pirozzolo, F.J., & Rayner, K. (1979). Cerebral organization and reading disability. *Neuropsychologica*, 17, 485–91.

Posner, M.I., Snyder, C.R., & Davidson, B.J. (1980). Attention and the detection of signals. *Journal of Experimental Psychology*, 109, 160–74.

Rayner, K. (1998). Eye movements in reading and information processing: 20 years of research. *Psychological Bulletin*, 124, 372–422.

Reichle, E.D., Pollatsek, A., Fisher, D.L., & Rayner, K. (1998). Toward a model of eye movement control in reading. *Psychological Review*, 105, 125–57.

Stein, J., & Walsh, V. (1997). To see but not to read; the magnocellular theory of dyslexia. *Trends in Neurosciences*, 20, 147–52.

Stein, J.F., Riddell, P.M., & Fowler, M.S. (1987). Fine binocular control in dyslexic children. *Eye*, 1(Pt 3), 433–8.

Stein, J.F., Riddell, P.M., & Fowler, S. (1988). Disordered vergence control in dyslexic children. *British Journal of Ophthalmology*, 72, 162–6.

Tzelepi, A., Lutz, A., & Kapoula, Z. (2004). EEG activity related to preparation and suppression of eye movements in three-dimensional space. *Experimental Brain Research*, 155, 439–49.

Vernet, M., Yang, Q., Daunys, G., Orssaud, C., Eggert, T., & Kapoula, Z. (2008). How the brain obeys Hering's law: A TMS study of the posterior parietal cortex. *Investigative Ophthalmology and Visual Science*, 49, 230–7.

Vitu, F., Kapoula, Z., Lancelin, D., & Lavigne, F. (2004). Eye movements in reading isolated words: evidence for strong biases towards the center of the screen. *Vision Research*, 44(3), 321–38.

Westheimer, G., & McKee, S.P. (1975). Visual acuity in the presence of retinal-image motion. *Journal of the Optical Society of America*, 65, 847–50.

Yang, Q., & Kapoula, Z. (2003). Binocular coordination of saccades at far and at near in children and in adults. *Journal of Vision*, 3, 554–61.

Yang, Q., Bucci, M.P., & Kapoula, Z. (2002). The latency of saccades, vergence, and combined eye movements in children and in adults. *Investigative Ophthalmology and Visual Science*, 43, 2939–49.

Ygge, J., Lennerstrand, G., Axelsson, I., & Rydberg, A. (1993a). Visual functions in a Swedish population of dyslexic and normally reading children. *Acta Ophthalmologica*, 71, 1–9.

Ygge, J., Lennerstrand, G., Rydberg, A., Wijecoon, S., & Pettersson, B.M. (1993b). Oculomotor functions in a Swedish population of dyslexic and normally reading children. *Acta Ophthalmologica*, 71, 10–21.

Zee, D.S., Fitzgibbon, E.J., & Optican, L.M. (1992). Saccade-vergence interactions in humans. *Journal of Neurophysiology*, 68, 1624–41.

Chapter 4

Origins of Visual Stress

Arnold Wilkins

The mathematics of uncomfortable images

The comfort with which visual images can be viewed depends in part on simple physical properties of the image, quite independently of what the images represent. This is the implication of recent studies by Juricevic et al. (2010) and by Fernandez and Wilkins (2008). Fourier analysis can be used to represent any image as a series of sine waves (Fourier components) with various frequencies, amplitudes, phases, and orientations. Most images, particularly those from nature, have a relatively high contrast of the lower spatial frequency Fourier components and the amplitude falls off as the spatial frequency increases. It falls off according to a power law, so that a graph of log amplitude (luminance contrast) against log spatial frequency is a straight line with a slope of approximately −1. If images do not have this simple relationship between spatial scale and contrast (larger spatial scales having larger contrast) they become uncomfortable to look at. Juricevic et al. (2010) generated meaningless artificial images from random noise and from randomly disposed rectangles of various sizes. The Fourier spectra of these two types of image were similar with respect to contrast amplitude, although they differed with respect to phase. The images were rated for comfort, and the comfort was found to be maximal when the slope of the amplitude spectrum was about −1, as it is in images from the natural world. When the curve was steeper (slopes in the range −1 to −2) the discomfort increased. When the curve was shallower (slopes in the range −1 to 0) the discomfort again increased. All of the images were novel and artificial and therefore equally unfamiliar, so the effect cannot be attributed to familiarity as such. The same result was obtained for both types of image, those from random noise and random rectangles. Evidently, images with unnatural spatial structure are uncomfortable to view, regardless of their content or meaning.

There are many ways in which the spatial structure of an image can differ from that found in images from nature, and some departures from the natural spatial structure are more uncomfortable than others. Images with unnatural Fourier spectra tend to be more uncomfortable if they have a relative excess of contrast energy at mid-range spatial frequencies, where the visual system is generally most sensitive. This has been shown by Fernandez and Wilkins (2008) who used a variety of images from works of contemporary non-representational art, photographs of everyday scenes, and artificial images generated from random noise. The images rated as comfortable had Fourier amplitude spectra similar to those for natural scenes; the uncomfortable images had the same average slope, but were not linear when plotted as log amplitude versus log frequency. They were curved, with an excess of contrast amplitude for mid-range spatial frequencies of about three cycles per degree. In a further study, Fernandez and Wilkins showed that decreasing the relative contrast amplitude at about three cycles per degree (whilst maintaining the overall contrast amplitude) increased the image comfort, even though the spectrum remained non-linear and unnatural. Evidently images were more uncomfortable if they had an unnatural excess of contrast amplitude at mid-range spatial frequencies relative to that elsewhere in the spectrum. Fernandez and Wilkins (2008) exchanged the Fourier phase and amplitude spectra of comfortable images with those of uncomfortable images. The ratings of comfort depended upon the amplitude spectra, even though the image appearance was more affected by the phase spectra.

Very uncomfortable stimuli—visual and non-visual effects

If all the contrast in an image is concentrated only at mid-range spatial frequencies, the image becomes intensely uncomfortable, even dangerous (Wilkins, 1995). Fig. 4.1 shows a pattern of stripes in which all the energy is concentrated at mid-range spatial frequencies. It is a photograph of the stair tread of an escalator. Images of this kind can induce headaches and seizures, so you are advised to cover this figure if you have migraine or epilepsy.

Images such as the stripes in Fig. 4.1 are not only uncomfortable to look at, they induce illusions of colour, shape, and motion. The number of illusions you see is related to the number of headaches you have: (1) people who see many distortions tend to have frequent headaches; (2) they see more distortions on days when they have a headache; (3) if the headache is on one side of the head the distortions are asymmetric; (4) people with migraine have a greater aversion to the pattern than others; (5) those with aura see more distortions on the side of the aura, between headaches. The parameters of patterns that induce illusions and discomfort are similar to those that provoke photosensitive seizures (Wilkins et al., 1984; Nulty et al., 1987; Marcus & Soso, 1989).

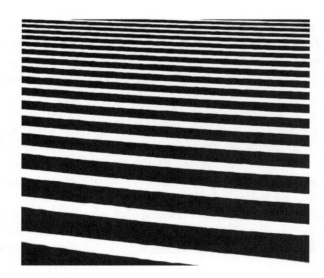

WARNING: COVER THIS PATTERN IF YOU HAVE MIGRAINE OR EPILEPSY

Fig. 4.1 The stair tread of an escalator. At typical viewing distances the spatial frequency is close to 3 cycles per degree.

The listed relationships between headaches and illusions occur only with respect to patterns that can cause seizures. Other patterns show no such relationships (Wilkins et al., 1984). It is possible that the illusions reflect a hyperexcitability of the visual cortex, because there is diverse but convergent evidence that in migraine the visual cortex is hyperexcitable, even between headaches (Palmer et al., 2000; Antal et al., 2005; Bowyer et al., 2005). This possibility will be explored later.

The photoparoxysmal electroencephalogram response

The susceptibility to seizures can be estimated without actually provoking them using the electroencephalogram (EEG). The brain's electrical activity shows a distinctive change involving spiked waveforms (a photoparoxysmal response) when the patient is exposed to stressful visual stimulation. In Fig. 4.2 the solid lines show the probability of this EEG response in patients with photosensitive epilepsy when they look at a pattern of stripes. Similar functions (broken lines) describe the number of illusions of colour, shape, and motion seen by normal observers when they look at the patterns. The similarity between the parameters that induce illusions and those that induce seizures is obvious. (Note that all graphs have the same scales and that the curves have not been adjusted in vertical position.) Patterns that give rise to the illusions of motion, shape, and colour and to seizures in patients with photosensitive epilepsy are usually uncomfortable (Wilkins et al., 1984).

The relationships between illusions, discomfort, and seizures apply not only to spatial properties of visual stimulation but also to temporal properties. Diffuse flicker can also give illusions, seizures, and discomfort, and the frequency at which it does so is similar, and close to the frequency at which flicker at threshold contrast is most readily perceived in large fields.

Therefore the visual stimuli that at high contrasts provoke illusions in most people, and in people with photosensitive epilepsy provoke seizures, have spatial and temporal characteristics very similar to those stimuli that are most readily seen at low contrasts. They are also stimuli that at higher contrasts interfere with the perception of other stimuli. Chronicle and Wilkins (1996) presented letters at low contrast at the centre of gratings and measured the contrast required to identify the letters as the gratings varied in spatial frequency, in size (angular subtense) and in shape (ratio of bar width to bar separation). The masking of the letter was maximal for spatial parameters in the range that was most strongly associated with the induction of illusions and seizures: in particular the masking increased with the area of the visual cortex to which the pattern projected, just as does the probability of seizures in patients with photosensitive epilepsy. The stimuli that have these properties can be said to be 'strong' stimuli.

Colour contrast

The colour contrasts that occur in nature tend not to be extreme and they tend to involve contrasts of particular hues. Juricevic et al. (2010) showed that meaningless patterns are rated as comfortable to the extent that the chromatic contrast resembles that found in natural images.

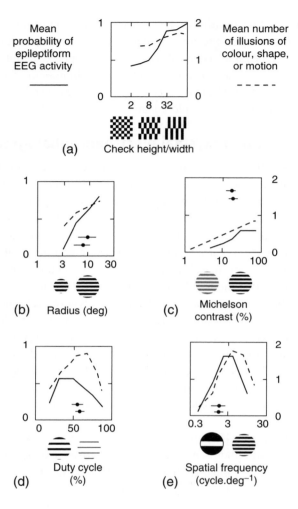

Fig. 4.2 Probability of epileptiform EEG activity in patients with pattern-sensitive epilepsy, shown as a function of several spatial characteristics of the pattern (solid curves). The broken lines show the number of illusions of colour, shape, or motion reported by normal observers. The horizontal points and bars show the mean ± 1 standard deviation of characteristics of text, when considered as a striped pattern, the lower bars for clear text and the upper bars for less clear text. Icons beneath each graph represent variation in the relevant spatial characteristic. Reproduced from Arnold J. Wilkins, *Visual Stress*, p. 40, © 1995, Oxford University Press, with permission from Oxford University Press.

If the spatial characteristics of a coloured pattern are reduced in complexity to the simplest spatial configuration—a pattern of stripes—a surprisingly simple relationship emerges between the characteristics of the pattern and how unpleasant it is. The unpleasantness depends mainly on how different the colours are—that is, how far apart their chromaticities are in the Commission Internationale de l'Elairage (CIE) Uniform Chromaticity Scale (UCS) diagram. People were asked to judge discomfort from patterns of stripes with two alternate colours, and in four experiments a consistent correlation was found between ratings of unpleasantness and the separation of the colours (chromaticities) in the CIE UCS diagram. This relationship was obtained for gratings in which the bars had the same luminance, and also in gratings in which the bars differed in luminance (Wilkins et al., 2008).

The haemodynamic response of the visual cortex to these coloured gratings was measured in four studies (in preparation) using near infrared spectroscopy (NIRS). NIRS is a technique in which low-power laser light is shone on the scalp, penetrates the skull, reflects from the surface of the brain, and re-emerges from the scalp, to be picked up by sensitive photodiodes. Changes in the concentration of oxyhaemoglobin and deoxyhae-moglobin can be calculated by comparing the signal reflected at two different wave-lengths. Both the discomfort from patterns of stripes and the haemodynamic response in the brain increased with the difference in colour between the stripes. This finding is con-sistent with the idea that coding in the brain is efficient for naturally occurring stimuli, which rarely show strong chromatic contrasts (Juricevic et al., 2010).

In short, we can now describe mathematically what makes images uncomfortable to look at. We can do so for both meaningless and meaningful images. Images that are uncomfortable tend to be those that are strong visual stimuli, and that induce a large haemodynamic response in the visual cortex. When we apply the mathematics to images from the contemporary urban environment, it transpires that the environment has many 'uncomfortable' images with unnatural image statistics. One of these is text.

Text as an uncomfortable image

Text has an unnatural spatial structure with an excess of contrast energy at mid-range spatial frequencies. This is particularly true of Western text: Arabic and Chinese text have less such energy. The high-contrast energy is due to the stripes from the lines of text. They are in the critical ranges of the parameters shown in Fig. 4.2. The spatial parameters of the stripes of text are shown by the horizontal bars.

Text is clearer if it has a relatively large spacing between the words, breaking up the 'grating' structure, and if the spacing between the lines is relatively large, decreasing the spatial frequency of the grating. In an experiment by Wilkins and Nimmo-Smith (1987) books were selected by students as having 'clear' or 'less clear' text. The 'clearer' text had more space, particularly space between the lines.

Reducing the luminance and contrast of the lines of text you are *not* reading, using a mask, can make the text you *are* reading clearer to see. Masks of this kind are known as *typoscopes* and they cover the lines below and above the lines that are being read. The mask can reduce eye strain (Wilkins & Nimmo-Smith, 1984) and also reduce seizures in photosensitive patients (Wilkins & Lindsay, 1985). People who report improvements in clarity with a typoscope tend to be those who report more illusions in patterns of stripes (Wilkins & Nimmo-Smith, 1984).

Stripes in letter strokes

In text it is not only the lines of words that are spatially repetitious, the strokes of letters can also form stripes. These stripes can interfere with reading as well, so much so that words such as *mum* take longer to read than words such as *dad* (Wilkins et al., 2007a). The stripes can be measured in terms of the first peak in the horizontal autocorrelation function. The first peak measures the extent to which the neighbouring strokes of letters resemble each other. The peak is far greater for the striped word *mum* than for the more rounded word *dad*. There are several possible reasons why spatially periodic words take longer to read. One is due to the adjustments in the alignment of the two eyes that occur when reading. When you read, your eyes make a series of jerks from left to right called saccades. After each saccade the alignment of the eyes has to be re-adjusted to bring the retinal images of the word into correspondence. The readjustment has to be more accurate when the eyes land on a word with a high autocorrelation perhaps because of the potential for false alignment of similar letter strokes, and this requirement for greater accuracy takes extra time. The above effects are not seen when reading is monocular. In any event, the time taken to fixate a striped word is greater, and reading takes longer (Jainta et al., 2010). The effect on ocular motor control may not be the only reason: the effect on reading speed is large relative to the increase in fixation duration. Be that as it may, the interference with ocular motor control as a result of spatial periodicity would be likely to increase the neural computation involved in reading, consistent with the proposal that strong excitation results in discomfort.

Font design

The average of the first peak in the horizontal autocorrelation of 1000 words was measured in various fonts. Times New Roman was among those with the highest spatial periodicity and Verdana among those with the least. Sassoon, a font widely used in primary education was similar to Times New Roman with respect to its high spatial periodicity. Studies comparing the reading speed for various fonts generally show that the fonts with higher spatial periodicity are read more slowly. One such study compared children's speed of reading passages printed in Sassoon with those printed in Verdana and found that children read more quickly with Verdana even though they were more familiar with Sassoon (Wilkins et al., 2010).

One way of reducing the effects of stripes, and decreasing the destructive effects of small errors of alignment of the eyes, is to increase the size of the letters. Increasing the size of the typeface has dramatic effects on children's reading speed, comprehension, and general reading ability. This is generally recognized to be the case, and text for young children is therefore printed in a large typeface. The height of the central body of the letters, known as x-height, begins at about 4 mm at age 5 and decreases to the adult size of about 2 mm over the course of the subsequent 5 years or so. Hughes and Wilkins (2000) created meaningless passages of randomly ordered common words that they asked children to read aloud as quickly as they could. The speed of reading the passages was measured for text with a variety of x-heights. Surprisingly, the speed of reading was *not* greatest with text of a size that the children were normally required to read and with which they were familiar. Instead the children (aged 5–9 years) read more quickly with text of a size normally used by younger children. In other words, text for children decreases in size at too early an age.

These findings have been replicated with more meaningful material. Wilkins et al. (2010) measured the speed with which 7–8-year-olds could silently read short sentences and classify them as true ('Fish live under the water') or false ('People have two noses'). The speed of comprehension (sentence verification) increased by 9% when the x-height was increased by 10%.

Wilkins et al. (2010) then made a version of the Salford Sentence Reading Test in which the text remained at the size of the initial sentences instead of decreasing in size as the test progressed, as is usual. The reading age increased by an average of 4 months when assessed by the version of the test in which the text remained large throughout. Evidently reading speed, comprehension speed, and reading age are all increased by increasing the size of text young children are required to read.

Environmental concerns

The task of classroom reading is made more difficult than it needs to be not only by the small size of text but by the way in which classrooms are lit. In a recent survey, 80% of UK classrooms were found to be lit with conventional fluorescent lighting that flickers 100 times per second (Winterbottom & Wilkins, 2007). The flicker is imperceptible but is resolved by the human retina (Berman et al., 1991), interferes with the control of eye movements (Wilkins, 1986), impairs visual performance (Veitch & McColl, 1995), and causes headaches (Wilkins et al., 1989). It is regrettable that low-frequency fluorescent ballasts, which are unhealthy and more expensive to operate than electronic ballasts, continue to be fitted into new school buildings because of their lower initial cost.

Typical classroom lighting not only flickers, but it is excessively and wastefully bright: in 84% of classrooms lighting levels exceed those at which visual discomfort starts to increase (Winterbottom & Wilkins, 2007).

In summary, we have seen that images with an unnatural spatial, temporal, and chromatic structure are more uncomfortable to look at, and that text is intrinsically an uncomfortable image. We have reviewed some of the consequences of the design of (Western) text. We now turn to the physiological reasons for the discomfort.

Neurological response to uncomfortable visual stimuli

It has long been held that visual systems are suited to the tasks they are required to carry out (e.g. Barlow, 1989) and that their resources are efficiently used. It has been shown that principal component filters (which sensory processes have been shown to emulate, e.g. Buchsbaum & Gottschalk (1984)) result in a sparse coding of natural scenes in which few neurons are active at any one time, conserving energy (Willmore & Tolhurst, 2001). It is quite possible that natural images are coded sparsely, and that unnatural images result in inefficient processing and excessive neuronal activity, as reflected in the haemodynamic response in the visual cortex (Juricevic et al., 2010). The excessive neuronal activity may have little consequence for most people, but may have adverse consequences for the 10% or so of the normal population whose cerebral cortex is already hyperexcitable (Aurora et al., 1999), a proportion that includes individuals who suffer migraine.

Individuals with migraine differ from matched controls in that their physiological response to sensory stimulation is abnormally large. Individuals with migraine: (1) see more illusions of colour, shape, and motion when they look at gratings, particularly gratings that would induce seizures in patients with photosensitive epilepsy (Wilkins et al., 1984); (2) they show a larger amplitude haemodynamic response to these gratings, as measured using functional magnetic resonance imaging (fMRI) blood oxygen level-dependent (BOLD) (Huang et al., 2003); (3) when measured using NIRS, the haemodynamic response can be shown to have a shorter latency (Coutts et al., in preparation); (4) the amplitude of the evoked potential fails to show the usual reduction in amplitude with repeated stimulation (Schoenen, 1996) and (5) when the occipital cortex is stimulated with a magnetic pulse the threshold current at which spots of light (phosphenes) first appear is lower (Aurora & Welch, 1998).

The over-responsiveness to sensory stimulation may reflect a cortical hyperexcitability because (1) the sensory stimulation to which patients with migraine are particularly susceptible is similar to the stimulation that induces seizures in patients with photosensitive epilepsy; (2) migraine and epilepsy are comorbid conditions (Brinciotti et al., 2000); (3) four antiepileptic drugs have been shown to prevent migraine in double-masked trials (Tfelt, 1996); and (4) DC-magnetoencephalography during visual stimulation reveals large-amplitude signals, reduced by the anticonvulsant, sodium valproate (Bowyer et al., 2005).

Coloured filters and reading

There is now considerable evidence that coloured filters can improve reading speed, although the reasons have proved to be elusive. There is no single colour that is generally beneficial, but each person seems to need their own individually selected colour (Wilkins & Neary, 1991; Wilkins et al., 1991, 1992a; 1992b, 1994, 1996, 2005a, 2005b, 2007b; Wilkins, 1992, 2003; Maclachlan et al., 1993; Evans et al., 1995, 1996a, 1996b, 1999, 2002; Tyrrell et al., 1995; Jeanes et al., 1997; Wilkins & Lewis, 1999; Bouldoukian et al., 2002; Scott et al., 2002; Huang et al., 2004; Waldie & Wilkins, 2004; Ludlow et al., 2006; Newman Wright et al., 2007; Smith & Wilkins, 2007; Allen et al., 2010).

Hollis and Allen (2006) separated individuals into two groups: those who reported many illusions when they looked at a striped pattern (a grating with spatial frequency close to three cycles/degree) and those who reported few. The former group reported an improvement in clarity of text with a coloured overlay, and read more quickly with the overlay. The latter group showed no such effect. The illusions reported in response to a striped pattern predicted the increment in reading speed better than the reports of visual discomfort in a symptom questionnaire.

Many individuals who use overlays for reading find that it is more convenient to use coloured lenses. The lenses have the advantage that they can be used for writing and for reading at distance. The colour optimal for use in overlays differs from that optimal for use in lenses, perhaps because the eyes are adapted to coloured light when coloured lenses are worn (Lightstone et al., 1999).

The *Intuitive Colorimeter* is an instrument that allows the colour that suits an individual to be selected. It shines coloured light on text and permits the separate manipulation of hue, saturation, and brightness. The chosen chromaticity is matched using combinations of tinted trial lenses. The combinations of trial lenses enable the tint to be tried out in natural viewing conditions and they guide the dyeing of spectacle lenses. The prescription is made up by dipping spectacle lenses into two dyes with hue similar to that of the desired tint. One advantage of the colorimeter is that the entire visual field is coloured so the eyes are adapted to coloured light. This is the simplest method of studying colour and its effect is similar to a coloured lens, not an overlay.

To check on the specificity and reliability of the optimal colour, Wilkins et al. (2005b) asked five observers who had used coloured lenses to read without their lenses. They read randomly ordered words repeatedly under light of different colours (Wilkins et al., 2005b). A computer algorithm was used to plot iso-reading speed contours in the CIE UCS diagram. The contours were similar from one test session to the next a few weeks later, and they showed no evidence of colour opponency. Although reading was usually slowest with white light and there was a large change in reading speed with colour, each individual had a different optimum. Despite the differences in optimal colour, the functions for all participants were similar when the data were plotted in terms of the difference in colour between the colour of light the individual was using for reading and the colour at which the text was perceived to be clearest. The reading speed decreased progressively with the difference in colour until the separation in CIE UCS chromaticity was about 0.06 when reading speed became similar to that under white light (Wilkins et al., 2005b).

These findings help predict how many different tints are necessary in an ophthalmic tinting system. To achieve an increment in reading speed within 95% of that obtainable with an optimum tint, about 6000 tints are necessary (Wilkins et al., 2005a). It is not necessary to offer 6000 trial lenses. Trial lenses can be placed one upon another to create different colours, and so it is not necessary to have more than about 35 trial lenses to achieve the requisite number of tints, provided the spectral transmissions are appropriately chosen.

Clinical indications

Tinted spectacles have shown clinical benefits in a variety of disorders. These disorders include not only reading difficulty, but photosensitive epilepsy (Wilkins et al., 1999, 2003), migraine (Wilkins et al., 2002), autism (Ludlow et al., 2006), and multiple sclerosis (Newman Wright et al., 2007). In all these disorders there is evidence (direct or indirect) for a hyperexcitability of the brain, particularly the visual cortex. There is direct evidence for a hyperexcitability in migraine, described earlier. In both autism and multiple sclerosis, the evidence is indirect: these disorders are comorbid with epilepsy (Sullivan, 1975; Kinnunen & Wikstrom, 1986; Levinson, 2007) and migraine (Gee et al., 2005; Casanova, 2009), and there is electrophysiological evidence for a hyperexcitability of the (motor) cortex in multiple sclerosis (Reddy et al., 2002; Caramia et al., 2004).

Strong stimulation

High-contrast stripes may be assumed to stimulate neurons strongly. Most visual neurons are responsive to the moderate contrasts found in natural scenes (Clatworthy et al., 2003) and their firing rate is likely to be close to maximal at contrasts above about 10%. With high-contrast stripes, the responsive neurons are likely to be firing strongly.

Stripes will stimulate columns of neurons with the appropriate orientation specificity, and the resulting excitation will presumably be concentrated within limited regions of the visual cortex, that is, the columns in which cells with the appropriate orientation specificity are to be found. There are at least two reasons for supposing that such a dense firing of neurons within the cortical network is detrimental: (1) when neurons fire, the concentration of ions in the extracellular space increases and excitatory effects can cause activation of adjacent neurons (Jefferys, 1991); (2) the orientationally selective pyramidal neurons are interconnected by inhibitory interneurons which are responsible for orientation tuning, and may help to prevent any strong excitation spreading through the cortical network. Because the interneurons are shared between pyramidal neurons, strong firing of neighbouring neurons might deplete the local availability of an inhibitory neurotransmitter such as gamma-aminobutyric acid, decreasing the inhibition and allowing a discharge to spread within the network (Meldrum & Wilkins, 1984).

Any spread of excitation might cause neurons to fire inappropriately, giving illusions of motion, shape, and colour. (The visual patterns that produce such illusions are curiously similar to the patterns seen as hallucinations when viewing bright (epileptogenic) flickering lights. The patterns can be inferred to arise as a result of lateral connectivity when the resting state of the visual cortex becomes unstable, see Bressloff et al. (2002).)

In rhesus monkeys the neurons in V2 show a topographic representation of colour. Neurons that respond to a red–black grating are found in areas that are next to areas in which the neurons respond to yellow–black gratings, and these in turn are next to areas in which the neurons respond to green–black gratings and so on. The colour selectivity is distributed across the cortex in much the same way as colours are distributed within the CIE UCS diagram (Xiao et al., 2003). For this reason, coloured filters are likely to redistribute the cortical excitation that results from a visual stimulus, at least in V2, one of the visual areas in which migraineurs show an abnormally large fMRI BOLD response (Huang et al., 2011). Colours that make visual stimuli more comfortable may be those that result in a redistribution of activity that avoids areas that are hyperexcitable.

We have already seen that the BOLD response is abnormally large in patients with migraine and this abnormality is most pronounced in visual areas V2 and V3 (Huang et al., 2011). With the appropriately coloured filter, the abnormal response in V2 and V3 is reduced in size and is normalized in terms of its spatial frequency tuning. There is no effect of the coloured filters in controls (Huang et al., 2011).

The latency of the haemodynamic response to visual stimuli can also be measured using a different technique, near infrared spectroscopy. With this technique it is evident that the response has an abnormally rapid decline in individuals with migraine. The decline is lessened (normalized) with filters selected to improve visual comfort. There is no such increase with control colours (Coutts et al., in press).

The imaging studies referred to previously indicate that (1) the over-responsiveness of the visual cortex seen in migraine is reduced with coloured filters, and (2) the reduction is dependent on the colour of the filters in a different way for each individual.

Peripheral consequences of central effects?

The effects of coloured filters are not exclusively central. Indeed, the individuals who respond to coloured filters show an underfocusing of the eyes (a lag of accommodation) that is greater than that seen in controls. The underfocusing is reduced by a coloured filter, one with a colour that individuals report as improving comfort, but is unaffected by other colours. There is no association between the focusing error and the particular colour that has this effect, as might be expected if the reduction in accommodative lag were due to the chromatic aberration of the eye. Instead it is possible that the underfocusing acts to slightly blur the retinal image so as to reduce the extent of cortical activation, thereby improving visual comfort (Allen et al., 2010).

Individual differences

The large individual differences in the therapeutic colour are difficult to explain. It is possible that they reflect differences in the distribution of hyperexcitability across the cortex in anterior cortical areas. It is also possible that the differences reflect peripheral effects. They may be a consequence of differences between individuals in the proportion of long-, middle-, and short-wavelength cones (L, M, and S cones) in the retina. The differences are large (the ratio of L:M cones can be as great as 16:1 (Hofer et al., 2005; Roorda & Williams, 1999)), but they do not appear to give rise to large perceptual differences between people. Perhaps the perceptual normalization that occurs is the result of a larger 'gain' being applied to the less numerous cones, and if so, the greater gain may have greater 'noise' associated with it. It is possible that the chosen filter colour acts to reduce the effects of the noise by increasing the relative activation of the less numerous cone type. However, the S cones are the least numerous (about 1 for every 20 L or M cones) and the large individual differences that have been observed pertain mainly to the ratio of L to M cones. We would therefore expect the individual differences to occur mainly along the L–M confusion line, and the differences do not appear to favour any particular axis of confusion (Wilkins et al., 2005b).

A synthesis

It is now possible to bring the very disparate components of this discourse together. It is possible to conceive of visual stress as arising from strong sensory stimulation. When the cortex is normally excitable, this strong stimulation is without adverse consequence. When, however, the cortex is hyperexcitable, visual illusions are experienced, together with discomfort. The discomfort can be seen as providing for homeostasis: individuals will avoid sensory stimulation that is bad for them. *In extremis*, the neural discharge that usually results in no more than visual illusions has more adverse consequences, resulting in a large discharge that may trigger migraine, or end in a seizure.

Reading can be a stressful activity—it is one for which the visual system was not designed. Text can be improved in design to reduce visual stress, but where individual susceptibility is extreme it may be helpful to use appropriately coloured filters that appear to act to reduce an overexcitation of the visual cortex. The reasons for the individual differences in the colour optimal for achieving this reduction remain an enigma.

Acknowledgements

The author thanks Dr Peter Allen, Dr David Tolhurst, and Professor Frances Wilkinson for comments.

References

Allen, P.M., Hussain, A., Usherwood, C., & Wilkins, A.J. (2010). Pattern-related visual stress, chromaticity and accommodation. *Investigative Ophthalmology and Visual Science*, 51, 6843–9.

Antal, A., Temme, J., Nitsche, M.A., Varga, E.T., Lang, N., & Paulus, W. (2005). Altered motion perception in migraineurs: evidence for interictal cortical hyperexcitability. *Cephalalgia*, 25, 788–94.

Aurora, S.K., Cao, Y., Bowyer, S.M., & Welch, K.M. (1999). The occipital cortex is hyperexcitable in migraine: experimental evidence. *Headache*, 39, 469–76.

Aurora, S.K. & Welch, K.M. (1998). Brain excitability in migraine: evidence from transcranial magnetic stimulation studies. *Current Opinion in Neurology*, 113, 205–9.

Barlow, H.B. (1989) Unsupervised learning. *Neural Computation*, 1, 295–311.

Berman, S.M., Greenhouse, D.S., Bailey, I.L., Clear, R., & Raasch, T.W. (1991). Human electroretinogram responses to video displays fluorescent lighting and other high frequency sources. *Optometry and Vision Science*, 68, 645–62.

Bouldoukian, J., Wilkins, A.J., & Evans, B.J.W. (2002). Randomised control trial of the effect of coloured overlays on the rate of reading of people with specific learning difficulties. *Ophthalmic and Physiological Optics*, 221, 55–60.

Bowyer, S., Mason, K.M., Moran, J.E., Tepley, N., & Mitsias, P.D. (2005). Cortical hyperexcitability in migraine patients before and after sodium valproate treatment. *Journal of Clinical Neurophysiology*, 22, 65–7.

Bressloff, P.C., Cowan, J.D., Golubitsky, M., Thomas, P.J., & Wiener, M.C. (2002). What gemometric visual halluminations tell us about the visual cortex. *Neural Computation*, 14, 473–91.

Brinciotti, M., Di Sabato, M., Matricadi, M., & Guidetti, V. (2000). Electroclinical features in children and adolescents with epilepsy and/or migraine, and occipital epileptiform EEG abnormalities. *Clinical Electroencephalography*, 31, 76–82.

Buchsbaum, G., & Gottschalk, A. (1984). Chromaticity coordinates of frequency-limited functions. *Journal of the Optical Society of America*, 1, 885–7.

Caramia, M.D., Palmieri, M.G., Desiato, M.T., Boffa, L., Galizia, P., and Rossini, P.M. (2004). Brain excitability changes in the relapsing and remitting phases of multiple sclerosis: A study with transcranial magnetic stimulation. *Clinical Neurophysiology*, 115, 956–65.

Casanova, M.F. (2009). The minicolumnopathy of autism: a link between migraine and gastrointestinal symptoms. *Medical Hypotheses*, 70, 73–80.

Chronicle, E., & Wilkins, A.J. (1996). Gratings that induce perceptual distortions mask superimposed targets. *Perception*, 25, 661–8.

Clatworthy, P.L., Chirimuuta, M., Lauritzen, J.S., & Tolhurst, D.J. (2003). Coding of the contrasts in natural images by populations of neurons in primary visual cortex (V1). *Vision Research*, 43, 1983–2001.

Coutts, L., Cooper, C., Elwell, C., & Wilkins A.J. (in press). The haemodynamic response to visual stimulation in migraine measured using near infrared spectroscopy Cephalalgia.

Evans, B.J.W., Busby, A., Jeanes, R., & Wilkins, A.J. (1995). Optometric correlates of Meares-Irlen syndrome: a matched group study. *Ophthalmic and Physiological Optics*, 15, 481–7.

Evans, B.J.W., Wilkins, A.J., Brown, J., Busby, A., Wingfield, A., Jeanes, R., *et al.* (1996a). A preliminary investigation into the aetiology of Meares-Irlen syndrome. *Ophthalmic and Physiological Optics*, 164, 286–96.

Evans, B.J.W., Wilkins, A.J., Busby, A., & Jeanes, R. (1996b). Optometric characteristics of children with reading difficulties who report a benefit from coloured filters. In: I.J.C.M. Dickinson, Murray, & D. Garden (Eds.) *John Dalton's Colour Vision Legacy*, pp. 709–15. London: Taylor and Francis.

Evans, B.J.W., Lightstone, A., Eperjesi, F., Duffy, J., Speedwell, L., Patel, R., *et al.* (1999). A review of the management of 323 consecutive patients seen in a specific learning difficulties clinic. *Ophthalmic and Physiological Optics*, 196, 454–66.

Evans, B.J.W., Patel, R., & Wilkins, A.J. (2002). Optometric function in visually sensitive migraine before and after treatment with tinted spectacles. *Ophthalmic and Physiological Optics*, 22, 130–42.

Fernandez, D., & Wilkins, A.J. (2008). Uncomfortable images in art and nature. *Perception*, 37, 1098–113.

Gee, J.R., Chang, J., Dublin, A.B., & Vijayan, N. (2005). The association of brainstem lesions with migraine-like headache: An imaging study of multiple sclerosis. *Headache*, 45, 670–7.

Hofer, H., Carrol, J., Neitz, J., Neitz, M., & Williams, D.R. (2005). Organization of the human trichromatic cone mosaic. *Journal of Neuroscience*, 25, 9669–79.

Hollis, J., & Allen, P.M. (2006). Screening for Meares-Irlen sensitivity in adults: can assessment methods predict changes in reading speed? *Ophthalmic and Physiological Optics*, 26, 566–71.

Huang, J., Cooper, T.G., Satana, B., Kaufman, D.I., & Cao, Y. (2003). Visual distortion associated with hypervisual neuronal activity in migraine. *Headache*, 43, 664–71.

Huang, J., Wilkins, A.J., & Cao, Y. (2004). Mechanisms whereby precision spectral filters reduce visual stress: an fMRI study. Tenth Annual Meeting of the Organization for Human Brain Mapping, June 13–17, 2004, Budapest, Hungary.

Huang, J., Zong, X., Wilkins A.J., Jenkins, B., Bozoki, A., & Cao, Y. (2011). A neurological basis for reducing cortical hyperactivation in migraine with precision ophthalmic tints. *Cephalalgia*, 31, 925–36.

Hughes, L.E., & Wilkins, A.J. (2000). Typography in children's reading schemes may be suboptimal: evidence from measures of reading rate. *Journal of Research in Reading*, 23, 314–24.

Jainta, S., Jaschinski, W., & Wilkins A.J. (2010). Periodic letter strokes within a word affect fixation disparity during reading. *Journal of Vision*, 10(13), 2.

Jeanes, R., Busby, A., Martin, J., Lewis, E., Stevenson, N., Pointon, D., *et al.* (1997). Prolonged use of coloured overlays for classroom reading. *British Journal of Psychology*, 88, 531–48.

Jefferys, J.G.R. (1991). Non-synaptic modulation of neuronal activity in the brain: electric currents and extracellular ions. *Physiological Reviews*, 75, 689–723.

Juricevic, I., Land, L., Wilkins, A.J., & Webster, M.A. (2010). Visual discomfort and natural image statistics. *Perception*, 39, 884–99.

Kinnunen, E., & Wikstrom, J. (1986). Prevalence and prognosis of epilepsy in patients with multiple sclerosis. *Epilepsia*, 27, 729–33.

Levinson, P.M. (2007). The autism-epilepsy connection. *Epilepsia*, 48, 33–5.

Lightstone, A., Lightstone, T., & Wilkins, A. (1999). Both coloured overlays and coloured lenses can improve reading fluency, but their optimal chromaticities differ. *Ophthalmic and Physiological Optics*, 19, 279–85.

Ludlow, A.K., Wilkins, A.J., & Heaton, P. (2006). The effect of coloured overlays on reading ability in children with autism. *Journal of Autism and Developmental Disorders*, 36, 507–16.

Maclachlan, A., Yale, S., & Wilkins, A.J. (1993). Open trials of precision ophthalmic tinting: 1-year follow-up of 55 patients. *Ophthalmic and Physiological Optics*, 13, 175–8.

Marcus, D.A., & Soso, M.J. (1989). Migraine and stripe-induced visual discomfort. *Archives of Neurology*, 46, 1129–32.

Meldrum, B.S., & Wilkins, A.J. (1984). Photosensitive epilepsy: integration of pharmacological and psychophysical evidence. In P. Schwatzkroin & H.V. Wheal (Eds.) *Electrophysiology of Epilepsy*, pp. 51–77. London: Academic Press.

Newman Wright, A., Wilkins, A., & Zoukos, Y. (2007). Spectral filters can improve reading and visual search in patients with multiple sclerosis. *Journal of Neurology*, 254, 1729–35.

Nulty, D., Wilkins, A.J., & Williams, J.M. (1987). Mood, pattern sensitivity and headache: a longitudinal study. *Psychological Medicine*, 17, 705–13.

Palmer, J.E., Chronicle, E.P., Rolan, P., & Mulleners, W.M. (2000). Cortical hyperexcitability is cortical under-inhibition: evidence from a novel functional test of migraine patients. *Cephalalgia*, 20, 525–32.

Reddy, H., Narayanan, S., Woolrich, M., Mitsumori, T., Lapierre, Y., Arnold, D., *et al.* (2002). Functional brain reorganisation for hand movement in patients with multiple sclerosis: Defining distinct effects of injury and disability. *Brain*, 125, 2646–57.

Roorda, A., & Williams, D.R. (1999). The arrangement of the three cone classes in the living human eye. *Nature*, 397, 520–2.

Schoenen, J. (1996). Deficient habituation of evoked cortical potentials in migraine: a link between brain biology, behavior and trigeminovascular activations? *Biomedicine and Pharmacotherapy*, 50, 71–8.

Scott, L., McWhinnie, H., Taylor, L., Stevenson, N., Irons, P., Lewis, E., *et al.* (2002). Coloured overlays in schools: orthoptic and optometric findings. *Ophthalmic and Physiological Optics*, 22, 156–65.

Smith, L., & Wilkins, A. (2007). How many overlay colours are necessary to increase reading speed? A comparison of two systems. *Journal of Research in Reading*, 30, 332–43.

Sullivan, R. (1975). Hunches on some biological factors of autism. *Journal of Autism and Childhood Schizophrenia*, 5, 177–86.

Tfelt, H.P. (1996). Drug treatment of migraine: acute treatment and migraine prophylaxis. *Current Opinion in Neurology*, 9, 211–13.

Tyrrell, R., Holland, K., Dennis, D., & Wilkins, A.J. (1995). Coloured overlays, visual discomfort, visual search and classroom reading. *Journal of Research in Reading*, 181, 10–23.

Veitch, J.A., & McColl, S.L. (1995). Modulation of fluorescent light: flicker rate and light source effects on visual performance and visual comfort. *Lighting Research and Technology*, 27, 243–56.

Waldie, M., & Wilkins, A. (2004). How big does a coloured overlay have to be? *Ophthalmic and Physiological Optics*, 24, 55–60.

Wilkins, A. (1986). Intermittent illumination from visual display units and fluorescent lighting affects movements of the eyes across text. *Human Factors*, 28, 75–81.

Wilkins, A. (1992). *A System for Precision Ophthalmic Tinting: Manual for the use of the Intuitive Colorimeter and Trial Lenses*, p. 27. Kent: Cerium Visual Technologies.

Wilkins, A.J. (1994). Overlays for classroom and optometric use. *Ophthalmic and Physiological Optics*, 14, 97–9.

Wilkins, A.J. (1995). *Visual Stress*. Oxford: Oxford University Press.

Wilkins, A.J. (2003). *Reading Through Colour. How coloured filters can reduce reading difficulty, eye strain, and headaches*. Chichester: John Wiley and Sons.

Wilkins, A.J. & Lewis, E. (1999). Coloured overlays, text and texture. *Perception*, 28, 641–50.

Wilkins, A.J. & Lindsay, J. (1985). Common forms of reflex epilepsy: physiological mechanisms and techniques for treatment. In Pedley, T.A., & Meldrum, B.S. (Eds.) *Recent advances in epilepsy II*, pp. 239–71. Edinburgh: Churchill Livingstone.

Wilkins, A.J. & Neary, C. (1991). Some visual, optometric and perceptual effects of coloured glasses. *Ophthalmic and Physiological Optics*, 11, 163–71.

Wilkins, A., & Nimmo-Smith, I. (1984). On the reduction of eye-strain when reading. *Ophthalmic and Physiological Optics*, 4, 53–9.

Wilkins, A.J., & Nimmo-Smith, M.I. (1987). The clarity and comfort of printed text. *Ergonomics*, 3012, 1705–20.

Wilkins, A.J., Nimmo-Smith, M. I., Tait, A., McManus, C., Della Sala, S., Tilley, A., *et al.* (1984). A neurological basis for visual discomfort. *Brain*, 107, 989–1017.

Wilkins, A.J., Nimmo, S.I., Slater, A.I., & Bedocs, L. (1989). Fluorescent lighting, headaches and eyestrain. *Lighting Research and Technology*, 21, 11–18.

Wilkins, A.J., Nimmo-Smith, I., & Jansons, J.E. (1991). A colorimeter for the intuitive manipulation of hue saturation and brightness. *Ophthalmic and Physiological Optics*, 12, 381–5.

Wilkins, A., Milroy, R., Nimmo-Smith, I., Wright, A., Tyrrell, R., Holland, K., *et al.* (1992a). Preliminary observations concerning treatment of visual discomfort and associated perceptual distortion. *Ophthalmic and Physiological Optics*, 12, 257–63.

Wilkins, A.J., Nimmo-Smith, I., & Jansons, J.E. (1992b). Colorimeter for the intuitive manipulation of hue and saturation and its role in the study of perceptual distortion. *Ophthalmic and Physiological Optics*, 12, 381–5.

Wilkins, A.J., Evans, B.J.W., Brown, J.A., Busby, A.E., Wingfield, A.E., Jeanes, R.J., *et al.* (1994). Double-masked placebo-controlled trial of precision spectral filters in children who use coloured overlays. *Ophthalmic and Physiological Optics*, 144, 365–70.

Wilkins, A.J., Jeanes, R.J., Pumfrey, P.D., & Laskier, M. (1996). Rate of Reading Test: its reliability, and its validity in the assessment of the effects of coloured overlays. *Ophthalmic and Physiological Optics*, 16, 491–7.

Wilkins, A.J., Baker, A., Smith, S., Bradford, J., Zaiwalla, Z., Besag, F.M., *et al.* (1999). Treatment of photosensitive epilepsy using coloured glasses. *Seizure*, 8, 444–9.

Wilkins, A.J., Patel, R., Adjamian, R., & Evans, B.J.W. (2002). Tinted spectacles and visually sensitive migraine. *Cephalalgia*, 22, 711–19.

Wilkins, A., Huang, J., & Cao, Y. (2003). Visual stress theory and its application to reading and reading tests. *Journal of Research in Reading*, 27, 152–62.

Wilkins, A., Sihra, N., & Nimmo-Smith, I. (2005a). How precise do precision tints have to be and how many are necessary? *Ophthalmic and Physiological Optics*, 25, 269–76.

Wilkins, A., Sihra, N., & Myers, A. (2005b). Increasing reading speed using colours: issues concerning reliability and specificity, and their theoretical and practical implications. *Perception*, 34, 109–20.

Wilkins, A.J., Smith, J., Willison, C.K., Beare, T., Boyd, A., Hardy, G., *et al.* (2007a). Stripes within words, reading speed and reading difficulty. *Perception*, 36, 1788–803.

Wilkins, A.J., Huang, J., & Cao, Y. (2007b). Prevention of visual stress and migraine with precision spectral filters. *Drug Development Research*, 68, 469–75.

Wilkins, A.J., Tang, P., Irabor, J., Baningham, L., & Coutts, L. (2008). Cortical haemodynamic response to coloured gratings. *Perception*, 37, 144.

Wilkins, A.J., Cleave, A., Grayson, N., & Wilson, L. (2010). Text for children may be inappropriately designed. *Journal of Research in Reading*, 32, 402–12.

Willmore, B., & Tolhurst, D. (2001). Characterising the sparseness of neural codes. *Network*, 12, 255–70.

Winterbottom, M. & Wilkins, A. (2007). Lighting and visual discomfort in the classroom. *Journal of Environmental Psychology*, 29, 63–75.

Xiao, Y., Wang, Y., & Felleman, D.J. (2003). A spatially organized representation of colour in macaque cortical area V2. *Nature*, 421, 535–9.

Chapter 5

Visual Discomfort and Reading

Elizabeth G. Conlon

Introduction

Efficient reading, comprising good fluency and comprehension, is essential to maximize educational and employment opportunities. The contribution of visual processing to reading and reading difficulties has a long and controversial history, with reports of impaired visual processing as explanations of reading difficulties appearing for over a century. During the 1980s, reports appeared that some individuals experience symptoms of visual fatigue (eye strain, headache, sore/tired eyes) and perceptual distortions (illusions of colour, pattern, and motion) when exposed to bright or flickering light and repetitive striped patterns with spatial frequencies of 1–4 cycles per degree (c/deg) (Wilkins et al., 1984; Marcus & Soso, 1989). Referred to as visual discomfort, evidence was presented that similar difficulties occur in sensitive individuals when viewing the pattern formed by a page of single-spaced text (Wilkins & Nimmo-Smith, 1984, 1987). An example of this stimulus configuration is shown in Fig. 5.1. Independent of this research, similar difficulties were reported in children (Meares, 1980) and adults referred to reading assessment clinics (Irlen, 1983). A reduced span of focus, difficulties in sustained concentration, eye strain, and headache were described together with reports of words and letters moving, shimmering, flickering, or disappearing (Meares, 1980; Irlen, 1983). Still controversial, it was additionally reported that these difficulties could be alleviated with the use of coloured perspex overlays (Meares, 1980; Irlen, 1983; Wilkins, 1995). This claim has led to much research activity to determine both the causes of visual distress and its effect on performance on reading and reading-like tasks.

Terminology and assessment

Those who have investigated this phenomenon all report similar perceptual, somatic, and functional difficulties induced by viewing a page of text. Many different terms, based on alternative assessment procedures or conceptualizations, have been used to describe these symptoms. While Wilkins and colleagues (1984) used the terms visual discomfort or pattern glare to describe sensitivity to bright light and pattern, Irlen (1983) introduced the term scotopic sensitivity syndrome, currently referred to as Irlen syndrome (Irlen, 1991) to describe difficulties specifically related to reading. When introduced, visual discomfort was characterized by anomalous effects induced by viewing certain patterns, but no formal criteria were provided to diagnose individuals. The term visual stress was then

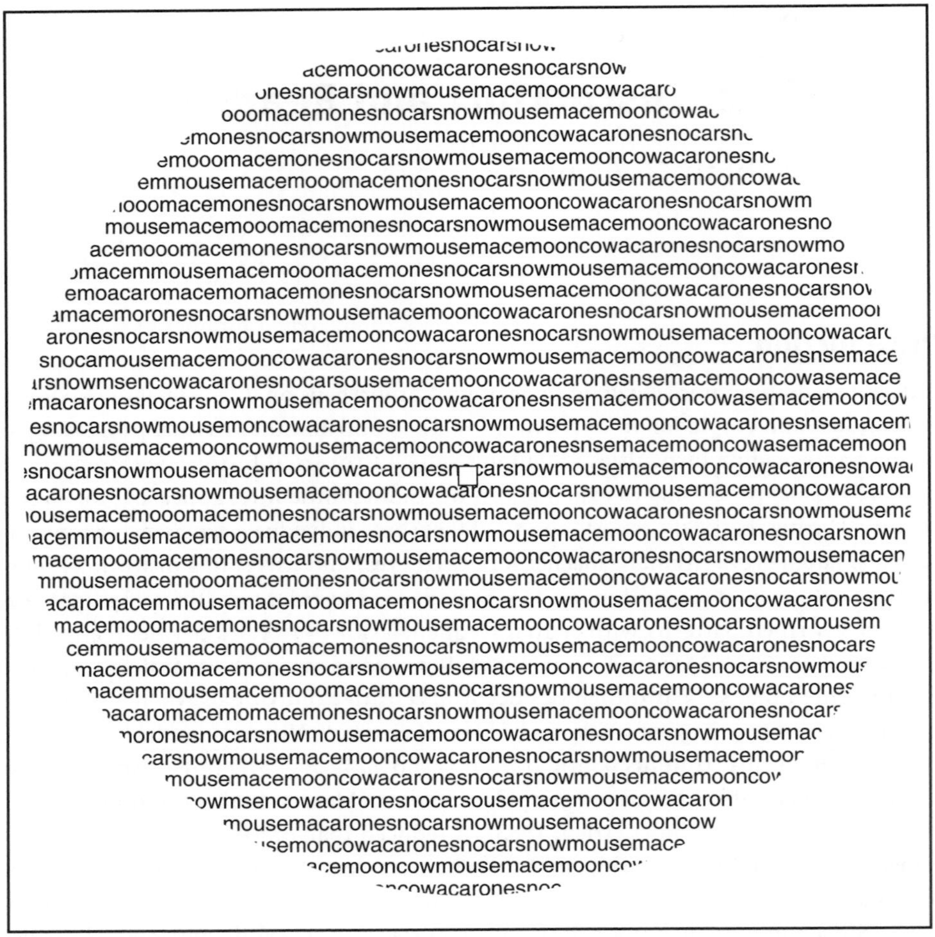

Fig. 5.1 Representation of the way lines of single spaced text can form a repetitive striped pattern.

introduced to describe these somatic, perceptual, and functional difficulties induced by reading text, together with poor fluency when reading high-frequency words presented in lines (Wilkins, 1995; Singleton & Trotter, 2005). Irlen syndrome was diagnosed using the Irlen Perceptual Schedule, which also provided evidence of the functional difficulties that occur when reading and on performance in one or more perceptual tasks (Irlen, 1991; Noble et al., 2004). Both Irlen and Wilkins reported that individually selected coloured overlays could reduce the symptoms and that selection of the correct colour is a critical component of assessment procedures. Individuals reporting visual stress symptoms who fail to improve performance with coloured overlays, either in terms of reading fluency or increased accuracy on perceptual tasks, are considered not to have the syndrome (Evans et al., 1996; Kruk et al., 2008). The similarity between the descriptions has led some researchers to label the anomaly Meares–Irlen syndrome (Evans et al., 1996;

Evans & Joseph, 2002; Kriss & Evans, 2005) or more recently Meares–Irlen visual stress syndrome (Evans, 2005).

Other terms used to describe these symptoms that have not included the effectiveness of colour in reducing them as part of the assessment, include pattern-related visual stress (Allen et al., 2008), reading discomfort (Ridder et al., 2008), and visual discomfort (Conlon et al., 1999; Borsting et al., 2007). The larger the number of endorsements on the self-report Visual Discomfort Scale or other symptom checklist (Hollis & Allen, 2006; Singleton & Henderson, 2008), the greater the severity of the condition. Individuals with higher scores on these measures were more likely to report the following difficulties: shorter effective reading time, frequent headaches, and a greater number of somatic and perceptual side effects when either viewing a 2.5-c/deg high-contrast square-wave grating or a page of single-spaced small text (Conlon et al., 1999).

One challenge that has faced researchers in this area is to assess the significance of adverse responses to specific environmental stimuli such as flickering lights, high-contrast repetitive patterns, or poorly presented text. Wilkins and Nimmo-Smith, (1984, 1987) found that everybody finds that some single-spaced text formats presented in continuous lines on an A4 page, are more comfortable to view than others. This shows that the way that text is presented can increase or decrease viewing comfort when reading. For individuals who report high levels of sensitivity to the textual format, reducing the number of lines visible within a reading mask increases reading comfort (Wilkins & Nimmo-Smith, 1984).

When groups of children used individually selected coloured overlays, their reading speed increased over a 3–6-month period (Jeanes et al., 1996; Wilkins et al., 2001; Noble et al., 2004). Even good readers may experience unpleasant effects with presentation of repetitive stripes on text pages. It has been estimated that at least 5% of children in school populations (Wilkins, 2002) and up to 20% of adults have some symptoms of visual discomfort (Conlon et al., 1999; Borsting et al., 2007). The proportion is higher in individuals with migraine headache, with up to 50% reporting symptoms (Shepherd, 2001). Up to 35% of children and adults with dyslexia also report some symptoms of visual discomfort (Evans & Joseph, 2002; Kriss & Evans, 2005).

Although continuous use of colour as a remedial strategy has been considered strong evidence of the presence of visual discomfort (Wilkins, 1995; Evans & Joseph, 2002), colour has not always proven effective (Allen et al., 2008). In addition, although increased reading speed has been consistently found, colour, while improving reading comprehension in some studies (Noble et al., 2004), has not been seen in others (Wilkins, 2002; Kruk et al., 2008). Differences in symptom severity and type may provide an explanation of these different outcomes.

Using the visual discomfort scale, a number of different symptom profiles have been obtained (Conlon et al., 1999, 2001; Borsting et al., 2007). Rasch analysis of items in the scale has shown that the most frequently reported effects are functional difficulties, such as poor concentration or unintentionally re-reading lines of text. Somatic difficulties such as eye strain and headache when reading are next most common, while perceptual difficulties, such as the words on the page shimmering, flickering, or disappearing were reported only when the other symptomatology was more severe. Correspondingly, quantitative and qualitative differences have been obtained in groups reporting moderate or severe symptomatology. When subjects were asked to report somatic and perceptual effects following 3-s exposures to repetitive patterns with spatial frequencies of 1–16 c/deg, the group reporting most severe symptomatology of visual discomfort also reported significantly more perceptual and somatic effects than other groups (Conlon et al., 1999). When these same groups made comparative judgements of difficulty, the group with severe visual discomfort reported greatest difficulty when viewing patterns with spatial frequencies of 2–4 c/deg. This finding is consistent with Wilkins et al. (1984), who reported that these spatial frequencies are the ones producing the strongest effects in affected individuals. In contrast to this, the group reporting moderate symptomatology reported greatest somatic and perceptual difficulties when viewing patterns with a much higher spatial frequency of 12 c/deg. In addition, the qualitative reports of the perceptual difficulties induced with pattern viewing differed between groups. Those with the most severe visual discomfort consistently reported illusions of motion, colour, and pattern, while those with a moderate number of symptoms reported greater difficulties with pattern flicker, blur, and double images (Conlon et al., 2001).

One explanation for the different symptom profiles found with subjective measures of visual discomfort, concerns the influence of optometric difficulties, such as uncorrected refractive errors or disorders of accommodation or vergence. Such anomalies are associated with visual discomfort in many individuals (Evans et al., 1995), so that their optometric abnormalities may explain their symptoms (Evans, 2005). However, one recent study that evaluated accommodation and vergence in adults with and without visual discomfort measured using the visual discomfort scale, found that their difficulties could not be explained by optometric problems (Borsting et al., 2010). Nevertheless because uncorrected optometric difficulties can contribute to visual discomfort, it is critical that careful visual assessment is conducted as part of the assessment process (Evans, 2005).

Visual discomfort and visual search

Subjective reports of difficulty with pattern and text viewing have been extended to performance in groups reporting different levels of symptom severity on reading-like visual search tasks. Tasks that have required observers to count the number of stimuli such as letters with a specific orientation in a square-wave-like pattern, a checkerboard-like pattern, or a plaid pattern have been used (see Fig. 5.2). Regardless of the presentation format, the group with severe visual discomfort performed less efficiently than groups with moderate or low visual discomfort (Conlon et al., 1998). The square-wave-like configuration produced the greatest subjective and objective difficulties; mean correct response times were longest and they caused the greatest subjective difficulty. Although the group with moderate visual discomfort reported greater subjective symptomatology when performing the visual search task, there was no evidence of performance difficulties. These results suggest two things. First, the immediate effects of pattern sensitivity did not produce performance difficulties in all observers reporting symptoms of visual discomfort, and individuals reporting severe symptomatology showed evidence of poorer performance efficiency regardless of the global pattern structure used.

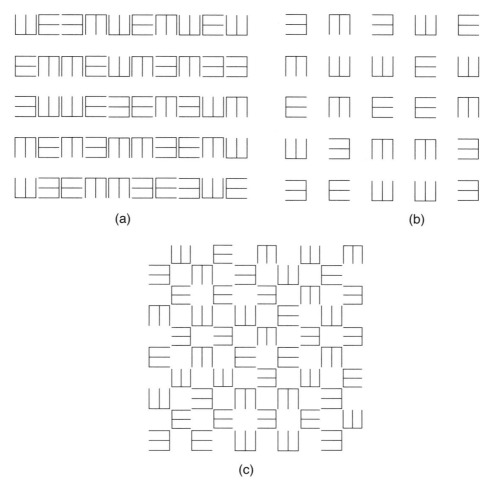

Fig. 5.2 Representation of different pattern structures used in assessing visual search performance in groups with visual discomfort.

In two further studies we studied whether the effects that occurred were the result of the square-wave-like structure used being insufficiently repetitive to induce strong effects in observers with moderate or severe visual discomfort, or whether the difficulties found in observers with more severe symptomatology extend to non-striped patterns. In the first, we used a pop-out search task, where automatic attention was deployed to a target stimulus. Stimuli were either embedded in a 2-c/deg square-wave, a series of lines, or on a uniform grey background (Conlon & Hine, 2000). The poorest performance was found for the group with visual discomfort when stimuli were embedded in the 2-c/deg square-wave, with no group differences in accuracy found when other backgrounds were used. The second study used a serial search task. Observers were required to consciously search among individual distractors for a less salient target feature. The group with high visual discomfort had significantly slower response times than the low visual discomfort group in the absence of a pattern background and regardless of whether four, eight, or

16 distractor stimuli were presented (Conlon & Humphreys, 2001). Together these findings suggest poorer efficiency in individuals with visual discomfort on visual search tasks. This occurs under two circumstances. First, in tasks where automatic attention can be deployed to a highly salient stimulus, poor performance only occurs in the presence of repetitive patterns that produce immediate perceptual difficulties. Second, in tasks requiring deployment of conscious serial visual attention to each stimulus in the visual array, the demands required when searching a large number of stimuli, produce poor performance regardless of whether a pattern background is presented.

These findings suggest that the visual complexity of the display used, regardless of whether this is a repetitive striped pattern or not, increases the processing difficulties of people with visual discomfort. Further evidence of poorer performance on tasks with increasing perceptual demands supports this explanation. Studies have been conducted where groups with high or low visual discomfort were asked either to match the same digit, presented in rows (Conlon & Sanders, 2011) or to count the number of times a prespecified single digit was presented in text-like rows of digits (Allen et al., 2008). On both tasks, the group with high visual discomfort was found to have significantly poorer performance than the other groups. In the digit matching study, significantly fewer digits were matched in a 2-min period and in the digit counting study, a higher error rate was found, regardless of whether a pattern surround was present or absent (Allen et al). Groups with either moderate or severe visual discomfort were also significantly less efficient than a control group when performing a copying task on a grid like pattern (Conlon, et al. 1999; Kruk et al., 2008). The attentional requirements of the task used in each of these studies, regardless of the pattern background used, suggests that those with visual discomfort have difficulty consciously attending to target stimuli when presented in cluttered visual arrays. The extent that this is true in cognitively demanding reading tasks has also been investigated.

Visual discomfort and reading

Many of the studies that have investigated reading in groups with visual discomfort have evaluated oral reading fluency using high-frequency unrelated words, presented in single-spaced lines of text. The test used in much of this research is the Wilkins Rate of Reading Test (Wilkins et al., 1996), developed to distinguish the cognitive or language difficulties seen in individuals with dyslexia from the visual perceptual difficulties induced by text. This task has shown that people with visual discomfort make more errors and have a slower reading rate than controls (Wilkins et al., 1996; Evans & Joseph, 2002; Singleton & Trotter, 2005; Hollis & Allen, 2006). Singleton and Henderson (2008), used the response speed of individuals on a visual search task, referred to as a visual stress screener, to classify individuals as having high or low visual discomfort. Individuals with slower visual search times in the presence of a repetitive patterned background (high visual discomfort) were shown to have a slower reading rate on the Wilkins Rate of Reading Test than those with faster speeds in the task (low visual discomfort). The reading rate of the group with high visual discomfort improved more using an individually selected coloured overlay than the group with low visual discomfort. These findings show that performance on the rate of reading test and difficulties found on a visual search task with a pattern background, are related. On both the Rate of Reading Test and on the visual stress screener task, high frequency words are used (Wilkins et al., 1996; Singleton & Henderson, 2008). The cognitive resources required on both tasks, where only the presentation format was manipulated, show that colour can be effective in reducing visual stress symptoms.

Most studies have assessed reading fluency using closely-spaced letters and single-spaced text. Few have investigated the impact of visual discomfort on reading comprehension. However, one study measured both the reading rate and comprehension of groups of adults with or without visual discomfort using double-spaced text; the text difficulty was consistent with adult reading skills (Conlon et al., 1999). Oral reading was used to ensure that each word could be correctly identified, as problems with the legibility of text occur in individuals with visual discomfort. Using this task, a group with visual discomfort was found to have a slower reading rate, but equivalent comprehension, to controls (Conlon et al., 1999). While the slower reading rate of those with visual discomfort could be caused by interference from the global repetitive pattern formed by the lines of text on the page, the use of double-spaced text should have minimized this source of interference; double spacing text has been reported to decrease visual discomfort (Wilkins & Nimmo-Smith, 1987). However, as a slower speed of processing was also found in groups with visual discomfort, particularly when cognitive tasks demands were high (Conlon et al., 1999; Allen et al., 2008), the cognitive complexity of the text used may also have contributed to the poorer reading rate found. In addition, group differences in reading skills or IQ may have contributed.

Possible alternative explanations for the poorer performance of those with visual discomfort were addressed in a study that contrasted the reading rate and comprehension of three groups of adults, all matched for cognitive ability using the vocabulary and block design tasks from the Wechsler Adult Intelligence Scales (Wechsler, 1998). Groups with visual discomfort, dyslexia, and normal readers with no symptoms of visual discomfort were studied, and the cognitive difficulty of the text passages was manipulated (Conlon & Sanders, 2011). The visual discomfort and the control groups had similar accuracy on measures of word reading, phonological and orthographic processing, and verbal and visual short-term memory. Both groups read at Grade 12 level. The group with dyslexia had poorer skills on all reading measures and verbal short-term memory than the other groups. Visual processing speed, measured using a visual matching task was similar in the visual discomfort and dyslexia groups. Both these groups had significantly slower processing speeds than the controls.

Silent reading rate and comprehension were assessed for two levels of text difficulty, namely Grade 9 text to match the average reading level of the dyslexics and Grade 12 text to match the average reading ability of the other groups. Texts were all about 14 lines with approximately 200 words and presented on single pages in single-spaced format using Times New Roman 12-point font. On the Grade 9 level text the control and visual discomfort groups did not differ on either reading rate or comprehension, whereas the group with dyslexia had a slower reading rate and poorer comprehension. When the

Grade 12 level text was presented, even though those with visual discomfort had a reading rate equivalent to that of the controls, they had significantly poorer comprehension, even after any differences in word decoding ability and estimated ability were controlled for statistically. The reading comprehension of the groups with visual discomfort and dyslexia was equivalent, whereas the group with dyslexia also read the text significantly more slowly (Conlon & Sanders, 2011).

These findings have three important implications. First, the cognitive resources needed to read the words in a text and extract the meaning may overload or distract sustained conscious attention when a combination of cognitive skills is required for efficient performance. Added to the perceptual difficulties induced by visual stress, combining salient features in an appropriate way may have influenced performance in the group with visual discomfort. When reading text below their assessed reading level for good comprehension, fewer cognitive resources were required, so greater resources could be allocated to extracting the words from the perceptually unstable text. When reading the more linguistically difficult Grade 12 text, reading rate dropped from 180 words/minute to 145 words/minute. This was a speed/accuracy trade-off, but reading rate slowed insufficiently to achieve good comprehension. There are two possible reasons for this. First, the longer reading time may have produced increased somatic and perceptual difficulties with text viewing, causing further difficulties with the extraction of individual words because of the interference of the global pattern. This would have reduced the allocation of automatic attention to individual words (McKonkie & Zola, 1987). Supporting this explanation, reading comprehension has been found to be reduced in normally reading adults when the text is distorted (Dickinson & Rabbitt, 1991). Second, high-functioning individuals with visual discomfort may allocate the attentional resources available to them in task-dependent ways. In more difficult reading tasks, skim reading may have been used to balance the demands required from the text that was both perceptually and linguistically difficult to read, resulting in poorer comprehension. The strategy of trading speed for accuracy has been found to alleviate the symptoms of pattern glare (Garcia & Wierwille, 1985). This strategy differed from that shown in a previous study that required oral text reading (Conlon et al., 1999) where a slower reading rate but comparable comprehension to other groups was found. In that study, cognitive resources were allocated to decoding individual words, not to comprehension. In high functioning individuals with visual discomfort, cognitive resources may be allocated based on the immediate task demands.

The second reason why these findings are important is because of the differences found between the performance of those with visual discomfort and dyslexia. The linguistic demands of the texts presented produced decoding difficulties for the group with dyslexia, shown by a persistently slow reading rate and poor comprehension at both the levels of text difficulty used. In contrast, the group with visual discomfort had no difficulty in word decoding, but poorer comprehension when reading text at their assessed reading level, a finding that cannot be explained by poor reading skills. Although both groups had poorer processing speed which is a defining characteristic of adults with dyslexia (Hatcher et al., 2002), the pattern of performance of the two groups was quite different, showing that the two types of difficulty produce independent effects. It should be noted that there were four individuals with dyslexia and high levels of visual discomfort. These individuals could not be distinguished from individuals in the group with dyslexia who did not have visual discomfort on either reading rate or comprehension at either level of text difficulty.

The third important outcome from this reading study shows that the reading performance of the group with visual discomfort differed based on the linguistic difficulty of the text presented. As the same format was used at both levels of text difficulty, other visual anomalies such as problems with vergence, binocular stability, or refractive errors cannot explain the performance of the group with visual discomfort. If these effects had explained the effects induced, poor comprehension would have been found in the group with visual discomfort at both levels of text difficulty.

Why does visual discomfort produce difficulties with reading?

Taking all the findings from different studies that have investigated the consequences of visual discomfort together, poorer performance is consistently found on pop-out search tasks in the presence of a patterned background and on serial search tasks with or without a pattern background. In addition, as the cognitive resources required to successfully complete these tasks increases, performance efficiency decreases, regardless of the pattern background presented. It has been suggested that extreme sensitivity to specific features in environmental stimuli such as the pattern of a page of printed text can cause cortical hyperexcitability (Wilkins, 1995). Although this explanation is consistent with difficulties found when viewing striped repetitive patterns with spatial frequencies of 2–4 c/deg, as is found on most text pages, this does not explain the more generalized difficulties found in adult groups with severe visual discomfort. Constant lifelong assault on the visual system by particular environmental patterns to which these individuals are especially sensitive may lead to more generalized visual problems. These effects may increase the internal noise present in the visual system, producing increased difficulty with discriminating signal from noise in cluttered visual environments. This may occur regardless of the way that multiple stimuli are presented, particularly when the cognitive demands of a task are high.

That groups with visual discomfort have difficulties excluding irrelevant visual noise has some support. One recent study that used a visual discrimination task in adults with or without visual discomfort and dyslexia found that those with symptoms had significantly poorer discrimination thresholds than a non-symptomatic control group when identifying visual symbols in the presence of dynamic Gaussian noise, but not in its absence. When individually selected coloured lenses were used to alleviate the visual discomfort, the discrimination thresholds of the clinically symptomatic group normalized, so that no group differences were now found (Northway et al., 2010). In addition, with little practice a group of adults with visual discomfort had difficulty discriminating the direction of motion from noise in a dynamic visual display. However, after many trials had been conducted, direction discrimination accuracy in the group with visual discomfort normalized. Furthermore, when the discrimination task used static images only, there was no impairment in pattern discrimination in the group with visual discomfort

(Conlon et al., 2009). A recent study did not find discrimination difficulties in groups with visual discomfort using psychophysical threshold detection or event-related potential recordings (Ridder et al., 2008). However, in that study stimuli were not presented in noise and the spatial frequency of 0.5 c/deg used was not in the range that induces anomalous perceptual effects in most symptomatic individuals. A further study that investigated motion discrimination in children with or without visual discomfort also found no evidence of poorer motion discrimination in the group with visual discomfort (Simmers et al., 2001). Together these studies suggest that impaired performance is only found in those with visual discomfort, when added noise is dynamic and task difficulty is high.

Although it is clear that many individuals with visual discomfort have difficulty excluding irrelevant visual stimuli regardless of its form, the few psychophysical studies that have been conducted have produced inconsistent evidence about the underlying neural causes. This is not surprising considering the heterogeneous nature of visual discomfort. Given that visual discomfort occurs in individuals with photosensitive epilepsy (Wilkins et al., 1980), migraine headache (Wilkins et al., 1984; Conlon & Humphreys, 2001; Shepherd, 2001), dyslexia (Kriss & Evans, 2005; Singleton & Trotter, 2005), and in otherwise normally functioning individuals (Wilkins, 1995; Conlon et al., 1999; Borsting et al., 2007), the processing difficulties experienced by these different groups may differ, according to severity and according to the underlying aetiology.

The use of individually selected coloured overlays to alleviate symptoms when reading might have different impacts on the underlying neural processes. For example, for many individuals with dyslexia and visual discomfort a yellow overlay alleviates difficulties. This colour may act to enhance processing in the magnocellular processing system, a deficit found in some individuals with dyslexia (Ray et al., 2005). The neural underpinnings of visual discomfort when occurring in normal readers or individuals with other coexisting neural difficulties may differ based on the characteristics of these additional difficulties. While difficulties due to hyperexcitability to environmental stimuli and poor reading efficiency are commonly reported, the heterogeneous nature of this disorder suggests that not only should the severity of visual discomfort be considered when investigating neural correlates, but also whether the individual has a history of migraine or dyslexia.

Future directions

The scepticism of many researchers and clinicians to early reports of visual discomfort when reading has been replaced by a growing body of evidence that in sensitive individuals unpleasant perceptual and somatic effects may be induced by pages of text. This visual discomfort impairs reading efficiency in these individuals. At a cognitive level, these effects may be explained by a reduced capacity to allocate attention to the letters and words on the page in an efficient manner, as attentional resources are wasted in reducing the perceptual impact of the anomalies. At a neural level, cortical hyperexcitability from a failure of inhibitory mechanisms (Wilkins, 1995) or increased internal noise may provide an explanation for these effects. In order to elucidate further the neural underpinnings of these anomalous effects, future research should carefully investigate the individual differences among those experiencing visual discomfort. Although those with high scores on the visual discomfort scale or whose reading speed increases on the Rate of Reading Test, show clear visual discomfort, the underlying reasons may differ. Examination of the specific sensitivities of individuals with visual discomfort and migraine, visual discomfort and dyslexia, and visual discomfort alone, may reveal different patterns of neural performance. The outcome of such research may enable us to develop a causal model to explain how visual discomfort occurs in different individuals and whether reading is affected differently in the different groups.

References

Allen, P.M., Gilchrist, J.M., & Hollis, J. (2008). Use of visual search in the assessment of pattern-related visual stress (PRVS) and its alleviation by colored filters. *Investigative Ophthalmology and Visual Science*, 49, 4210–18.

Borsting, E., Chase, C.H., & Ridder, W.H. (2007). Measuring visual discomfort in college students. *Optometry and Visual Science*, 84, 745–51.

Borsting, E., Tosha, C., Chase, C., & Ridder, W.H. (2010). Measuring near-induced transient myopia in college students with visual discomfort. *Optometry and Visual Science*, 87, 760–6.

Conlon, E., & Hine, T. (2000). The influence of pattern interference on performance in migraine and visual discomfort groups. *Cephalalgia*, 20, 708–13.

Conlon, E., & Humphreys, L. (2001). Visual search in migraine and visual discomfort groups, *Vision Research*, 41, 3063–8.

Conlon, E.G., & Sanders, M.A. (2011). The reading rate and comprehension of adults with impaired reading skills or visual discomfort. *Journal of Research in Reading*, 34, 193–214.

Conlon, E.G., Lovegrove, W., Hine, T., Chekaluk, E., Piatek, K., & Hayes-Williams, K. (1998). The effects of visual discomfort and pattern structure on visual search. *Perception*, 27, 21–33.

Conlon, E.G., Lovegrove, W., Chekaluk, E., & Pattison, P.E. (1999). Measuring visual discomfort. *Visual Cognition*, 6, 637–63.

Conlon, E., Sanders, M., & Wright, C. (2009). Relationships between global motion and global form processing, practice, cognitive and visual processing in adults with dyslexia or visual discomfort. *Neuropsychologia*, 47, 907–15.

Dickinson, C.M., & Rabbitt, P.M.A. (1991). Simulated visual impairment: effects on text comprehension and reading speed. *Clinical Visual Sciences*, 4, 301–8.

Evans, B.J.W. (2005). The need for optometric investigation in suspected Meares-Irlen syndrome or visual stress. *Ophthalmic and Physiological Optics*, 25, 363–70.

Evans, B.J., & Joseph, R. (2002). The effect of coloured filters on the rate of reading in an adult student population. *Ophthalmic and Physiological Optics*, 22, 535–45.

Evans, B.J.W., Busby, A., Jeanes, R., & Wilkins, A.J. (1995). Optometric correlates of Meares-Irlen syndrome: a matched group study. *Ophthalmic and Physiological Optics*, 15, 481–7.

Evans, B.J.W., Wilkins, A.J., Brown, J., Busby, A., Wingfield, A., Jeanes, R., *et al.* (1996). A preliminary investigation into the aetiology of Meares-Irlen syndrome. *Ophthalmic and Physiological Optics*, 16, 286–96.

Garcia, K.D., & Wierville, W.W. (1985). Effect of glare on performance in a VDT reading-comprehension task. *Human Factors*, 27, 163–73.

Hatcher, J., Snowling, M. J., & Griffiths, Y. M. (2002). Cognitive assessment of dyslexic students in higher education. *British Journal of Educational Psychology*, 72, 119–33.

Hollis, J., & Allen, P.M. (2006). Screening for Meares-Irlen sensitivity in adults: can assessment methods predict changes in reading speed. *Ophthalmic and Physiological Optics*, 26, 566–71.

Irlen, H. (1983). Successful Treatment of Learning Disabilities. Paper presented at the 91st annual convention of the American Psychological Association. Anaheim, CA.

Irlen, H. (1991). *Reading by the colors*. New York: Avery Publishing Co.

Kriss, I., & Evans, B. J. (2005). The relationship between dyslexia and Meares-Irlen Syndrome. *Journal of Research in Reading*, 28, 350–64.

Kruk, R., Sumbler, K., & Willows, D. (2008). Visual processing characteristics of children with Meares-Irlen syndrome. *Ophthalmic and Physiological Optics*, 28, 35–46.

Marcus, D.A., & Soso, M.J. (1989). Migraine and striped induced visual discomfort. *Archives in Neurology*, 46, 1129–32.

McConkie, G W., & Zola, D. (1987). Visual attention during eye-fixations while reading. In: M. Coltheart (Ed.) *Attention and Performance XII*, pp. 385–401. Hillsdale, NJ: Lawrence Earlbaum.

Meares, O. (1980). Figure/ground, brightness, contrast and reading disabilities. *Visible Language*, XIV, 13–29.

Noble, J., Orton, M., Irlen, S., & Robinson, G. (2004). A controlled field study of the use of coloured overlays on reading achievement. *Australian Journal of Learning Disabilities*, 9, 14–22.

Northway, N., Manahilov, V., & Simpson, W. (2010). Coloured filters improve exclusion of perceptual noise in visually symptomatic dyslexics. *Journal of Research in Reading*, 33, 223–30.

Ray, N.C., Fowler, S., & Stein, J.F. (2005). Yellow filters can improve magnocellular function: Motion sensitivity, convergence, accommodation and reading. *Annals of the New York Academy of Sciences*, 1039, 283–92.

Ridder, W.H., Borsting, E., Tosha, C., Dougherty, R., & Chase, C. (2008). ERGs and psychophysical thresholds in students with reading discomfort, *Optometry and Visual Science*, 85, 180–6.

Shepherd, A.J. (2001). Increased visual after-effects following pattern adaptation in migraine: a lack of intracortical excitation? *Brain*, 124, 2310–18.

Simmers, A., Bex, P.J., Smith, F.K.H., & Wilkins, A.J. (2001). Spatiotemporal visual function in tinted lens wearers. *Investigative Ophthalmology and Visual Science*, 42, 879–84.

Singleton, C., & Henderson, L. (2008). Computerised screening for visual stress in reading. *Journal of Research in Reading*, 30, 316–31.

Singleton, C., & Trotter, S. (2005). Visual stress in adults with and without dyslexia. *Journal of Research in Reading*, 28, 365–78.

Wechsler, D. (1998). *Wechsler Adult Intelligence Scale – Third Edition – Australian Adaptation*. The Psychological Corporation. Adapted by Harcourt Brace & Company, New York.

Wilkins, A.J. (1995). *Visual stress*. Oxford: Oxford University Press.

Wilkins, A.J. (2002). Coloured overlays and their effects on reading speed: a review. *Ophthalmology and Physiological Optics*, 22, 448–54.

Wilkins, A.J., & Nimmo-Smith, J. (1984). On the reduction of eye-strain when reading. *Ophthalmology and Physiological Optics*, 4, 53–9.

Wilkins, A.J., & Nimmo-Smith, J. (1987). The clarity and comfort of printed text. *Ergonomics*, 30, 1705–20.

Wilkins, A.J., Binnie, C.D., & Darby, C.E. (1980). Visually induced seizures. *Progress in Neurobiology*, 15, 85–117.

Wilkins, A.J., Nimmo-Smith, I., Tait, A., McManus, C., Sala, S.G., Tilley, A., *et al.* (1984). A neurological basis for visual discomfort. *Brain*, 107, 989–1017.

Wilkins, A. J., Jeanes, R. J., Pumfrey, P. D., & Laskier, M. (1996). Rate of reading test: its reliability, and its validity in the assessment of the effects of coloured overlays. *Ophthalmic & Physiological Optics*, 16, 491–7.

Wilkins, A.J., Lewis, L., Smith, F., & Rowland, E. (2001). Coloured overlays and their benefits for reading. *Journal of Research in Reading*, 24, 41–64.

Wilkins, A.J., Huang, J., & Cao, Y. (2004). Visual stress theory and its application to reading and reading tests. *Journal of Research in Reading*, 27, 152–62.

Chapter 6

Visual Stress and its Relationship to Dyslexia

Chris Singleton

Ever since the first descriptions of developmental dyslexia over 100 years ago there has been controversy regarding the aetiological role of visual factors in the condition. The earliest writers on the subject—neurologists as well as ophthalmologists—regarded dyslexia primarily as a visual problem, a view that persisted for over 70 years. The notion that letter reversals in reading and writing are a defining feature of the condition became established during this period and the term 'word blindness' was in common use in both medical and educational circles (Critchley, 1970; Miles & Miles, 1999). However, significant advances in teaching were made following the realization that difficulties in phonology and verbal memory are fundamental characteristics of the disorder, regardless of any visual problems the child might have. A teaching programme devised by Gillingham and Stillman (1946), in which the dyslexic child is taught to build words from their sounds rather than memorize their visual appearance, became the forerunner of almost all subsequent dyslexia teaching systems and is also the historical antecedent of the modern approach known as 'synthetic phonics' (for review of evidence on dyslexia teaching systems, see Singleton, 2009a). After an influential series of studies by Vellutino (1979), which concluded that visual-perceptual factors do not play a significant role in dyslexia, the focus of psychological research in the field shifted firmly away from vision to language. Evidence steadily amassed for the theory that dyslexics have a phonological deficit, i.e. poor phonological representations of words (Snowling, 2000), and today this theory of dyslexia enjoys the widest (but by no means universal) support (Ramus, 2001; Ramus et al., 2003; Vellutino et al., 2004; Vellutino & Fletcher, 2005; White et al., 2006).

Nevertheless, a handful of researchers out of the mainstream continued to investigate visual factors in dyslexia. Visual stress is but one of these strands of research, which also include eye movements (e.g. Rayner, 1998), visual attention (e.g. Fischer et al., 2000; Valdois et al., 2004), eye dominance (e.g. Stein & Fowler, 1985, 1993; Bishop, 1989), photoreceptor distribution (e.g. Grosser & Spafford, 1989), as well as motion perception and the magnocellular system (e.g. Lovegrove et al., 1986; Cornellisen et al., 1995; Stein, 2001). Each of these approaches has uncovered evidence of visually-related deficits or anomalies in dyslexic individuals, and although some (e.g. eye movements) are probably a consequence rather than a cause of dyslexia, others (e.g. the magnocellular system) are at least strongly suggestive of a causal role, albeit one that is far from being understood at the present time. Perhaps most importantly, the findings across these areas of visual research run counter to the commonly held view that at neurological and cognitive levels dyslexia can be understood solely in phonological terms.

Visual stress: a brief overview

Visual stress is the subjective experience of unpleasant visual symptoms when reading (especially for prolonged duration) and in response to some other visual stimuli. The symptoms of the condition fall into two main categories: (1) Visual-perceptual distortions and illusions, including illusions of shape, motion, and colour in the text, blurring, and double vision; (2) aesthenopia (discomfort; sore or tired eyes; headaches; photophobia) (Sheedy et al., 2003; Borsting et al., 2007). These symptoms, which were first noted independently by Meares (1980) and Irlen (1983), tend to persist over time (Borsting et al., 2008) and are not due to visual-perceptual deficits (Kruk et al., 2008) or optometric dysfunction (Evans et al., 1995; Scott et al., 2002). Meares and Irlen both noted that such symptoms can frequently be alleviated by using colour, either in the form of acetate sheets placed over the text ('coloured overlays'), or tinted spectacles (see Irlen, 1991). The condition has been given various labels, including 'Meares–Irlen syndrome', 'visual discomfort', 'visual dyslexia', and 'scotopic sensitivity syndrome'. Arguably, some of these terms are less appropriate than others but 'visual stress' is now the generally preferred label (Evans, 2001; Wilkins, 2003; Singleton & Henderson, 2007a).

Diagnosis of visual stress is most commonly made on the basis of reported symptoms or by determining (by means of overlay screening or colorimeter test) whether use of colour makes reading more comfortable (Wilkins et al., 1992; Wilkins, 2002, 2003; Hollis & Allen, 2006; Singleton, 2008). These subjective methods have notable limitations and can result in unacceptably large numbers of false positives and false negatives, especially in children (see Northway, 2003, Singleton & Henderson, 2007a). An alternative approach is the Pattern Glare Test (Wilkins & Evans, 2001; Evans & Stevenson, 2008) which, although also subjective, has the merit of presenting stimuli that are most likely to provoke symptoms in those who are susceptible; however, norms for the general population are not yet available. A more objective method is to calculate the increase in rate of reading when using a tint (Tyrrell et al., 1995; Wilkins et al., 2001; Hollis & Allen, 2006) but this only evaluates the treatment over a short duration and does not reliably predict long-term benefits. Recently, however, an objective computer-based screening system for visual stress (ViSS) that compares visual processing under varying conditions of symptom provocation has become available, and this can be used with children and adults (Singleton & Henderson, 2007c). ViSS employ a visual search task, which individuals with visual stress tend to find particularly difficult (Tyrell et al., 1995; Conlon et al., 1998; Conlon & Hine, 2000). Individuals are required to locate a simple three-letter word in a matrix of distractor three-letter words, where the background is either visually unstressful (grey) or visually stressful (alternating black/white horizontal stripes of equal duty cycle). Children classified as having high susceptibility to visual stress by ViSS showed significantly larger increases in reading rate with a coloured overlay compared with those classified as having low susceptibility to visual stress, and also reported more unpleasant symptoms (Singleton & Henderson, 2007a). Singleton and Henderson (2007b) showed that the program is equally capable of identifying susceptibility to visual stress in children with dyslexia, because it is not significantly influenced by reading ability. Visually stressful stimuli were found to cause significantly more disruption of visual search in the dyslexics compared with controls, but on visually unstressful stimuli there were no differences between the groups. This not only demonstrates the effectiveness of ViSS for objective screening for visual stress in dyslexic as well as non-dyslexic children, but also indicates that ViSS is not simply measuring other cognitive abilities, such as memory or attention, which are clearly required for visual search but which may also be deficient in dyslexia. Similar results were obtained with adults by Allen et al. (2008), who found that, compared with controls, participants with visual stress made significantly more errors in a multiple-target number visual search task in the presence of a visually stressful background. However, no differences in search time were found in this study, most probably because a slightly different search task was used and participants were adults rather than children.

Visual stress interferes with the ability to read for any reasonable duration and hence children who experience visual stress symptoms tend to avoid reading. Consequently they lack the amount of practice that is essential for the development of fluent decoding of text and good reading comprehension (Tyrrell et al., 1995). Practice enables decoding to become automatic, reading eye movements to become smooth and disciplined, and the brain to cope with processing and understanding large amounts of text (Rayner, 1998). If visual stress is not identified and addressed early on it is likely that children will remain unskilled readers, particularly when trying to cope with more advanced texts (Singleton, 2008). Many adults who suffer from visual stress tend to steer clear of activities involving reading, which can have implications for education and employment (Singleton & Trotter, 2005). Unsurprisingly, therefore, visual stress is most frequently observed amongst children and adults who have relatively poor reading skills (Jeanes et al., 1997) although considerable numbers of educationally successful individuals also experience symptoms. Visual stress has been noted to be an increasingly common problem that interferes with students' studies at college and university (Evans & Joseph, 2002; Grant, 2004; Singleton & Trotter, 2005).

The most widely used treatment for visual stress is use of coloured tints, either in the form of acetate overlays or tinted lenses (Evans and Drasdo, 1991; Wilkins, 2002, 2003). However, symptoms can also be alleviated by enlarging font size (Wilkins et al., 2004a, 2009) or by masking the lines of text above and below the lines being read, which eliminates the striped pattern of printed text and stops pattern glare (Hughes & Wilkins, 2000). Extreme lighting conditions, including both low illumination and excessive illumination, as well as flicker from fluorescent lighting, have been found to exacerbate symptoms (Winterbottom & Wilkins, 2009). During the 1980s, Irlen became a champion of coloured tints but until the 1990s dearth of well-conducted scientific trials fuelled widespread scepticism regarding the existence of the condition and the putative benefits of treatment. Since then, however, accumulating evidence of symptom reduction and gains in rate of reading using coloured overlays and filters in children (e.g. Evans et al., 1994, 1996; Wilkins et al., 1994, 2001; Tyrrell et al., 1995; Jeanes et al., 1997; Wilkins & Lewis, 1999; Bouldoukian et al., 2002) as well as adults (e.g. Robinson & Conway, 2000), together with more modest evidence regarding gains in reading accuracy and comprehension (e.g. Robinson & Foreman, 1999; Evans & Joseph, 2002) has resulted in the approach becoming more widely accepted in schools (Whiteley & Smith, 2001), colleges, and universities (Evans & Joseph, 2002; Singleton & Trotter, 2005). It is claimed that the effects of colour are specific and different for each individual (Wilkins et al., 2004b, 2005).

Prevalence of visual stress and dyslexia

The prevalence of visual stress in the general population is generally estimated at about 20%, although figures vary according to the criteria and type of sample used (Wilkins et al., 1996; Jeanes et al., 1997; Kriss & Evans, 2005). This makes visual stress considerably more common than dyslexia, for which rates of around 5% are most typically quoted, although from time to time rather higher figures for dyslexia have been suggested (see Miles, 1991; Shaywitz et al., 1990; Shaywitz & Shaywitz, 2001).

A number of studies have revealed that the prevalence of visual stress is considerably higher in children and adults with dyslexia than in the rest of the population (Singleton & Trotter, 2005; Singleton, 2008). Whiteley and Smith (2001) estimated the prevalence of visual stress in dyslexics to be in the region of 50%, which turned out to be not far from recently reported figures. Using percentage increase in rate of reading with a coloured overlay as the criterion for assessing susceptibility to visual stress, Kriss and Evans (2005) found that 45% of dyslexic children read 5% faster with an overlay, compared with 25% of non-dyslexic control children; when a more conservative criterion of 8% increase in reading speed with an overlay was applied, these figures dropped to 34% and 22%, respectively. Using ViSS, a computer-based screening tool for visual stress, Singleton and Henderson (2007b) found that 41% of dyslexic children in their sample showed high susceptibility to visual stress; the corresponding figure for the non-dyslexic control group was 23%. White et al. (2006) found that 35% of their sample of dyslexic children aged 8–12 years met criteria for visual stress while only 18% of the non-dyslexic control group matched for non-verbal IQ met these criteria. Grant (2004) reported that of a sample of 377 university students referred for psychological assessment for dyslexia 42% showed strong evidence of visual stress and a further 34% reported some visual stress symptoms. A recent study of 80 dyslexic and 306 non-dyslexic university students using a detailed rating scale revealed high symptoms of visual stress in 18.6% of the non-dyslexics compared with 58.8% of the dyslexics (Singleton, unpublished data).

The increased prevalence of visual stress in dyslexics compared with other members of the population clearly requires an explanation. One possibility is that dyslexia and visual stress have closely related aetiologies, i.e. the neurological impairments or anomalies that give rise to the symptoms of dyslexia also cause visual stress. An alternative perspective is that dyslexia, in effect, *causes* visual stress. While this cannot be true in all cases (since at least half of dyslexics do not seem to be troubled by visual stress and most individuals who suffer from visual stress are not dyslexic) one of the many consequences of dyslexia could be that it makes the person more sensitive to the types of stimuli that can trigger visual stress, i.e. increasing susceptibility to visual stress. A third logical possibility is that susceptibility to visual stress could be one of the causes of dyslexia. However, this explanation seems less plausible: despite the fact that visual stress can result in reading difficulties the determining features of dyslexia are considerably more than poor reading skills. Dyslexia is characterized by weaknesses in phonological awareness, verbal memory and speed of processing verbal information (Snowling, 2000; Vellutino et al., 2004), which in turn give rise to problems in recognizing and spelling words. Hence an essential part of the diagnostic process for dyslexia is the identification of deficits in underlying cognitive processing (Turner, 1997; Thomson, 2009). Furthermore, unlike dyslexia, visual stress is not fundamentally a difficulty that emerges at the level of the *word*; rather, it is mainly when the reader is confronted by *lines of text* (or similar visual patterns) that the symptoms of visual stress are most likely to be experienced (Tyrrell et al., 1995). (Note, however, recent evidence that intraword characteristics—specifically, the degree of 'stripedness' of the word—can contribute to legibility and reading speed and hence may give rise to visual stress symptoms in some individuals; Wilkins et al., 2007.) Nevertheless, it remains possible that in some cases of dyslexia the root cause (or, at least, part of the cause) is visual rather than phonological.

Cortical hyperexcitability

A widely supported theory of visual stress is that it is the result of general overexcitation of the visual cortex triggered by hypersensitivity to contrast or pattern glare (Wilkins, 1995, 2003; see also Evans, 2001). Wilkins has hypothesized that the visual cortex functions normally until strong physiological stimulation results in excitation of neurons that are close together. These neurons share inhibitory neurons and therefore normal inhibitory processes are likely to be compromised if they all fire together because amounts of inhibitory neurotransmitter will be depleted. The outcome is the triggering of other neurons signalling movement or colour that are consequently experienced as subjectively disturbing illusions or hallucinations. In other words, the visual cortex works normally until stimulation is too strong, whereupon a catastrophic non-linear failure of inhibition occurs, which spreads to other neurons (Wilkins, 1995; Wilkins et al., 2004a).

Any stimulus that creates square-wave on-off signals in the visual cortex can potentially trigger these neural effects, the most obvious examples being high contrast, rapidly flashing or flickering illumination such as strobe lighting, fluorescent lighting, cathode ray tube (CRT) computer monitors with low refresh rate, and bright sunlight viewed through trees when moving in a vehicle. All these stimuli cause headaches in many people, especially those suffering from migraine (Hay et al., 1994; Aurora et al., 1999; Welch et al., 2001; Huang et al., 2003; Harle & Evans, 2004; Harle et al., 2006; Friedman & De Ver Dye, 2009). They can also trigger seizures in people with photosensitive epilepsy (Wilkins, 1995). The most dramatic case of epileptic seizures being triggered by flashing stimuli occurred in Japan in 1997, when a cartoon transmitted on TV resulted in

685 people (most of them children) being admitted to hospital—560 were found to have had epileptic seizures and of these 76% of these had no previous history of epilepsy. The seizures were subsequently shown to be attributable to intense, rapidly flashing colour changes, viewed under conditions of high contrast (Harding, 1998; Furusho et al., 2002). Similar effects, including epileptic seizures, have been reported with some computer and video games (Quirk et al., 1995; Wilkins et al., 2004b). Geometric repetitive patterns, such as stripes, create square-wave on-off neural signals similar to those causes by flashing lights, especially when there is a strong light/dark contrast. This explains why such patterns, even though stationary, can also cause unpleasant somatic and perceptual side effects (McKay, 1957; McKay et al., 1979; Wilkins & Nimmo-Smith, 1987), including triggering seizures in some people who suffer from photosensitive epilepsy (Harding & Jeavons, 1995; Fisher et al., 2005).

Text can resemble a pattern of stripes with visually stressful characteristics and the visual grating created by moving the eyes across lines of print, especially where contrast is strong and the pattern is glaring, can generate similar physiological effects to those created by flashing lights (Wilkins & Nimmo-Smith, 1987). These findings suggest a continuum of photosensitivity for people suffering from photosensitive epilepsy, migraine, and visual stress (Aurora et al., 1999). Individuals who suffer from visual stress (but not photosensitive epilepsy or migraine) would be regarded as 'moderately photosensitive', so that their symptoms are not as extreme or easily triggered as those of individuals who suffer from photosensitive epilepsy or migraine.

Why then, does colour usually have a palliative effect on the symptoms of visual stress? Wilkins (1995, 2003) suggests that because the wavelength of light is known to affect neuronal sensitivity, the use of colour could reduce overexcitation, redistributing cortical hyperexcitability and thus reducing perceptual distortion and headaches. Tints have been found to reduce the amount of accommodative lag seen in patients who suffer from visual stress but not in controls (Allen et al., 2010). Tinted filters have been shown to reduce headaches in patients who suffer from migraine provoked by visual stimuli (Wilkins et al., 2002; Riddell et al., 2006), and the incidence of a family history of migraine in children who benefit from coloured filters has been found to be twice that of children who do not (Maclachlan et al., 1993). These findings are consistent with Wilkins's hypothesis that the therapeutic effects of coloured filters derives from a reduction in cortical hyperexcitability (Wilkins, 1995, 2003).

Visual stress and the magnocellular system

An alternative perspective on visual stress comes from researchers investigating the magnocellular pathways in the visual system. There are two principal cell types found in primate neural tracts between the retina and the visual cortex: *magnocells* are large cells that are sensitive to fast temporal resolution, low contrast, and low spatial frequencies, and which code information about contrast and movement; *parvocells* are smaller, sensitive to moderate temporal resolution, high contrast, medium and high spatial frequencies, and code information about colour, form, and texture (Merigan & Maunsell, 1993).

The magnocellular system plays several important roles in visual functioning, including binocular control of eye movements, selective attention and visual search (Stein & Walsh, 1997; Steinman et al., 1997; Vidyasagar, 1998; Vidyasagar & Pammer, 1999; Iles et al., 2000; Facoetti et al., 2003). Cooperation between the magnocellular system (sometimes referred to as the M pathway or transient system) and the parvocelluar system (sometimes referred to as the P pathway or sustained system) enables perception of a stationary image during saccadic movement of the eyes across a scene or a page of text, as vision is suppressed during saccades, thus avoiding blurring (Breitmeyer, 1993).

Accumulating studies reporting deficits in M functioning in poor readers and dyslexics gave rise to the magnocellular deficit theory of dyslexia (Lovegrove et al., 1986). This theory was originally predicated on the belief that the M system suppresses the P system when a saccade is initiated, thus preventing the image from one fixation becoming confused with that from the next fixation. It was postulated that in dyslexic readers this suppression process is depressed or absent (Livingstone et al., 1991; Lovegrove et al., 1986, 1990; Lovegrove, 1991). However, this explanation is not particularly convincing, since failure of suppression would be expected to cause difficulties in perception across a wide range of everyday tasks, not just reading. Moreover, subsequent evidence that it is actually the M system rather than the P system that is suppressed during saccades rendered the magnocellular deficit theory untenable, at least in its original form (Burr et al., 1994, 1996).

Stein and his colleagues (Stein & Talcott, 1999; Stein & Walsh, 1997; Stein et al., 2000, 2001) proposed a modification of this theory, in which deficiencies in the M system are claimed to result in poor binocular control such that the dyslexic's reading would suffer from misperception of words and inefficient saccadic targeting. This deficiency could be caused by disorganization of the M layer and smaller M cells, for which there is some physiological and anatomical evidence (Livingstone et al., 1991). According to Stein and his colleagues (see Stein & Walsh, 1997; Stein & Talcott, 1999) the effects of this problem include letters seeming to move on the page, jumbling up, merging and crossing over each other. Since the impact of the presumed M deficit is described in terms more-or-less identical to those attributed to visual stress, it is clear, therefore, that these authors regard visual stress as part of the effects of dyslexia, although they acknowledge that phonological and motor symptoms are concomitants of the disorder. Support for this hypothesis come from a variety of studies: for example, Cornelissen et al. (1995) found dyslexics to be significantly poorer than controls in perception of moving stimuli, and Talcott et al. (1998) found dyslexics to have significantly higher thresholds for perception of coherent motion using random dot kinematograms. Eden et al. (1996) found that dyslexics did not show activation of certain critical areas of the visual cortex that are normally activated by moving stimuli, and Evans et al. (1994) reported a number of anomalies in the M processing of dyslexics, including in contrast sensitivity. Subsequent studies have widened the scope of the M deficit theory to include spatial attention and higher levels of visual processing along the dorsal stream (e.g. Vidyasagar & Pammer, 1999; Hari & Renvall, 2001; Facoetti et al., 2003).

However, reviewing 22 different studies of M functioning in dyslexics, Skotton (2000) found that only four were clearly in support of the hypothesis that dyslexia could be attributed to M deficits. More recently, Schulte-Körne and Bruder (2010) reviewed physiological studies of the M system and failed to uncover clear evidence that would support a magnocellular cause of dyslexia mediated by motion processing or contrast sensitivity. Deficits in motion perception are certainly not found in all dyslexics (e.g. Everatt et al., 1999) or with all motion-perception tasks (e.g. Raymond & Sorensen, 1998). White et al. (2006) found that M tasks did not significantly discriminate dyslexic from control children; only two out of 23 dyslexic children showed deficits in visual motion while three out of 22 control children showed deficits in visual motion. Thus while it remains a possibility that a minority of dyslexics have deficits in M functioning, the evidence for the magnocellular theory of dyslexia is far from compelling (Parke & Skottun, 1999; Skoyles & Skottun, 2004; Skottun, 2005). Skottun and Skoyles (2004, 2006) have also argued that coherent motion tasks—which rely on the ability to identify direction of movement—are unsatisfactory for assessing M function because directional sensitivity is largely a function of neurons in the visual cortex and not the M system, and hence other systems can influence perception of coherent motion. Furthermore, similar perceptual deficiencies have been found in association with autism, Williams's syndrome, hemiplegia, and schizophrenia (Skottun & Skoyles, 2008), indicating that they are by no means unique to dyslexia.

Shovman and Ahissar (2006) assessed the performance of dyslexics and controls in reading-like visual conditions in which letter size, crowding (i.e. inclusion of adjacent distracting letters) were varied. Previous investigations that have reported significant effects of letter size and crowding on dyslexics' letter identification have failed fully to eliminate the effects of real word recognition and memory, both of which are known to be deficient in dyslexia (Cornelissen et al., 1991; Enns et al., 1995; Hawelka & Wimmer, 2005). In other words, findings of differences between dyslexics and non-dyslexics in these studies that have been attributed to visual processing could actually have been due to non-visual factors. Shovman and Ahissar used a subset of Georgian letters that were graphically similar to both English and Hebrew and found no significant differences in letter recognition between dyslexics and controls when letter size was decreased and crowding increased. Hutzler et al. (2006) also found that dyslexic readers do not have difficulties in the accurate perception of letters or in control of eye movements during reading, hence their reading difficulties cannot be explained in terms of oculomotor and visuo-perceptual problems.

The magnocellular deficit theory also needs to explain how coloured filters might alleviate visual stress, given that the M system is relatively insensitive to colour. M cells probably receive input from red, green, and blue cones in proportion to their density in the retina (Roorda & Williams, 1999) thus coloured filters could selectively block the light in a zone of the spectrum, effectively redistributing those proportions (Stein, 2003, 2007). Ray et al. (2005) reported that wearing yellow filters increased sensitivity to motion in a small group of children with reading difficulties. Yellow filters also enhanced vergence and accommodation, and reading accuracy was slightly improved, although

Ciuffreda et al. (1997) did not find that Irlen filters had any effect on accommodation. Ray et al. (2005) suggest that highly saturated yellow filters may boost M activity by eliminating blue light. Elsewhere, however, Stein (2007) has presented evidence suggesting that highly saturated *blue* filters may also have similar beneficial effects, which seems contradictory given that blue and yellow are 'opposing' colours: yellow filters will cut out blue light and blue filters will cut out yellow light (Mollon et al., 2003). The position is further complicated by the finding that red light impairs reading performance under normal luminance contrast conditions, but also that isoluminant text (i.e. green text on a red background of the same luminance as the text) is easier to read under red light (Chase et al., 2003). Since there is evidence that isoluminant text selectively activates the P pathway (Legge et al., 1990), Chase et al. argue that red light suppresses function in the M pathway, which they suggest is the dominant visual pathway for text perception. Chase (1996) has proposed a model of dyslexia in which red light is assumed to disrupt orthographic processing at the prelexical stage, affecting perception of letters and words, with the P pathway adding finer details in order to resolve ambiguity. The implications of this theory for dyslexia are that disruption of the faster M pathway may result in the child learning to rely more on the slower P pathway, giving rise to a variety of reading impairments, including slower reading.

Given the range of apparently contradictory results in connection with the magnocellular deficit theory probably the safest conclusion to draw at the present time is that it remains unproven. Much is still to be done to resolve disputed issues in the field, including appropriate identification of dyslexic participants (see Schulte-Körne & Bruder, 2010), selection of experimental tasks that activate M and P pathways (see Skotun & Skoyles, 2006), and clarifying the effects of colour on the component systems (see Chase et al., 2003). Differences between dyslexics and non-dyslexics in tasks that are presumed to activate the M system could simply be correlational and not causal of reading difficulties (see Hutzler et al., 2006), mediated by a genetic deviation that is responsible for disruption in several neural systems (see Frith & Frith, 1996; Ramus, 2004). On current evidence it looks increasingly unlikely that the M system plays a major aetiological role in either visual stress or dyslexia but it remains possible that M deficits could predominate in certain subtypes of dyslexia (see Heim et al., 2008). This would not be inconsistent with results obtained by White et al. (2006), who found that 13% of their sample of dyslexic children met criteria for visual stress but had no other cognitive deficits, while a further 22% had visual stress together with other cognitive deficits, including phonological, auditory and motor problems. Similarly, Reid et al. (2006) found that 7% of a sample of dyslexic adults exhibited a visual magnocellular deficit, while a further 7% had a visual magnocellular deficit and phonological deficit. Stein's (2001) assumption that the wider system of M cells in the brain is recruited by a variety of cognitive functions, including attention and auditory processing as well as visual processing finds support from recent functional magnetic resonance imaging studies, leading to the hypothesis that distinct subtypes of dyslexia may have different patterns of brain activation: e.g. dyslexics with phonological deficits having reduced left frontal activation and dyslexics with magnocellular deficits probably having enhanced right frontal activation (see Heim et al., 2010).

Hence it may turn out that some individuals who have been diagnosed as dyslexic, rather than having phonological difficulties as the root cause of their literacy problems, might have impaired M pathway which, among other consequences, impedes the rapid attentional shifts essential for fluent reading (see Simmers & Bex, 2001; Laycock & Crewther, 2008). This would not only disrupt the reading process but also give rise to symptoms of visual stress.

Threshold shift theory

If we accept—at least, for the time being—that dyslexia and visual stress are probably different conditions with separate aetiologies, an explanation still has to found for the increased prevalence of visual stress amongst dyslexics compared with the general population. Wilkins's exposition of cortical hyperexcitability and the role it plays in causing symptoms of visual stress portrays it as an *abnormal response* of the visual system: a visual disorder found in certain individuals. On this basis, visual stress is a developmental disorder that, like several other conditions, can be comorbid with dyslexia, possibly because of an overlapping genetic nexus (see Frith and Frith, 1996; Pennington & Olson, 2005). On the other hand, an alternative perspective is that cortical hyperexcitability could be a *normal response* of the visual cortex when subjected to certain exceptional visual stimuli. It follows from this that everyone is potentially susceptible to visual stress, at least to some degree: a conclusion that is supported by the aversion that many people have to rapidly flashing lights, and widespread experience of illusions of movement and colour reported by individuals confronted with certain high contrast regular striped patterns in clothing, wallpaper, or window blinds (McKay, 1957; McKay et al., 1979; Wilkins & Nimmo-Smith, 1987).

It is obvious that some people are more susceptible to visual stress than others and that dyslexics belong to the higher susceptibility group. To account for this, Singleton (2008, 2009b) has suggested that the link between dyslexia and visual stress may not necessarily be causal. Visual stress discourages inclination to practice reading, which will create a 'Matthew effect' (i.e. the gap between good and poor readers progressively widening as a function of differences in reading experience; Stanovich, 1986). It is likely that the dyslexic person's lack of automaticity in word recognition (e.g. due to underlying deficits in phonology or memory) forces them to adopt techniques for processing text (e.g. detailed scrutiny of individual 'problem' words) that increase their sensitivity to the physical characteristics of the print. In turn, this will naturally tend to make symptoms or effects of visual stress worse. A similar conclusion was drawn by Shovman and Ahissar (2006): although finding no evidence that the reading difficulties of their dyslexic subjects were due to oculomotor or visuo-perceptual problems they did find that many more dyslexic participants complained of visual discomfort during the experimental tasks. They surmised that:

> Dyslexics probably need to acquire more accurate visual information, compared with controls, to compensate for their phonological deficits, perhaps due to impoverished phonological representations. Hence, for dyslexics, the task of reading may put a heavier load on visual attention compared to their peers. It may resemble the experience of 'expert' readers when trying to read foreign names

with unfamiliar syllabic structure. While skilled readers typically scan the text in what 'feels' like effortless fluency, when encountering such words, they need to visually focus, and more accurately identify each letter in the sequence. It becomes a visually more demanding task, which may perhaps induce discomfort when such words are the main components of the text.

(Shovman & Ahissar, 2006, pp. 3523–4.)

A key feature of the threshold shift theory is that susceptibility to visual stress varies from person to person: the majority of the population is only mildly susceptible (i.e. they have a *high threshold*); at the other end of the spectrum, individuals who suffer from photosensitive epilepsy or from migraine tend to be highly susceptible to visual stress (i.e. they have a *low threshold*). Singleton (2008, 2009b) has hypothesized that there is a continuum of physiological excitation (sensitivity) to visually stressful stimuli from low sensitivity to high sensitivity, which may be assumed (for the time being, at least) to be approximately normally distributed. All individuals will lie at a theoretical point somewhere on this continuum of physiological sensitivity as a consequence of availability of inhibitor neurotransmitters, determined by a combination of genetic, developmental and environmental factors. This point may be called the *physiological threshold for visual stress*. Individuals who suffer from migraine or photosensitive epilepsy will be near to the upper (high sensitive) end of this distribution and hence will have a low threshold. This theory also posits another point on the continuum of physiological sensitivity that constitutes a *clinical threshold for visual stress*, i.e. a point above which individuals find that symptoms of visual stress interfere significantly and substantially with everyday functioning such that aversive action to mitigate symptoms is called for. For any given individual, there will be a difference (on the continuum of physiological sensitivity) between their physiological threshold for visual stress and their clinical threshold for visual stress. This difference is the amount to which the threshold for visual stress has been shifted as a result of nonphysiological factors. It is anticipated that in almost every person the clinical threshold will be lower than the physiological threshold, because various factors will tend to increase sensitivity. The degree of *threshold shift* will be determined by the following factors:

1. *Cognitive factors* (e.g. dyslexia, reading problems; working memory). The greater the difficulty in decoding text and in holding the information in working memory while deriving meaning, the greater the sensitivity and lower the threshold.

2. *Demand factors* (e.g. demands created by education or employment circumstances). The greater the amount of reading the person has to do and the higher the cognitive load placed on the person by that reading, the greater the sensitivity and lower the threshold.

3. *Ophthalmic and orthoptic factors* (e.g. amblyopia, astigmatism, diplopia, hypermetropia, nystagmus, detached retina, cataracts). The presence and severity of these visual problems will tend to increase sensitivity and lower the threshold.

4. *Optical factors* (e.g. lighting conditions, font type and size, line spacing, contrast, glare, flicker). The more that these factors diverge from the ideal, the greater the sensitivity and the lower the threshold.

5. *Subjective factors* (e.g. personality type and personal tolerance of discomfort).

This theory of the relationship between dyslexia and visual stress can be called '*threshold shift*'. In a nutshell, this view is that dyslexia tends to increase a person's susceptibility to visual stress because the effect of dyslexia is to shift the threshold for visual stress from higher to lower. The threshold shift theory is consistent with much of the current evidence on visual stress. It predicts that visual stress will be more prevalent in dyslexics and in other poor readers than in the rest of the population, which has been shown in many studies (e.g. Kriss & Evans, 2005; White et al., 2006; Singleton & Henderson, 2007b). Connah (unpublished) tested undergraduate students with dyslexia using the computerized screening system ViSS (Singleton & Henderson, 2007c) and found that the average increase in visual search time for this group on visually stressful items compared to that on non-visually stressful items was 33%; the corresponding figure for non-dyslexic controls was 11%.

The threshold shift theory also predicts that the more severe the reading/dyslexic difficulties, greater the sensitivity to visual stress and lower the threshold. This prediction has some support: Connah (unpublished) found that severity of dyslexia accounts for a significant proportion (11%) of the variance in severity of visual stress. The threshold shift theory also predicts that in situations where intensive reading is called for (e.g. at university), visual stress will be more prevalent. Evans and Joseph (2002) studied 113 unselected university students and found that 89% reported beneficial perceptual effects of a chosen coloured overlay and these students read significantly faster with an overlay than without it. Eighty-one of the students experienced headaches, of which 44% said they were associated with reading. These figures are higher than in studies of school children. In addition, the threshold shift theory predicts that people with ophthalmic and orthoptic problems are more likely to display symptoms of visual stress, which has been reported (Garzia & Nicholson, 1990; Evans, 2001). There is also evidence that personality factors (specifically, neuroticism and high sensitivity to external stimuli) influences susceptibility to visual stress (Hollis et al., 2007).

Optical factors have also been found to influence susceptibility to visual stress. Hughes and Wilkins (2000) not only found that children's reading speed is a function of font size and characteristics of the text, but those children who were susceptible to visual stress were disproportionately affected by font size and text characteristics. Wilkins (2002) has observed that the levels of illumination often found in classrooms is up to four times that recommended by European standards, with the result that contrast is increased and children become more vulnerable to visual stress. Winterbottom and Wilkins (2009) examined 90 classrooms in 11 different secondary schools and found that in most of these illumination (including quality and intensity of fluorescent lighting, glare from whiteboards, and high contrast patterns created by Venetian blinds) was visually uncomfortable. Adjustment of lighting conditions, font size and viewing distance have been found to induce aesthenopia and other symptoms of visual stress such as blurring of text and diplopia during reading in adults without any previous history of visual stress (Sheedy et al., 2003; Nahar et al., 2007).

A further prediction of the threshold shift theory is that the distribution of reported symptoms of visual stress in unselected samples would not be normal, but would be positively skewed (i.e. an elongated right tail with mode <median <mean) because the

non-physiological factors listed earlier will shift the threshold and extend the number of cases in the right (higher) tail of the distribution. There is some evidence for this: Singleton and Trotter (2005) and Singleton (unpublished data) found that the distribution of reported symptoms of visual stress in unselected samples [number of symptoms × severity of symptoms] has a positive skew. However, the threshold shift theory raises some unanswered questions. For example, we do not know whether the use of coloured tints (1) *lowers the physiological threshold* making the person less sensitive and less likely to experience symptoms of visual stress, or (2) *lowers the clinical threshold*, thus reducing threshold shift and bringing the clinical threshold closer to the physiological threshold, or (3) a combination of these two effects.

Conclusions

The organization of the various components involved in reading, including eye movements, letter perception, word recognition, working memory, and comprehension, develop and become integrated as an efficient system as a result of the experience of learning to read. This underlines the educational requirement for adequate and appropriate practice in text reading in order to discipline eye movements, attain fluency in decoding, and provide a firm basis for competent reading comprehension. There is a strong case for screening for visual stress in all children because the condition disrupts the reading process, which, in turn, has detrimental effects on the development of fluency and comprehension. Remedial action to alleviate the symptoms of visual stress is important in order to minimize negative consequences of the condition throughout schooling, in further and higher education, as well as in employment (Wilkins, 2002; Grant, 2004; Singleton and Trotter, 2005).

Where individuals have visual stress comorbid with dyslexia there is likely to be a multiplicative detrimental effect on reading (Singleton, 2008). As combined result of lack of reading experience and the reading style that dyslexics are forced to adopt, the sensitivity threshold for visual stress is likely to be shifted, making them more sensitive to the physical characteristics of text (such as contrast, glare, stripedness, and font size) and increasing their risk of experiencing the unpleasant symptoms of visual stress. It is therefore particularly important that children who are already known to have dyslexia are also screened for visual stress, since not only is their risk of visual stress much greater than that found in other individuals but, also, if they do suffer from visual stress, the repercussions of remaining untreated are likely to be of more profound. The identification of visual stress in schools is now a straightforward task for teachers using a choice of readily accessible methods that include objective computer-based screening, and the availability of efficacious treatment with coloured tints provides cost-effective solutions that are easy to use in the classroom and at home.

References

Allen, P.M., Gilchrist, J.M., & Hollis, J. (2008). Use of visual search in the assessment of pattern-related visual stress (PRVS) and its alleviation by colored filters. *Investigative Ophthalmology and Vision Science, 49*, 4210–18.

Allen, P.M., Hussain, A., Usherwood, C., & Wilkins, A.J. (2010). Pattern-related visual stress, chromaticity and accommodation. *Investigative Ophthalmology and Vision Science,* 10, 1167.

Aurora, S.K., Cao, Y., Bowyer, S.M., & Welch, K.M.A. (1999). The occipital cortex is hyperexcitable in migraine: Experimental evidence. *Headache,* 39, 469–76.

Biship, D.V.M. (1989). Unfixed reference, monocular occlusion, and developmental dyslexia— a critique. *British Journal of Ophthalmology,* 73, 209–15.

Borsting, E., Chase, C.H., & Ridder, W.H. (2007). Measuring visual discomfort in college students. *Optometry and Vision Science,* 84, 745–51.

Borsting, E., Chase, C.H., Tosha, C., & Ridder, W.H. (2008). Longitudinal study of visual discomfort symptoms in college students. *Optometry and Vision Science,* 85, 992–8.

Bouldoukian, J., Wilkins, A.J. and Evans, B.J.W. (2002). Randomized controlled trial of the effect of coloured overlays on the rate of reading of people with specific learning difficulties. *Ophthalmic and Physiological Optics,* 22, 55–60.

Breitmeyer, B.G. (1993). Sustained (P) and transient (M) channels in vision: a review and implications for reading. In: D.M. Willows, R.S. Kruk, & E. Corcos (Eds.) *Visual processes in reading and reading disabilities,* pp. 95–110. Hillsdale, NJ: Lawrence Erlbaum Associates Inc.

Burr, D.C., Morone, M.C., & Ross, J. (1994). Selective suppression of the magnocellular visual pathway during saccadic eye movements. *Nature,* 371, 511–13.

Chase, C.H. (1996). A visual deficit model of developmental dyslexia. In: C.H. Chase, G.D. Rosen, & G.F. Sherman (Eds.) *Developmental dyslexia: neural cognitive and genetic mechanisms,* pp. 127–156. Timonium, MD: York Press.

Chase, C., Ashourzadeh, A., Kelly, C., Monfette, S., & Kinsey, K. (2003). Can the magnocellular pathway read? Evidence from studies of colour. *Vision Research,* 43, 1211–22.

Ciuffreda, K.J., Scheiman, M., Ong, E., Rosenfield, M., & Solan, H.A. (1997). Irlen lenses do not improve accommodative accuracy at near. *Optometry & Vision Science* 74, 298–302.

Conlon, E., & Hine, T. (2000). The influence of pattern interference on performance in migraine and visual discomfort groups. *Cephalagia,* 20, 708–13.

Conlon, E., Lovegrove, W., Hine, T., Chekaluk, E., Piatek, K., & Hayes-Williams, K. (1998). The effect of visual discomfort and pattern structure on visual search. *Perception,* 27, 21–33.

Connah, A. (unpublished). Investigating the relationship between dyslexia and visual stress in adults. Unpublished Research Project Report, Department of Psychology, University of Hull, May 2008.

Cornelissen, P., Bradley, L., Fowler, M.S., & Stein, J.F. (1991). What children see affects how they read. *Developmental Medicine and Child Neurology,* 33, 755–62.

Cornelissen, P., Richardson, A., Mason, A., & Stein, J.F. (1995). Contrast sensitivity and coherent motion detection measured at photopic luminance levels in dyslexics and controls. *Vision Research,* 35, 1483–94.

Critchley, M. (1970). *The Dyslexic Child.* London: Heinemann.

Eden, G.F., VanMeter, J.W., Rumsey, J.W., Maisog, J., & Zeffiro, T.A. (1996). Functional MRI reveals differences in visual motion processing in individuals with dyslexia. *Nature,* 382, 66–9.

Enns, J. T., Bryson, S., & Roes, C. (1995). Search for letter identity and location by disabled readers. *Canadian Journal of Experimental Psychology,* 49, 357–67.

Evans, B.J.W. (2001). *Dyslexia and Vision.* London: Whurr.

Evans, B.J.W., & Drasdo, N. (1991). Tinted lenses and related therapies for learning disabilities— a review. *Ophthalmic & Physiological Optics,* 11, 206–17.

Evans, B.J.W., & Joseph, R. (2002). The effect of coloured filters on the rate of reading in an adult student population. *Ophthalmic & Physiological Optics,* 22, 535–45.

Evans, B.J.W., & Stevenson, S.J. (2008). The Pattern Glare Test: a review and determination of normative values. *Ophthalmic & Physiological Optics,* 28, 295–309.

Evans, B.J.W., Drasdo, N., & Richards, I. (1994). An investigation of some sensory and refractive visual factors in dyslexia. *Vision Research*, 34, 1913–26.

Evans, B.J.W., Busby, A., Jeanes, R., & Wilkins, A.J. (1995). Optometric correlates of Meares-Irlen Syndrome: a matched group study. *Ophthalmic & Physiological Optics*, 15, 481–7.

Evans, B.J.W., Wilkins, A.J., Brown, J., Busby, A., Wingfield, A.E., Jeanes, R., *et al.* (1996). A preliminary investigation into the aetiology of Meares–Irlen Syndrome. *Ophthalmic & Physiological Optics*, 16, 286–96.

Everatt, J., Bradshaw, M.F., & Hibbard, P.B. (1999). Visual processing and dyslexia. *Perception*, 28, 243–54.

Facoetti, A., Lorusso, M.L., Paganoni, P., Cattaneo, C., Galli, R., & Mascetti, G.G. (2003). The time course of attentional focusing in dyslexic and normally reading children. *Brain and Cognition*, 53, 181–4.

Fischer, B., Hartnegg, K., & Miklet, A. (2000). Dynamic visual perception of dyslexic children. *Perception*, 29, 523–30.

Fisher, R.S., Harding, G., Erba, G., Barkley, G.L., & Winkins, A. J. (2005). Photic- and pattern-induced seizures: a review for the Epilepsy Foundation of America working group. *Epilepsia*, 46, 1426–41.

Friedman, D.I., & De Ver Dye, T. (2009). Migraine and the environment. *Headache*, 49, 941–52.

Frith, C., & Frith, U. (1996). A biological marker for dyslexia. *Nature*, 382, 19–20.

Furusho, J., Suzuki, M., Tazaki, H., Yamaguchi, K., Iikura, Y., Kumagi, K., *et al.* (2002). A comparison survey of seizures and other symptoms of Pokemon phenomena. *Pediatric Neurology*, 27, 350–5.

Garzia, R.P., & Nicholson, S.B. (1990). Optometric factors in reading disability. In: D.M. Willows, R.S. Kruk, & E. Corcos (Eds.) *Visual processes in reading and reading disabilities*, pp. 419–34. Hillsdale, NJ: Lawrence Erlbaum Associates Inc.

Gillingham, A., & Stillman, B.E. (1946). *Remedial training for children with specific disability in reading spelling and penmanship*. Cambridge, MA: Educator's Publishing Service.

Grant, D. (2004). From myths to realities: Lessons to be drawn from over 600 student assessments. Paper presented at the 6th International Conference of the British Dyslexia Association, University of Warwick, March 2004.

Grosser, G.S., & Spafford, C.S. (1989). Perceptual evidence for an anomalous distribution of rods and cones in the retinas of dyslexics: a new hypothesis. *Perceptual and Motor Skills*, 68, 683–98.

Harding, G.F.A. (1998). TV can be bad for your health. *Nature Medicine*, 4, 265–7.

Harding, G.F.A., & Jeavons, P.M. (1995). Photosensitive epilepsy. *Clinics in Developmental Medicine, No. 133*. Cambridge: Cambridge University Press.

Hari, R., & Renvall, H. (2001). Impaired processing of rapid stimulus sequences in dyslexia. *Trends in Cognitive Sciences*, 5(12), 525–32.

Harle, D.E., & Evans, B.J.W. (2004). The optometric correlates of migraine. *Ophthalmic and Physiological Optics*, 24, 369–83.

Harle, D. E., Shepherd, A.J., & Evans, B.J.W. (2006). Visual stimuli are common triggers of migraine and are associated with pattern glare. *Headache*, 46, 1431–40.

Hawelka, S., & Wimmer, H. (2005). Impaired visual processing of multi-element arrays is associated with increased number of eye movements in dyslexic reading. *Vision Research*, 45(7), 855–63.

Hay, K.M., Mortimer, M.J., Barker, D.C., Debney, L.M., & Good, P.A. (1994). 1044 women with migraine: the effect of environmental stimuli. *Headache*, 34, 166–8.

Heim, S., Grande, M., Pape-Neumann, J., Erminen, M. van, Meffert, E., Grabowska, A., *et al.* (2010). Interaction of phonological awareness and 'magnocellular' processing during normal and dyslexic reading: Behavioural and fMRI investigations. *Dyslexia*, 16, 258–82.

Heim, S., Tschierse, J., Amunts, K., Vossel, S., Wilms, M., & Willmes, K., *et al.* (2008). Cognitive subtypes of dyslexia. *Acta Neurobiologiae Experimentalis*, 68, 73–82.

Hollis, J., & Allen. P.M. (2006). Screening for Meares–Irlen sensitivity in adults: can assessment methods predict changes in reading speed? *Ophthalmic and Physiological Optics*, 26, 566–71.

Hollis, J., Allen. P.M., Fleischmann, D., & Aulak, R. (2007). Personality dimensions of people who suffer from visual stress. *Ophthalmic and Physiological Optics*, 27, 603–10.

Huang, J., Cooper, T.G., Satana, B., Kaufman, D. I., & Cao, Y. (2003). Visual distortion provoked by a stimulus in migraine associated with hyperneuronal activity. *Headache*, 43, 664–71.

Hughes, L.E., & Wilkins, A.J. (2000). Typography in children's reading schemes may be suboptimal: Evidence from measures of reading rate. *Journal of Research in Reading*, 12, 314–24.

Hutzler, F., Kronbichler, M., Jacobs, A.M., & Wimmer, H. (2006). Perhaps correlational but not causal: No effect of dyslexic readers' magnocellular system on their eye movements during reading. *Neuropsychologia*, 44, 637–48.

Iles, J., Walsh, V., & Richardson, A. (2000). Visual search performance in dyslexia. *Dyslexia*, 6, 163–177.

Irlen, H. (1983). Successful treatment of learning difficulties. Paper presented at the *Annual Convention of the American Psychological Association*, Anaheim, CA.

Irlen, H. (1991). *Reading by the colours*. New York: Avery.

Jeanes, R., Busby, A., Martin, J., Lewis, E., Stevenson, N., Pointon, D., & Wilkins, A. (1997). Prolonged use of coloured overlays for classroom reading. *British Journal of Psychology*, 88, 531–48.

Kriss, I., & Evans, B.J.W. (2005). The relationship between dyslexia and Meares-Irlen syndrome. *Journal of Research in Reading,* 28, 350–64.

Kruk, R., Sumbler, K., & Willows, D. (2008). Visual processing characteristics of children with Meares–Irlen syndrome. *Ophthalmic and Physiological Optics*, 28, 35–46.

Laycock, R., & Crewther, S.G. (2008). Towards an understanding of the role of the 'magnocellular advantage' in fluent reading. *Neuroscience and Biobehavioral Reviews,* 32, 1494–506.

Legge, G.E., Parish, D.H., Luebker, A., & Wurm, L.H. (1990). Psychophysics of reading: XI. Comparing color contrast and luminance contrast. *Journal of the Optical Society of America,* 7(10), 2002–10.

Livingstone, M., Rosen, G.D., Drislane, F., & Galaburda, A. (1991). Physiological and anatomical evidence for a magnocellular deficit in developmental dyslexia. *Proceedings of the National Academy of Sciences of the United States of America*, 88, 7943–7.

Lovegrove, W.J. (1991). Is the question of the role of visual deficits as a cause of reading disabilities a closed one? Comments on Hulme. *Cognitive Neuropsychology*, 8, 435–41.

Lovegrove, W.J., Garzia, R.P., & Nicholson, S.B. (1990). Experimental evidence of a transient system deficit in specific reading disability. *Journal of the American Optometric Association*, 61, 137–46.

Lovegrove, W.J. Martin, F., & Slaghuis, W.L. (1986). A theoretical and experiental case for a visual deficit in specific reading disability. *Cognitive Neuropsychology*, 3, 225–7.

Maclachan, A., Yale, S., & Wilkins, A.J. (1993). Open trials of precision ophthalmic tinting: 1-year follow-up of 55 patients. *Ophthalmic and Physiological Optics*, 13, 175–8.

McKay, D.M. (1957). Moving visual images produced by regular stationary patterns. *Nature*, 180. 849–50.

McKay, D.M., Gerrits, H.J.M., & Stassen, H.P.W. (1979). Interaction of stabilized retinal patterns with visual noise. *Vision Research*, 19, 713–16.

Meares, O. (1980). Figure/ground brightness contrast and reading disabilities. *Visible Language*, 14, 13–29.

Merigan, W.H., & Maunsell, J.H. (1993). How parallel are the primate visual pathways? *Annual Review of Neuroscience,* 16, 369–402.

Miles, T.R. (1991). On determining the prevalence of dyslexia. In: M. Snowling & M. Thomson (Eds.) *Dyslexia: Integrating theory and practice*, pp. 144–153. London: Whurr.

Miles, T.R., & Miles, E. (1999). *Dyslexia: A hundred years on.* (2nd edn.). Buckingham: Open University Press.

Mollon, J., Pokorny, J., & Knoblauch, K. (2003). *Normal and defective colour vision*. Oxford: Oxford University Press.

Nahar, N.K., Sheedy, J.E., Hayes, J., & Tai, Y-C. (2007). Objective measurement of lower-level visual stress. *Optometry and Vision Science*, 84, 620–9.

Northway, N. (2003). Predicting the continued use of overlays in school children—a comparison of the Developmental Eye Movement test and the Rate of Reading test. *Ophthalmic and Physiological Optics*, 23, 457–64.

Parke, L.A., & Skottun, B.C. (1999). The possible relationship between visual deficits and dyslexia: Examination of a critical assumption. *Journal of Learning Disabilities*, 32, 2–5.

Pennington, B.F., & Olson, R. K. (2005). Genetics of dyslexia. In: M. Snowling & C. Hulme (Eds.) *The Science of Reading*: A Handbook, pp. 453–472. Oxford: Blackwell.

Quirk, J.A., Fish, D.R., & Smith, S.J. (1995). First seizures associated with playing electronic screen games: a community-based study in Great Britain. *Annals of Neurology*, 37, 733–7.

Ramus, F. (2001). Outstanding questions about phonological processing in dyslexia. *Dyslexia*, 7, 197–216.

Ramus, F. (2004). Neurobiology of dyslexia: a reinterpretation of the data. *Tends in Neurosciences*, 27, 720–6.

Ramus, F., Rosen, S., Dakin, S.C., Day, B.L., Castellote, J.M., White, S., *et al.* (2003). Theories of developmental dyslexia: Insights from a multiple case study of dyslexic adults. *Brain*, 126, 1–25.

Ray, N.J., Fowler, S., & Stein, J.F. (2005). Yellow filters can improve magnocellular function: Motion sensitivity, convergence, accommodation, and reading. *Annals of the New York Academy of Science*, 1039, 283–93.

Raymond, J.E., & Sorensen, R. (1998). Visual motion perception in children with dyslexia: normal detection but abnormal integration. *Visual Cognition*, 5, 389–404.

Rayner, K. (1998). Eye movements in reading and information processing: 20 years of research. *Psychological Bulletin*, 124, 372–422.

Reid, A.A., Szczerbinski, M., Iskierka-Kasperek, E., & Hansen, P. (2006). Cognitive profiles of adult developmental dyslexics: Theoretical implications. *Dyslexia*, 13, 1–24.

Riddell, P.M., Wilkins, A.J., & Hainline, L. (2006). The effect of colored lens on the visual evoked response in children with visual stress. *Optometry and Vision Science*, 83, 299–305.

Robinson, G.L., & Conway, R.N.F. (2000). Irlen lenses and adults: a small-scale study of reading speed, accuracy comprehension and self-image. *Australian Journal of Learning Disabilities*, 5, 4–12.

Robinson, G.L., & Foreman, P.J. (1999). Scotopic sensitivity/Irlen Syndrome and the use of coloured filters: a long-term placebo-controlled and masked study of reading achievement and perception of ability. *Perceptual and Motor Skills*, 88, 35–52.

Roorda, A., & Williams, D.R. (1999). The arrangement of the three cone classes in the living human eye. *Nature*, 397, 520–2.

Ross, J., Burr, D., & Morrone, C. (1996). Suppression of the magnocellular pathways during saccades. *Behavioural Brain Research*, 80, 1–8.

Schulte-Körne, G., & Bruder, J. (2010). Clinical neurophysiology of visual and auditory processing in dyslexia. *Clinical Neurophysiology*, 121, 1794–809.

Scott, L., McWhinnie, H., Taylor, L., Stevenson, N., Irons, I., Lewis, E., *et al.* (2002). Coloured overlays in schools: orthoptic and optometric findings. *Ophthalmic and Physiological Optics*, 22, 156–65.

Shaywitz, S.E., & Shaywitz, B.A. (2001). The neurobiology of reading and dyslexia. *Focus on Basics*, pp. 11–15. NCSALL. Available at http://ncsall.gse.harvard.edu.

Shaywitz, S.E., Shaywitz, B.A., Fletcher, J.M., & Escobar, M.D. (1990). Prevalence of reading disability in boys and girls. *Journal of the American Medical Association*, 264, 998–1002.

Sheedy, J.E., Hayes, J., & Engle, J. (2003). Is all asthenopia the same? *Optometry and Vision Science*, 80, 732–9.

Shovman, M.M., & Ahissar, M. (2006). Isolating the impact of visual perception on dyslexics' reading ability. *Vision Research*, 46, 3514–25.

Simmers, A.J., & Bex, P.J. (2001). Deficit of visual contour integration in dyslexia. *Investigative Ophthalmology and Visual Science*, 42, 2737–42.

Singleton, C.H. (2008). Visual factors in reading. *Educational and Child Psychology*, 25, 8–20.

Singleton, C.H. (2009a). *Intervention for Dyslexia: A review of published evidence on the impact of specialist dyslexia teaching*. Bracknell, Berks: The Dyslexia-SpLD Trust.

Singleton, C.H. (2009b). Visual stress and dyslexia. In G. Reid (Ed.) *The Routledge Companion to Dyslexia*, pp. 43–57. London: Routledge.

Singleton, C.H., & Henderson, L.M. (2007a). Computerised screening for visual stress in reading. *Journal of Research in Reading*, 30, 316–31.

Singleton, C.H., & Henderson, L.M. (2007b). Computerised screening for visual stress in children with dyslexia. *Dyslexia*, 13, 130–51.

Singleton, C.H., & Henderson, L.M. (2007c). *Lucid Visual Stress Screener (ViSS)*. Beverley, East Yorkshire: Lucid Research Ltd.

Singleton, C.H., & Trotter, S. (2005). Visual stress in adults with and without dyslexia. *Journal of Research in Reading*, 28, 365–78.

Skottun, B.C. (2000). On the conflicting support for the magnocellular-deficit theory of dyslexia. *Trends in Cognitive Science*, 4, 211–12.

Skottun, B.C. (2005). Magnocellular reading and dyslexia. *Vision Research*, 45, 133–4.

Skottun, B. C., & Skoyles, J.R. (2004). Some remarks on the use of motion VEPs to assess magnocellular sensitivity. *Clinical Neurophysiology*, 115, 2834–6.

Skottun, B.C., & Skoyles, J.R. (2006). Is coherent motion an appropriate test for magnocellular sensitivity? *Brain & Cognition*, 61, 172–80.

Skottun, B.C., & Skoyles, J.R. (2008). Coherent motion, magnocellular sensitivity and the causation of dyslexia. *International Journal of Neuroscience*, 118, 185–90.

Skoyles, J., & Skottun, B.C. (2004). On the prevalence of magnocellular defcits in the visual system of non-dyslexic individuals. *Brain and Language*, 88, 79–82.

Smith, L., & Wilkins, A. (2007). How many colours are necessary to increase the reading of children with visual stress? A comparison of two systems. *Journal of Research in Reading*, 30, 332–43.

Snowling, M.J. (2000). *Dyslexia* (2nd edn.). Oxford: Blackwell.

Stanovich, K. E. (1986). Matthew effects in reading: Some consequences of individual differences in the acquisition of reading. *Reading Research Quarterly*, 21, 360–407.

Stein, J.F. (2001). The magnocellular theory of dyslexia. *Dyslexia*, 7, 12–36.

Stein, J.F. (2003). Visual motion sensitivity and reading. *Neuropsychologia*, 41, 1785–93.

Stein, J.F. (2007). *Blue or yellow filters can improve reading in dyslexic children*. Submission to the Enterprise and Learning Committee of the Welsh Assembly, Document EL(3) 09–07 (p. 4).

Stein, J.F., & Fowler, M.S. (1985). Effect of monocular occlusion on reading in dyslexic children. *Lancet*, 13 July, 69–73.

Stein, J.F., & Fowler, M.S. (1993). Unstable binocular control in children with specific reading retardation. *Journal of Research in Reading*, 16, 30–45.

Stein, J.F., & Talcottt, J. (1999). Impaired neuronal timing in developmental dyslexia—the magnocellular hypothesis. *Dyslexia*, 5, 59–77.

Stein, J.F., & Walsh, V. (1997). To see but not to read: the magnocellular theory of dyslexia. *Trends in Neuroscience*, 20, 147–52.

Stein, J.F., Talcottt, J., & Walsh, V. (2000). Controversy about the visual magnocellular deficit in developmental dyslexics. *Trends in Cognitive Science*, 4, 209–11.

Steinman, B., Steinman, S., & Lehmkuhle, S. (1997). Transient visual attention is dominated by the magnocellular stream. *Vision Research*, 37, 17–23.

Talcott, J.B., Hansen, P.C., Willis-Owen, C., McKinnell, I.W., Richardson, A.J., & Stein, J.F. (1998). Visual magnocellular impairment in adult developmental dyslexics. *Neuro-Ophthalmology*, 20, 187–201.

Thomson, M.E. (2009). *The psychology of dyslexia* (2nd edn.). Oxford: Wiley-Blackwell.

Turner, M. (1997). *Psychological Assessment of Dyslexia*. London: Whurr.

Tyrrell, R., Holland, K., Dennis, D., & Wilkins, A.J. (1995). Coloured overlays, visual discomfort, visual search and classroom reading. *Journal of Research in Reading*, 18(1), 10–23.

Valdois, S., Boss, M-L., & Taintuurier, M.-J. (2004). The cognitive deficits responsible for developmental dyslexia: Review of evidence for selection visual attentional disorder. *Dyslexia*, 10, 339–63.

Vellutino, F.R. (1979). *Dyslexia: Theory and Research*. Cambridge, MA: MIT Press.

Vellutino, F.R., & Fletcher, J.M. (2005). Developmental dyslexia. In M.J. Snowling & C. Hulme (Eds.) *The Science of Reading: A Handbook*, pp. 521–537. Oxford: Blackwell.

Vellutino, F.R., Fletcher, J.M., Snowling, M.J., & Scanlon, D.M. (2004). Specific reading disability (dyslexia): what have we learned in the past four decades? *Journal of Child Psychology and Psychiatry*, 45, 2–40.

Vidyasagar, T.R. (1998). Gating of neuronal responses in macaque primary visual cortex by an attentional spotlight. *NeuroReport*, 9, 1947–52.

Vidyasagar, T.R., & Pammer, K. (1999). Impaired visual search in dyslexia relates to the role of the magnocellular pathway in attention. *NeuroReport*, 10, 1283–7.

Welch, K.M.A., Bowyer, S.M., Aurora, S.K., Moran, J.E., & Tepley, N. (2001). Visual stress-induced migraine aura compared to spontaneous aura studied by magnetoencephalography. *Journal of Headache and Pain*, 2, S131–S136.

White, S., Milne, E., Rosen, S., Hansen, P., Swettenham, J., Frith, U., & Ramus, F. (2006). The role of sensorimotor impairments in dyslexia: a multiple case study of dyslexic children, *Developmental Science*, 9(3), 237–69.

Whiteley, H.E., & Smith, C.D. (2001). The use of tinted lenses to alleviate reading difficulties. *Journal of Research in Reading*, 24, 30–40.

Wilkins, A.J. (1995). *Visual Stress*. Oxford: Oxford University Press.

Wilkins, A.J. (2002). Coloured overlays and their effects on reading speed: a review. *Ophthalmic and Physiological Optics*, 22, 448–54.

Wilkins, A.J. (2003). *Reading Through Colour*. Chichester: Wiley.

Wilkins, A.J., & Nimmo-Smith, M.I. (1987). The clarity and comfort of printed text. *Ergonomics*, 3012, 1705–20.

Wilkins, A.J., Nimmo-Smith, I., & Jansons, J. (1992). A colorimeter for the intuitive manipulation of hue and saturation, and its application in the study of perceptual distortion. *Ophthalmic and Physiological Optics*, 12, 381–5.

Wilkins, A.J., Evans, B.J.W., Brown, J., Busby, A., Winfield, A.E., Jeanes, R., *et al.* (1994). Double masked placebo controlled trials of precision spectral filters in children who use coloured overlays. *Ophthalmic and Physiological Optics*, 14, 365–70.

Wilkins, A.J., Jeanes, R. J., Pumfrey, P.D., & Laskier, M. (1996). Rate of Reading Test: its reliability and its validity in the assessment of the effects of coloured overlays. *Ophthalmic and Physiological Optics*, 16, 491–7.

Wilkins, A.J., & Lewis, E. (1999). Coloured overlays, text and texture. *Perception*, 28, 641–50.

Wilkins, A.J., Lewis, E., Smith, F., Rowland, E., & Tweedie, W. (2001). Coloured overlays and their benefit for reading. *Journal of Research in Reading*, 24, 41–64.

Wilkins, A.J., Patel, R., Adjamian, R., & Evans, B.J.W. (2002). Tinted spectacles and visually sensitive migraine. *Cephalagia*, 22, 711–19.

Wilkins, A.J., Huang, J., & Cao, Y. (2004a). Visual stress theory and its application to reading and reading tests. *Journal of Research in Reading*, 27, 152–62.

Wilkins, A.J., Bonanni, P., Porciatti, V., & Guerrini, R. (2004b). Physiology of human photosensitivity. *Epilepsia*, 45(Supplement 1), 1–7.

Wilkins, A.J., Sihra, N., & Myers, A. (2005). Increasing reading speed by using colours: Issues concerning reliability and specificity, and their theoretical and practical implications. *Perception*, 34, 109–20.

Wilkins, A.J., Smith, J., Willison, C.K., Beare, T., Boyd, A., Hardy, G., *et al.* (2007). Stripes within words affect reading. *Perception*, 36, 1788–803.

Wilkins, A.J., Cleave, R., Grayson, N., & Wilson, L. (2009). Typography for children may be inappropriately designed. *Journal of Research in Reading*, 32, 402–11.

Winterbottom, M., & Wilkins, A.J. (2009). Lighting and discomfort in the classroom. *Journal of Environmental Psychology*, 29, 63–75.

Chapter 7

The Visual Nature of the Visual Attention Span Disorder in Developmental Dyslexia

Sylviane Valdois, Delphine Lassus-Sangosse, and Muriel Lobier

Introduction

Since the first reports of cases of developmental dyslexia at the beginning of the last century, the challenge has been to understand why some children with otherwise normal intellectual ability and appropriate environmental opportunities fail to learn to read. Because learning to read in an alphabetic system involves learning the relationships between sequences of visual symbols (i.e. relevant orthographic units such as graphemes, syllables, whole words) and the corresponding units of sounds (i.e. relevant phonological units such as phonemes, syllables, or whole words), problems in either visual or phonological processing, or in the matching of visual and phonological information might result in reading acquisition difficulties. Many studies have now shown that dyslexic individuals exhibit a visual (cf. the magnocellular theory; Stein & Walsh, 1997) or a visual attentional (e.g. sluggish attentional shifting; Hari & Renvall, 2001) disorder. However, the phonological theory of developmental dyslexia (DD) remains predominant because visual (attentional) problems are typically described in dyslexic individuals who also exhibit a phonological problem. Hence the phonological difficulties can be cited as the most probable proximal cause of their reading disorder (Ramus et al., 2003). Even the recent and rather provocative view that phonological problems might themselves follow from visual (attentional) problems (Vidyasagar & Pammer, 2010) acknowledges that phonological and visual disorders typically co-occur in developmental dyslexia.

The visual attention (VA) span theory alone differs from previous accounts in postulating that a VA span disorder can dissociate from phonological problems in developmental dyslexia and directly impact reading acquisition. The VA span theory of DD thus relates directly to the idea that there are different dyslexic subtypes characterized by different neurobiological and cognitive disorders (Peyrin et al., 2011). Another strength of the VA span deficit hypothesis is that the impact of a VA span disorder on reading acquisition can easily be explained within the framework of the multitrace memory model of reading we proposed in 1998 (Ans et al., 1998; Valdois et al., 2004).

In this chapter, we will first present the multitrace memory model of reading (hereafter, the MTM model) in order to understand the importance of the VA span and the role of visual attention in reading. We will then describe the letter report paradigms we use to assess VA span abilities and we will review evidence for a VA span disorder in DD. Because the report tasks involve letter-string processing and oral report of letter names, some authors (Ziegler et al., 2010) have questioned the 'visual' nature of the deficit, thus putting phonology back in the front row. We will review evidence for the visual nature of the VA span disorder in developmental dyslexia that argue strongly against any interpretation of this very specific parallel processing disorder in phonological terms.

The MTM reading model

The MTM model of polysyllabic word reading was the first theoretical model to incorporate a visual attentional process as part of the reading system (Ans et al., 1998). The model postulates that, in addition to the phonological component, a visual attentional component—called the visual attentional window—plays a crucial role in skilled reading and reading acquisition. The size of this window determines the amount of orthographic information that is extracted from the input letter string during reading and becomes available for processing.

The model, outlined in Fig. 7.1, postulates that reading relies on two types of reading procedures (global and analytic), that differ in the kind of visual attention and phonological processing they involve.

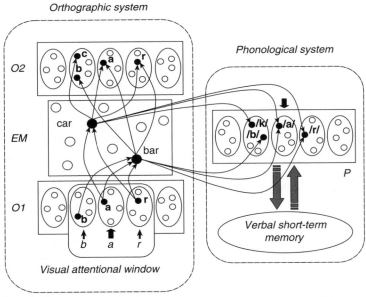

Fig. 7.1 Schematic representation of the multitrace memory model of polysyllabic word reading. The input word to be read is 'bar'. The figure depicts competition between 'bar' and 'car' (bus). *O1, O2* = input and output orthographic layers; *EM* = episodic memory; *P* = phonological output layer. The VAW encompasses the whole sequence of the input word.

In particular the two reading procedures differ in the size of the visual attentional window through which information from the orthographic input is extracted. In global reading mode, the visual attentional window extends over the whole sequence of the input letter string whereas it narrows down to focus attention successively on the different parts of the input when reading in analytic mode. In expert reading, familiar word processing is done in global mode, thus requiring the visual attentional window to be large enough to adapt to the input-word length. When the input sequence is an unknown word or pseudoword, processing is initiated in global mode as previously; but it typically fails and the system shifts into analytic mode. The visual attentional window then narrows down to focus in turn on the relevant sublexical units (graphemes or syllables) of the input letter string. Familiar word processing thus typically involves larger visual attentional windows than pseudoword processing.

Implementation of this theoretical model as a connectionist network showed that a reduction in the size of the visual attentional window primarily impacted familiar word processing. Irregular word reading was more specifically affected, and resulted in regularization errors. Regular words could be accurately read through a reduced attentional window, but reading speed was slowed down. A greater reduction of the visual attentional window size further affected regular word and pseudoword reading accuracy. A severely reduced attentional window does not allow simultaneous processing of all the letters of complex graphemes, resulting in poor analytic processing. The model thus predicts that a visual attentional window reduction would interfere with reading performance and potentially disturb the processing of any kind of item.

The MTM model remains novel. Even though a visual attention component has recently been added to dual route models, this only applies to the sublexical route of reading; so any disorder of visual attention in DD would be restricted to this procedure and only impact pseudoword reading performance (Perry et al., 2007). However, the MTM model postulates the existence of another kind of visual attentional process which contributes to both lexical (global) and sublexical (analytic) reading procedures for parallel processing of the letters that make up relevant orthographic units (the whole word in global mode; the syllables or graphemes in analytic mode). The model further includes a shifting mechanism specific to the analytic procedure for the sequential processing of sublexical orthographic units within unfamiliar strings. This later mechanism is similar to the mechanism of serial graphemic parsing postulated by the connectionist dual process plus (CDP+) model (Perry et al., 2007). The postulate of a shifting mechanism under the control of spatial attention within the analytic procedure is in accordance with behavioural data showing that those dyslexic individuals who suffer from sluggish attentional shifting further show poor pseudoword reading (Facoetti et al., 2006). Evidence for the independence of this attentional shifting mechanism from the VA span has been recently provided through a single case study of a young adult with phonological dyslexia who exhibited sluggish attentional shifting in the visual (and auditory) modality but preserved VA span (Lallier et al., 2010).

The MTM model further predicts that in DD the phonological and visual attentional components can be independently disturbed. Thus we showed that 'damage' at the phonological level of the skilled network had no impact on visual attentional processing. Conversely, a reduction of the visual attentional window did not affect the efficiency of phonological processing. It was thus inferred (Ans et al., 1998; Valdois et al., 2004) that a visual attentional deficit should result in a subtype of developmental dyslexia characterized by impaired processing of the input letter string but preserved phonological abilities. The VA span concept was proposed as a psychological counterpart of the visual attentional window.

Assessment of the visual attention span

The term 'visual attention span' refers to the number of distinct elements which can be processed simultaneously in a visual display (Bosse et al., 2007). In reading, the VA span corresponds to the number of orthographic units which can be simultaneously processed in a letter string. It is worth noting here that a VA span disorder in DD thus refers to a parallel processing disorder (Lassus-Sangosse et al., 2008). Accordingly, a VA span dysfunction in DD can only be assessed through tasks of multielement processing in which processing time is constrained to prevent eye movements and multiple extraction of orthographic information during processing.

At the behavioural level, the VA span is estimated using letter report tasks—flashing five-consonant strings (e.g. R H S D M) for 200 ms at the centre of the screen. Participants are asked to report either the whole letter string (global report condition; identity not location) or a single cued letter (partial report). The displayed strings are not random consonant strings formatted as in text; the strings do not include couples of letters that correspond to complex graphemes (e.g. PH) so that each single letter has to be processed as an independent orthographic unit. The five-consonant strings never match the skeleton of a real word (e.g. FLMBR for FLAMBER 'burn') in order to restrict performance to early visual analysis and avoid top-down influences. The centre-to-centre distance between adjacent letters is increased. As we know that dyslexic children show stronger crowding effects (Pernet et al., 2006; Martelli et al., 2009), increasing the distance between letters allows assessing VA span abilities while minimizing the potential influence of crowding. Up to now, VA span abilities have been mainly estimated through performance on multiletter string processing. Similar findings are nevertheless expected using other types of stimuli (such as digits or non-alphanumeric items) or other types of configurations. It is noteworthy here that a VA span disorder is not just a letter-string disorder and does not tap the visual attentional mechanisms specific to letter-string processing. On the contrary, the VA span is a general visual attention process specialized for parallel processing which existed before the cultural invention of reading and was adopted for reading as a special type of parallel processing task.

The two global and partial report paradigms have been administered to a large sample of typically developing children from the 1st to the 5th grade (Bosse & Valdois, 2009). Results show that the response pattern in global report is characterized by a slight left-to-right gradient (see Fig. 7.2). Letters are better named in the left than in the right visual field. This left-to-right gradient is not found in partial report; here performance does not

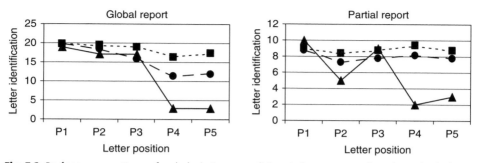

Fig. 7.2 Performance pattern of a dyslexic teenager (triangles) as compared to chronological age (squares) and reading age (circles) matched controls in the global and partial report tasks.

show any positional effect, but a similarly high performance whatever the position of the cued letter to be named. These findings suggest that the global report task is sensitive to the direction of reading, but not the partial report condition in which a letter position is randomly chosen as target at each new trial. Even if the global and partial report paradigms differ in some other way, the number of letters accurately named strongly correlates in global and partial report, so that VA span abilities are typically estimated from mean performance on both tasks. We estimated that 3.1 letters on average were simultaneously processed in first grade, against 4 in the third and 4.3 in the fifth grade.

The two report tasks are typically administered together with a control task estimating the threshold for single letter identification. In this control task, a single letter is presented at the centre of the screen during short presentation times varying from 33–101 ms. Each child's threshold is taken as the shortest presentation time required to accurately identify at least 80% of the target letters. Good performance on this task, but poor performance in letter report within strings, suggests that performance in global and partial report does not just reflect difficulties in single-letter processing but taps the visual attentional mechanisms involved in multielement simultaneous processing.

Evidence for a visual attention span disorder in developmental dyslexia

First evidence for a VA span disorder in DD was provided through the case study of a French teenager, Nicolas, who showed a pattern of surface dyslexia/dysgraphia (Valdois et al., 2003). A phonological cause of his poor reading seemed unlikely given that Nicolas performed as well as control children of the same chronological age on phoneme awareness and phonological decoding. Nicolas was thus administered the global and partial report tasks.

As illustrated in Fig. 7.2, Nicolas performed poorly and showed a very similar atypical pattern of performance in both the global and partial report conditions. He could only name a few letters displayed in position 4 and 5 and further showed poor performance in position 2 (which reached significance in global report when compared to chronological-age matched children). In sum, Nicolas could only identify two letters—the first letter of the string and the letter at the fixation point—at the expected level for his age, thus demonstrating a VA span reduction. Importantly, he performed worse than reading age matched controls on both tasks, showing that his poor performance was not just a consequence of his poor reading level.

Nicolas's report shows that phonological and VA span abilities can dissociate in DD. A case study of phonological dyslexia (Valdois et al., 2003) further showed that the reverse pattern could be found in a dyslexic participant with otherwise a very similar background, demonstrating double dissociation. However, case studies do not tell us how common VA span disorders are in the dyslexic population; they could be very rare. Large sample studies were later conducted to confirm the independence of phonological and VA span disorders in DD.

Bosse and colleagues (2007) investigated phonological and VA span abilities in two populations of French and British dyslexic participants of around 11 years of age. As a group, the dyslexic participants showed poor phoneme awareness and lower performance than the controls in both the global and partial report VA span tasks. They further exhibited a severe reading acquisition delay and poor reading performance on all types of item (regular, irregular, or pseudowords). Although the dyslexic group was characterized by a double deficit, the analysis revealed the existence of four dyslexic subgroups with different cognitive disorders: a phonological-deficit group, a VA-span-deficit group, a double-deficit group, and a 'no-deficit' group. Independence between the phonological and VA span disorders was found in the majority of dyslexic individuals (more than 60%). Moreover a high proportion of dyslexic individuals in both the French and British samples exhibited a VA span disorder (isolated or not), thus showing that this disorder is not at all rare in the dyslexic population. The number of dyslexic children with a VA span disorder was at least as high as the number with a phonological disorder. In accordance with the MTM model, these findings suggest that phonological and VA span disorders are separable sources of reading dysfunction. Such a conclusion, however, requires demonstrating that the global and partial letter report tasks do measure visual attention abilities, and that poor performance on these tasks cannot be attributed to some phonological disorder not involved in the phoneme awareness tasks typically used to address phonological skills in our dyslexic participants.

Evidence against a phonological account of the VA span disorder

The VA span tasks obviously induce verbal coding of the string letter names to be orally reported at the offset of the display. Moreover, five letters have to be named in global report, thus further taxing verbal short-term memory which is known to be deficient in DD. Moreover, no deficit was found in dyslexic individuals when they were given multi-element string processing tasks that avoided name coding (Hawelka & Wimmer, 2008) or used non-alphanumeric material (Ziegler et al., 2010) which contrasted with their poor performance when processing letter or digit strings. As a consequence, lower performance in the report tasks might be viewed as reflecting a problem with verbal material and verbal short-term memory rather than a purely visual attention dysfunction.

However, a phonological cause for the poor performance of dyslexic readers in letter report is unlikely. First, performance in global and partial reports typically correlate in dyslexic individuals showing that the two tasks share common processes. Given that a single letter has to be orally named in partial report against five in global report, it is unlikely that verbal short-term memory or a name coding problem is a major factor in the former condition. In any case, the memory load is higher in global report so that performance should be drastically lower on this task if primarily reflecting a verbal short-term memory dysfunction, which is not found.

Second, a verbal coding or verbal short-term memory interpretation does not fit well with the results of Lassus-Sangosse et al. (2008). These authors compared the performance of dyslexic readers in two conditions in which the participants were asked to report the names of five consonants which were either simultaneously presented in strings (global condition) or sequentially displayed (sequential condition). The two tasks were designed to require similar rapid letter naming and verbal short-term memory skill. As a consequence, the two tasks should have resulted in similarly poor performance if a verbal coding or verbal short-term memory disorder was responsible for the poor performance of dyslexic readers. Against this expectation, the dyslexic participants performed as well as the control participants in the sequential condition while exhibiting poor performance when the five consonants were simultaneously displayed. So it is clear from these results that dyslexic individuals suffered from a specific parallel processing disorder but were not sensitive to the task memory load.

Still against a phonological interpretation, Dixon and Shedden (1993) showed that partial report was only minimally affected by articulatory suppression. To assess how articulatory suppression affected performance in global report, dyslexic participants were administered two backward-masked global report tasks, one of which was carried out with concurrent articulation (Valdois et al., 2012). Concurrent articulation was expected to prevent online verbal encoding during processing, so that the performance of dyslexic children in global report was expected to improve and become more similar to that of the controls if their poor performance followed from a verbal encoding disorder. As shown on Fig. 7.3, dyslexic children performed worse than control children not only in the classic paradigm but also in the condition with concurrent articulation. Performance was worse in the global report task with concurrent articulation in both groups but no significant group by task interaction was found showing that performance in the condition with concurrent articulation decreased similarly in the dyslexic and skilled reader participants. These results show that the task is more difficult in the condition with concurrent articulation confirming that verbal encoding is used during processing and helps in performing the task.

However, dyslexic children suffered from articulatory suppression as normal readers do, suggesting they similarly used verbal rehearsal to perform the task. More importantly, however, their deficit remained apparent in both conditions and of similar magnitude whether concurrent articulation was present or not, showing that the disorder we were measuring was not affected by concurrent articulation. Accordingly, the current findings do not support any interpretation of the poor performance of dyslexic readers in global

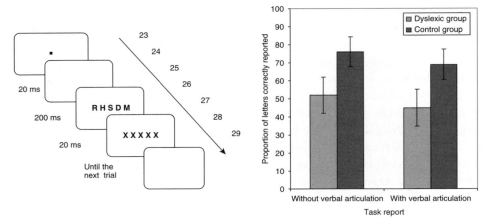

Fig. 7.3 Schematic representation of the global backward-masked report with concurrent articulation paradigm (left panel) and performance of dyslexic and control children in the two conditions of report with and without concurrent articulation (right panel).

report in terms of online verbal coding difficulty. It is further noteworthy that since verbal coding difficulties are primarily expected in the context of phonological problems (Vellutino et al., 2004), poor VA span abilities would then typically co-occur with phonological disorders in developmental dyslexia. Against this expectation, performance in global report is typically preserved in those dyslexic individuals with associated phonological problems (Valdois et al., 2003; Bosse et al., 2007; Lallier et al., 2010) but impaired in the children without phonological impairments (Lassus-Sangosse et al., 2008).

In summary, any phonological interpretation of the VA span disorder in developmental dyslexia is unlikely to be due to a phonological deficit, because the poor performance of dyslexic children in the letter report tasks cannot be attributed to a verbal encoding problem or a verbal short-term memory disorder. A phonological interpretation of this disorder is all the more unlikely since performance on the report tasks was found to correlate with eye movements in text reading but was unaffected by differences in phoneme awareness (Prado et al., 2007). Poor performance in letter report can no longer be viewed as just a consequence of poor reading experience. Indeed, dyslexic children with a similarly poor reading level can show quite contrasting (very poor or unimpaired) performance in the report tasks and younger but typically developing children of the same reading level show higher performance than dyslexic children on these tasks (Bosse & Valdois, 2003). Moreover, lack of reading experience might cause difficulties with letter-string processing but should not affect digit-string processing, whereas the evidence suggests similar difficulties in processing either kind of item (Hawelka & Wimmer, 2005; Ziegler et al., 2010).

It remains crucial, however, to demonstrate that a VA span disorder affects non-verbal as well as verbal material. A deficit restricted to alphanumeric material with no impact on non-verbal string processing could be interpreted as resulting only from deficient mapping between visual and phonological codes, in accordance with a phonological account of the disorder (Ziegler et al., 2010). In contrast, a general visual attention disorder affecting parallel processing would similarly impact on verbal and non-verbal material.

We addressed this issue in two experiments in which dyslexic and control children were asked to process strings of nameable (colour patches) or unnameable (pseudoletters and unfamiliar shapes) material in addition to alphanumeric strings (Lobier et al., 2011; Valdois et al., 2012). Results of the first experiment conducted with letters, digits, and colour patches, mainly replicated Ziegler et al.'s (2010) findings in showing impaired performance for letters and digits, but preserved performance for non-alphabetic material in a global and partial report paradigm. Interestingly enough, however, these findings are totally at odds with any interpretation of the disorder as a visual to phonology mapping problem since the colour report tasks do require the mapping of visual patches to phonological codes (colour names), exactly like letter- and digit-string processing. However, as for symbols, performance of skilled readers was very poor in colour-string processing with good identification of the item at the fixation point but rapid decay of performance with eccentricity, suggesting that colour report did not rely on parallel processing.

In a second experiment (Lobier et al., 2011), we used a multielement categorization task which required visual attention to spread over all the elements of the string to report the number of elements belonging to a target category. Target categories were either alphanumeric (letters and digits) or non-alphanumeric (unnameable characters). Dyslexic children showed similarly poor performance in the alphanumeric and non-alphanumeric condition, thus showing that their VA span disorder extended to non-verbal stimuli as well. Still in agreement with a purely visual attention disorder, we recently reported on a dyslexic child with very severe mixed dyslexia but an isolated VA span disorder. He also showed poor performance when engaged in a sequential reaching movement task which involved parallel processing of the targets to be reached (Valdois et al., 2011). Thus, far from being restricted only to alphanumeric string processing, the VA span disorder seems to affect all the situations that require multielement parallel processing.

Conclusion

Our letter report tasks were designed to assess VA span abilities and tap those visual attention mechanisms more specifically involved in parallel processing. Although the report tasks rely on various processing mechanisms including phonological ones, poor performance of dyslexic children is not sensitive to the task memory load and remains unchanged in conditions of articulatory suppression. More crucially, the disorder extends to the processing of unfamiliar unnameable items in strings, against any interpretation as a visual to phonology mapping disorder. Lastly, some data suggests the problem might spread to other conditions very different from reading but which also rely on parallel processing, as in the sequential reaching of multiple targets. Converging evidence thus suggests that in DD poor performance on these tasks does reflect a purely visual attention disorder which affects multielement parallel processing. Given the key role of parallel processing in reading, such a disorder has a strong impact on reading acquisition while not affecting phonological skills much. Although further research is required to establish that the relationship between VA span disorder and DD is causal, our findings suggest that VA span deficiencies play a key role in DD. It follows that in addition to phonological abilities, VA span tasks should be included in the clinical assessment of DD.

References

Ans, B., Carbonnel, S., & Valdois, S. (1998). A connectionist multiple-trace memory model for polysyllabic word reading. *Psychological Review*, 105, 678–723.

Bosse, M.-L., & Valdois, S. (2003). Patterns of developmental dyslexia according to a multi-trace memory model of reading. *Current Psychology Letters* (Special Issue on Language Disorders and Reading Acquisition), 10(1).

Bosse, M.-L., & Valdois, S. (2009). Influence of the visual attention span on child reading performance: a cross-sectional study. *Journal of Research in Reading*, 32, 230–53.

Bosse, M.-L., Tainturier, M.-J., & Valdois, S. (2007). Developmental dyslexia: the Visual Attention Span hypothesis. *Cognition*, 104, 198–230.

Dixon, P., & Shedden, J.M. (1993). On the nature of the span of apprehension. *Psychological Research*, 55, 29–39.

Facoetti, A., Zorzi, M., Cestnick, L., Lorusso, M.L., Molteni, M., Paganoni, P., *et al.* (2006). The relationship between visuo-spatial attention and nonword reading in developmental dyslexia. *Cognitive Neuropsychology*, 23, 841–55.

Hari, R., & Renvall, H. (2001). Impaired processing of rapid stimulus sequences in dyslexia. *Trends in Cognitive Sciences*, 5, 525–32.

Hawelka, S., & Wimmer, H. (2005). Impaired visual processing of multi-element arrays is associated with increased number of eye movements in dyslexic reading. *Vision Research*, 45, 855–63.

Hawelka, S., & Wimmer, H. (2008). Visual target detection is not impaired in dyslexic readers. *Vision Research*, 48, 850–2.

Lallier, M., Donnadieu, S., Berger, C., & Valdois, S. (2010). A case study of developmental phonological dyslexia: Is the attentional deficit in rapid stimuli sequences processing amodal? *Cortex Cortex*, 46, 231–41.

Lassus-Sangosse, D., N'Guyen-Morel, M.A., & Valdois, S. (2008). Sequential or simultaneous visual processing deficit in developmental dyslexia. *Vision Research*, 48, 979–88.

Lobier, M., Lassus-Sangosse, D., Zoubrinetzki, R., & Valdois, S. (in press). The visual attention span disorder in developmental dyslexia is visual not verbal. *Cortex*.

Martelli, M.L., Di Filippo, G., Spinelli, D., & Zoccolotti, P. (2009). Crowding, reading and developmental dyslexia. *Journal of Vision*, 9, 1–18.

Pernet, C., Valdois, S., Celsis, P., & Démonet, J.F. (2006). Lateral masking, levels of processing and stimulus category: A comparative study between normal and dyslexic readers. *Neuropsychologia*, 44, 2374–85.

Perry, C., Ziegler, J.C. & Zorzi, M. (2007). Nested incremental modelling in the development of computational theories: The CDP+ model of reading aloud. *Psychological Review*, 114, 273–315.

Peyrin, C., Démonet, J.F., Baciu, M., Le Bas, J.F., & Valdois, S. (2011). Superior parietal lobe dysfunction in a homogeneous group of dyslexic children with a single visual attention span disorder. *Brain & Language*, 118, 128–38.

Prado, C., Dubois, M., & Valdois, S. (2007). The eye movements of dyslexic children during reading and visual search: Impact of the visual attention span. *Vision Research*, 47, 2521–30.

Ramus, F., Rosen, S., Dakin, S.C., Day, B.L., Castellote, J.M., White, S., *et al.* (2003). Theories of developmental dyslexia: Insights from a multiple case study of dyslexic adults. *Brain*, 126, 841–65.

Stein, A., & Walsh, V. (1997). To see but not to read; the magnocellular theory of dyslexia. *Trends in Neurosciences*, 20, 147–52.

Valdois, S., Bosse, M.L., Ans, B., Carbonnel, S., Zorman, M., David, D., *et al.* (2003). Phonological and visual processing deficits can dissociate in developmental dyslexia: Evidence from two case studies. *Reading and Writing*, 16, 541–72.

Valdois, S., Bosse, M.L., & Tainturier, M.J. (2004). Cognitive correlates of developmental dyslexia: Review of evidence for a selective visual attentional deficit. *Dyslexia*, 10, 1–25.

Valdois, S., Bidet-Ildei, C., Prado, C., Lassus-Sangosse, D., Guinet, E., & Orliaguet, J.P. (2011). A visual processing but no phonological disorder in a child with mixed dyslexia. *Cortex*, 47, 1197–218.

Valdois, S., Lassus-Sangosse, D., & Lobier, M. (2012). Impaired letter-string processing in developmental dyslexia: what visual-to-phonological code mapping disorder? *Dyslexia*, Epub 21 March.

Vellutino, F.R., Fletcher, J.M., Snowling, M.J., & Scanlon, D.M. (2004). Specific reading disability (dyslexia): What have we learned in the past four decades? *Journal of Child Psychology and Psychiatry*, 45, 2–40.

Vidyasagar, T.R., & Pammer, K. (2010). Dyslexia: a deficit in visuo-spatial attention not in phonological processing. *Trends in Cognitive Sciences*, 14, 57–63.

Ziegler, J.C., Pech-Georgel, C., Dufau, S. & Grainger, J. (2010). Rapid processing of letters, digits and symbols: what purely visual attention deficit in developmental dyslexia? *Developmental Science*, 13, F8–F14.

Chapter 8

Spatial Attention Disorders in Developmental Dyslexia: Towards the Prevention of Reading Acquisition Deficits

Andrea Facoetti

Developmental dyslexia and phonological decoding

Developmental dyslexia (DD) is a neurobiological disorder (see Habib, 2000; Démonet & Reilhac, 2012 in the present book for reviews) characterized by difficulties in reading acquisition despite adequate intelligence, conventional education, and motivation (American Psychiatric Association, 1994). It is widely believed that impaired phonological processing characterizes individuals with DD (see Ramus, 2003; Vellutino et al., 2004; Shaywitz & Shaywitz, 2005; Gabrieli, 2009 for reviews). Thus children and adults with DD display poor phonological awareness, slow lexical retrieval, and poor phonological short-term memory. These phonological deficits interfere with one of the most critical skills for successful reading acquisition, that is, phonological decoding (e.g. Ziegler et al., 2003; Ziegler & Goswami, 2005). Phonological decoding is based on letter-to-sound conversion, allowing children to make the connection between novel letter strings and words that are already stored in their phonological (spoken word) lexicon (Share, 1995). Efficient phonological decoding requires accurate auditory representations at the phoneme level (e.g. Harm & Seidenberg, 1999; Perry et al., 2007). Since Italian letter-to-sound orthography is particularly regular, phonological decoding is crucial for learning to read. Nevertheless, it is also essential for learning to read in more irregular letter-to-sound orthographies, such as English (Share, 1995).

Developmental dyslexia and auditory processing

Many studies have sought to explain impaired phonological skills in terms of lower-level deficits, with special reference to sensory and attentional auditory processing. They indicate that auditory deficits impair speech perception, which, in turn, affects grapheme-to-phoneme mapping and phonological short-term memory (Ramus, 2003). Indeed, developmental deficits that affect speech perception do increase the risk of language and literacy problems. Recent biobehavioural evidence supports the idea that individuals with DD and/or with specific language impairment (SLI) are impaired in their perception of non-linguistic auditory information (see Wright et al., 2000 for a review). In particular, individuals with DD and/or SLI have difficulty with perceiving sequential sounds, in sound-frequency discrimination, and in the detection of target sounds in noise. Children with DD show deficits in speech perception when the stimuli are presented in noise (e.g. Geiger et al., 2008). Speech-in-noise perception deficits persist even when dyslexics' performance is compared to that of much younger children matched for reading level, suggesting that a perceptual noise exclusion deficit could possibly be a core deficit in DD (Ziegler et al., 2009). It is important to note that a similar speech-in-noise perception deficit is also present in younger children with SLI (Ziegler et al., 2005).

Goswami et al. (2002) reported that children with DD are relatively insensitive to the rise times of amplitude envelope onsets in acoustic signals compared to younger normally reading children matched for reading level. The ability to detect this acoustic feature provides a non-speech-specific mechanism for segmenting syllable onsets and rimes: a crucial precursor to the development of phoneme segmentation skills and, consequently, phonological awareness (Goswami et al., 2002).

More recently, matched samples of children with and without DD who were learning three very different spoken and written languages (English, Spanish, and Chinese) were compared in amplitude envelope onset. Despite phonological and orthographic differences, for each language, rise time sensitivity was a significant predictor of phonological awareness, and rise time was the only consistent predictor of reading acquisition (Goswami et al., 2011).

Experimental evidence has provided support for the idea that auditory attention—focusing the spotlight on sound—is crucially important for correctly ordering a sequence of sounds and for sound-frequency discrimination, as well as for the detection of target sounds in noise (see Fritz et al., 2007; Shamma & Micheyl, 2010 for recent reviews). This suggests that fine speech signal segmentation requires rapid orienting of auditory attention. It has been consistently demonstrated that auditory attention is impaired in children with DD (e.g. Asbjørnsen & Bryden, 1998; Renvall & Hari, 2002; Facoetti et al. 2010a; Lallier et al., 2010) as well as in children with SLI (e.g. Stevens et al., 2006). Thus, early difficulties in perceiving auditory sensory cues—caused by a basic attentional dysfunction—could developmentally lead to under-specialization (i.e. reduced neural tuning) of the left perisylvian phonological system. A dysfunction of sensory and attentional auditory temporal sampling controlled by temporo-parietal regions might therefore be the primary basis of the phonological deficits in DD.

Developmental dyslexia and orthographic processing

No evidence, however, definitively supports the role of phonological awareness in determining proficient reading (see Castles & Coltheart, 2004 for a review). Indeed it has been suggested that cause and effect may be the other way round, reading improvement increasing phonological performance. Phonological decoding requires precise mapping from orthographic to phonological representations; recent studies have shown that orthographic–phonological binding is impaired in adults and children with DD (see Blomert, 2011 for a recent review). Disorders of reading acquisition might therefore be associated not only with a weakened neural tuning of the left auditory-perisylvian system for phonological processing (e.g. Pugh et al., 2000), but also with under-specialization of the left visual-orthographic system, that is, the visual word form area (VWFA) in the left occipito-temporal cortex (see McCandliss et al., 2003 for a review). The development of the VWFA reflects a specialization of the object recognition system for letter-string processing (McCandliss et al., 2003). The VWFA seems to be hierarchically organized for visual orthographic processing: the posterior areas (in the occipital lobe) are specifically involved in low-level visual features and letter-shape processing, whereas the anterior areas (in the ventral temporal lobe) are linked to more abstract letter-string processing (McCandliss et al., 2003). Supporting a developmentally-based VWFA dysfunction (see Cohen & Dehaene, 2009 for a recent review), many studies have shown that DD children are impaired in low-level visual and/or attentional processing (e.g. Cornelissen et al., 1995; Hari et al., 2001; Sperling et al., 2005; Hawelka et al., 2006; Bosse et al., 2007; Martelli et al., 2009; Facoetti et al., 2010a).

Developmental dyslexia and visual perceptual processing

Letter strings must be segmented into their constituent graphemes (graphemic parsing) before phonological assembly. Evidence for a string processing deficit in dyslexia was obtained in a recent study in which participants were required to name a single element in digit strings in response to a position probe. The strings were briefly presented and then masked (Hawelka & Wimmer, 2005). For two-digit strings the dyslexics were about as fast as normal readers, requiring only about 20 ms. However, for four- and six-digit strings, dyslexic readers were much slower (for four-digit strings they required 80 ms versus 40 ms for the normal readers). Furthermore, slower recognition of the longer strings was associated with a larger number of fixations during phonological decoding (Hawelka & Wimmer, 2005). 'This general and massive string processing deficit speaks against the hypothesis that the slow reading of the dyslexic participants solely results from a failure to store or to use visual orthographic recognition units for frequently encountered words' (Hawelka et al., 2006, p. 772). Although these findings apply to nameable visual stimuli (see also Bosse et al., 2007), a deficit in the processing of strings of non-nameable symbols in dyslexic children has also been found (Pammer et al., 2004).

Martelli et al. (2009) tested the hypothesis that crowding effects are responsible for the characteristic letter-string processing deficit in DD. They measured contrast thresholds for identifying letters and words as a function of stimulus duration. At a limited time exposure, thresholds were higher in dyslexics than controls for words, but not for letters, confirming a letter-string processing deficit in DD. However, at the long time exposure, word thresholds were comparable in the two groups, suggesting that perceptual noise exclusion could depend on sluggish temporal sampling of letters in a cluttered condition. More importantly, the researchers measured the spacing between target letters and two flankers as a function of eccentricity. With eccentricity, the spacing to avoid crowding scaled in the good readers with 0.62 proportionality but with a greater proportionality (0.95) in the dyslexic children. Recently, we saw that a simple manipulation of letter spacing substantially improved text reading performance on the fly, without any training, in a large unselected sample of Italian and French dyslexic children (Zorzi et al., 2012).

Martelli et al. (2009) concluded that string processing is sluggish in dyslexics because of greater crowding, which limits letter identification in multiletter arrays across the peripheral visual field. Recently, we studied the crowding effect in a letter-string identification task by using progressive demasking (Montani et al., 2010). In this stimulus presentation, the letter string gradually emerges from the mask. Stimuli were familiar words or pronounceable non-words, and the spacing between the letters was manipulated. Our results showed that decreasing distance between letters impaired non-word more than word identification, implying a top-down modulation of the crowding effect. Since sublexical identification and phonological decoding are crucial for reading development, an increased degree of crowding could be an important factor underlying the reading difficulties typically displayed in dyslexic children.

Sperling et al. (2005) evaluated signal-to-noise discrimination in children with and without DD, using visual stimuli presented either with or without visual noise. Children with DD had elevated contrast thresholds when visual stimuli were presented in noise, but performed as well as normally reading children when the visual stimuli were displayed without noise. These findings confirm that deficits in perceptual noise exclusion might contribute to the weak neural tuning of the VWFA in DD. However, the massive string processing impairment shown in adults and children with DD probably reflects a primary visual attentional disorder (see Valdois et al., 2012 in the present book).

Developmental dyslexia and visual attentional processing

Visual spatial attention is particularly important for orthographic processing because graphemic parsing of the order of letter strings is essential for efficient phonological assembly. In particular, graphemic parsing requires rapid and accurate attentional orienting along the letter string. Computational models of reading assume that some graphemic parsing forms achieve the level of representation on which the spelling-to-sound conversion mechanisms operate (see Zorzi, 2005 for a recent review). Regardless of how this process is exactly conceived (e.g. Ans et al., 1998; Whitney & Cornelissen, 2005; Perry et al., 2007), it requires the serial orienting of visual attention onto each sublexical unit. Converging evidence for the hypothesis that a visual spatial attentional deficit could specifically impair sublexical processing in DD comes from both experimental and clinical studies, which have suggested that orienting of visual spatial attention—controlled by the frontoparietal attention system—is actually more important for non-word reading than for word reading (e.g. Sieroff et al., 1988; Ladavas et al., 1997; Auclair & Sieroff, 2002). Attentional orienting improves visual perception by intensifying the signal inside the focus of attention as well as by diminishing the effect of noise outside the focus of attention (see Reynolds & Heeger, 2009 for a recent review). Thus when letters are spatially close, letter identification accuracy is reduced (Bouma, 1970) because of massive competition for processing resources (see Pelli, 2008 for a review). However, almost no competition occurs if attention is rapidly engaged onto the visual object (e.g. Van der Lubbe & Keuss, 2001; see Enns & Di Lollo, 2000 for a review). Rapid orienting of spatial attention improves perception in many visual tasks, such as contrast sensitivity, texture segmentation, and visual search, by enhancing spatial resolution (Carrasco et al., 2002).

It allows decisions to be based on the selected stimulus alone, disregarding distracting stimuli by perceptual noise exclusion (Dosher & Lu, 2000).

A deficit of visual attentional orienting has been repeatedly described in DD (see Hari & Renvall, 2001; Valdois et al., 2004; Vidyasagar & Pammer, 2010 for reviews) and more specifically in dyslexics with poor phonological decoding skills (e.g. Cestnick & Coltheart, 1999; Buchholz & McKone, 2004; Kinsey et al., 2004; Roach & Hogben, 2007; Facoetti et al., 2008b, 2010a; Jones et al., 2008; Ruffino et al., 2010a). In our recent study, we investigated automatic orienting of attention in dyslexic children by measuring reaction times to visual and auditory stimuli in cued-detection tasks (Facoetti et al., 2010a). Dyslexics with poor non-word decoding accuracy showed a slower time course of visual and auditory spatial attention when compared with both chronological age and reading level controls as well as with dyslexics with slow but accurate non-word decoding abilities. Notably, individual differences in the time course of multisensory spatial attention accounted for 31% of unique variance in the non-word reading performance of the entire dyslexic sample, after controlling for age, IQ, and phonological skills. Our study suggests that multisensory sluggish attention-orienting selectively impairs the sublexical level of orthographic-to-phonological binding that are critical for reading development. Visual engagement and disengagement of non-spatial attention were studied in dyslexic children and for normally reading children by measuring 'attentional masking' (AM) and 'attentional blink' (AB) effects (Facoetti et al., 2008). AM refers to an impaired identification of the first (T1) of two rapidly sequential masked targets (i.e. attentional engagement). In contrast, AB refers to an impaired identification of the second target (T2) in the sequence (i.e. attentional disengagement).

Our results revealed a specific temporal deficit of non-spatial attention in dyslexic children and that the abnormality in AM and AB is large (77% and 54%, respectively). In addition, we showed that individual differences in non-spatial attention were specifically related to phonological decoding. In a more recent study, spatiotemporal distribution of attentional engagement onto three-pseudoletter strings was studied in dyslexic and normally reading children by measuring AM (Ruffino et al., 2010a). T1 was always centrally displayed, whereas the location of T2 (central or lateral) and the T1–T2 interval were manipulated. Dyslexic children showed a larger AM at the shortest T1–T2 interval and a sluggish AM recovery at the longest T1–T2 interval, as well as an abnormal lateral AM. More importantly, these spatiotemporal deficits of attentional engagement were selectively present in dyslexics with poor phonological decoding skills. In addition to a sluggish engagement of non-spatial attention (Facoetti et al., 2008), dyslexic children show an inefficient spatial selection of visual stimuli. Globally, these results suggest not only a 'longer temporal,' but also a 'larger spatial' window in which attentional engagement is labile (Potter et al., 2002), coherently with a perceptual noise exclusion deficit in DD (Sperling et al., 2005; Martelli et al., 2009). Thus, individuals with DD typically show a specific deficit in the ability to detect relevant stimuli (the signal object) when spatiotemporal irrelevant stimuli (the noise object) are closely presented. However, sluggish attentional orienting might be the crucial process involved in all of these perceptual noise exclusion deficits.

We measured the accuracy of target identification in dyslexic and normally reading children by using an experimental paradigm involving the use of two attentional (focused vs. unfocused) and two noise conditions (signal alone vs. signal with lateral noise) (Ruffino et al., 2010b). Our results confirmed that children with DD have a target identification deficit only when stimuli are displayed with lateral noise. More importantly, dyslexics are impaired in the perception of the signal with lateral noise only in focused attention, demonstrating that a disorder of automatic orienting of visual attention is associated with a perceptual noise exclusion deficit in DD.

Developmental dyslexia and the magnocellular dorsal visual pathway

A possible neurobiological substrate of sluggish attentional orienting and engagement deficits in DD could be a weakened or abnormal magnocellular (M) input to the dorsal (D) visual stream, and a consequent dysfunction of the frontoparietal attentional system (Livingstone et al., 1991; Stein & Walsh, 1997; see also Stein, 2012 and Pammer, 2012 in the present book). Deficits in the M pathway, albeit controversial (e.g. Amitay et al., 2002), could influence higher visual processing stages through the D stream, and, therefore, lead to reading difficulties through impaired attentional orienting (Hari & Renvall, 2001; Boden & Giaschi, 2007; Vidyasagar & Pammer, 2010; see also Vidyasagar, 2012 in the present book).

In a recent study, we investigated the visual MD and parvocellular ventral pathway in dyslexics and in normally reading children by measuring sensitivity to dynamic (the spatial frequency doubling illusion, SFDI) and static stimuli, respectively. The results revealed a specific deficit of the MD pathway in dyslexics. More importantly, the MD deficit was selectively present in poor non-word readers, suggesting a specific role for the MD pathway in phonological decoding. We further showed that in dyslexic children, individual differences in MD sensitivity accounted for 29% of unique variance in non-word reading fluency after controlling for age and IQ. This MD deficit appears to be frequent because 75% of the poor non-word readers were at least one standard deviation below the mean of the controls (Facoetti et al., 2009). This data suggests that MD deficits contribute to the aetiology of the phonological decoding disorder (new word and non-word reading), probably impairing serial attentional orienting on letter strings. Thus, a specific MD impairment causing an attentional orienting disorder in DD children with phonological decoding deficits was specifically predicted by this neurobiological hypothesis.

In another study, we investigated the MD pathway and attentional orienting in dyslexic (with or without phonological decoding deficits) by measuring SFDI and the time course of automatic orienting of visual attention, respectively. The results confirmed a specific deficit of the MD pathway in dyslexics with phonological decoding deficits (Facoetti et al., 2009). More importantly, the same group of dyslexics with MD deficits showed sluggish attentional orienting. In dyslexic children with phonological decoding deficits, attentional facilitation occurred at much longer cue-target stimulus onset asynchronies (SOAs) compared with normally reading children (Facoetti et al., 2010c). These results highlight the fact that an MD deficit linked to dysfunction of the orienting of visual attention might impair the phonological decoding mechanisms that are critical for reading acquisition.

At the neurobiological level, the role of visual attentional orienting in phonological decoding is emphasized by the additional activation of the corresponding brain regions when participants read long non-words (e.g. Valdois et al., 2006). Accordingly, neuroimaging studies of both typical and atypical reading development have consistently implicated regions that are known to subserve the orienting of visual attention (see Corbetta & Shulman, 2002 for a review of the functional anatomy of attention). For example, several studies employing phonological decoding tasks have shown deficient task-related activation in areas surrounding the bilateral frontoparietal attentional system in dyslexics (see Eden & Zeffiro, 1998 for a review). While the left frontoparietal system has been linked to auditory-phonological processing (Pugh et al., 2000), the right frontoparietal system is a crucial component of the network subserving the automatic orienting of attention (Corbetta & Shulman, 2002). Thus developmental changes in activation of the right frontoparietal system have been linked to reading acquisition in normally developing children (Turkeltaub et al., 2003), and some studies have observed a right frontoparietal system dysfunction in dyslexics (e.g. Hoeft et al., 2006; Grünling et al., 2004).

Developmental dyslexia and early identification of visual spatial attention deficits

According to multifactorial developmental cognitive models of reading acquisition (e.g. Pernet et al., 2009; Menghini et al., 2010; see Pennington, 2006 for a review), mastery of automatic grapheme-phoneme mappings is a crucial prerequisite for the development of skilled reading (Blomert, 2011). Multisensory phonological assembly—leading from a visual input to a linguistic output—requires, in addition to speech-sound segmentation, efficient serial attentional orienting that segments letter strings into separate graphemes.

Whether MD and attentional deficits are causally linked to reading disorders in dyslexic children has been hotly disputed (e.g. Goswami, 2003; Ramus, 2003; but see Vidyasagar & Pammer, 2010, Vidyasagar, Chapter 10, this volume). It has been argued that MD and attentional deficits are a consequence, rather than a cause of the reading difficulties that characterize DD. An important step towards the demonstration that impaired spatial attention is a core deficit in DD was provided by our previous study on dyslexic children (Facoetti et al., 2010b) because those with phonological decoding deficits showed abnormal deployment of spatial attention, even in comparison to much younger, typically developing children matched for reading level.

In a cross-sectional study on typically developing children, Bosse and Valdois (2009) have shown that visual attention contributes to phonological decoding skills, independently of auditory-phonological processing, even among first graders. Moreover, recent longitudinal studies have suggested that MD pathway sensitivity, as well as visual attentional orienting, in addition to phonological awareness, are important predictors of early reading abilities (e.g. Plaza & Cohen, 2006; Boets et al., 2008; Ferretti et al., 2008; Kevan & Pammer, 2009; Facoetti et al., 2010a). We measured the interference of global stimuli in preschooler children, on the processing of local stimuli, as well as the interference of local stimuli on the processing of global stimuli by using a variant of the Navon task. One year later, we tested the reading abilities in the same sample when the children were completing the first grade in primary school. Preschooler good readers presented the typical global interference effect during local processing (i.e. they see the 'forest before the trees'), whereas poor readers did not show this effect, suggesting that they had a global perception deficit. Interestingly, poor readers showed a larger local interference effect during global processing in comparison to good readers (Franceschini et al., 2010). These results demonstrate that children who present reading difficulties show a pre-existing atypical local perception precedence (i.e. they see the 'trees before the forest'), suggesting that visual MD efficiency plays a specific role even before reading acquisition. Accordingly, in their longitudinal studies, Boets et al. (2008) and Kevan and Pammer (2009), found that MD sensitivity (i.e. coherent dot motion and SFDI thresholds) in pre-reading children were related to their reading skills in first grade.

About half of all reading deficits can be attributed to genetic influences (Gayàn & Olson, 2001), and DD is known to frequently run in families (Fisher, 1905; Thomas, 1905; Hallgren, 1950). Note that familial transmission is necessary, but not sufficient evidence for a genetic aetiology because family members typically share both genes and environment (DeFries, 1985). What is important for our purposes, however, is that children with one dyslexic parent present a high risk in terms of developing reading difficulties. The hypothesis that impaired orienting of spatial attention is a core deficit in DD (Facoetti et al., 2010b) leads to the prediction that at least some of those at risk should manifest this dysfunction even before they begin to learn to read. An impairment of the MD stream in pre-readers at risk for DD has been described by Kevan and Pammer (2008), who found that both coherent dot motion and SFDI thresholds were higher in at-risk children in comparison to unselected pre-readers. However, their study did not explicitly investigate the orienting of spatial attention. A causal hypothesis suggests that the visual attentional orienting mechanism is already compromised in preschoolers at risk of developing DD.

To investigate this hypothesis, we measured the efficiency in orienting visual attention to a brief spatial peripheral cue when children were engaged in a task that required the identification of a target flanked by lateral noise. Our results show for the first time that children at risk of DD compared to controls, presented a marked disorder of visual attentional orienting, in addition to their typical syllabic segmentation deficit (Facoetti et al., 2010a). In particular, the defective automatic orienting of visual attention observed in the at-risk pre-readers was consistent with other neuropsychological studies of children with DD (see Hari & Renvall, 2001; Valdois et al., 2004; Vidyasagar & Pammer, 2010, Vidyasagar, Chapter 10, this volume, for reviews). The lack of the cueing effect at a short cue-target SOA (i.e. 100 ms) observed in our study of at-risk pre-reader children is predicted by the 'sluggish attentional shifting' (SAS) hypothesis (see Hari & Renvall, 2001 for a review) and is consistent with the finding that dyslexic children are slow at attention orienting (Facoetti et al., 2010b). At-risk pre-reader children were significantly less sensitive to peripheral transient and uninformative cues compared with the group without familial risk for DD. This attentional deficit could be specific to the DM stream because it is mainly involved in the processing of peripheral and transient stimuli (see Stein & Walsh, 1997; Boden & Giaschi, 2007; Vidyasagar & Pammer, 2010 for reviews).

These results support the idea that a deficit of multisensory (visual and auditory) attention actually causes DD. To investigate this causal hypothesis in a more stringent way, we measured the efficiency of orienting visual attention to a brief spatial peripheral cue in preschoolers. The pre-readers were followed-up and classified as either poor or normal readers on the basis of their reading ability development later during the first grade of primary school. Both linear regressions suggest that efficiency in the orienting of visual attention is an effective predictor of reading acquisition (Franceschini et al., 2012). All of these results support the hypothesis of a causal link between visual spatial attention deficits and disorders of reading acquisition.

Towards a more efficient prevention of developmental dyslexia

One of the most important aims of studies predicting future reading difficulties is to improve identification of at-risk children for treatment with preventive remediation programmes before they begin to fail at learning to read (Gabrieli, 2009). Recent studies have confirmed that reading abilities can be improved by specific pre-reading programmes (e.g. Gormley et al., 2008), suggesting that preventive programmes could reduce the incidence of DD. Overall, this review supports the prediction that, in children at familial risk for DD, visual attentional impairment—in addition to the typically observed speech segmentation deficit—exists prior to the beginning of formal reading instruction. Thus the combination of visual spatial attention and syllabic segmentation scores was more reliable than either single measure alone for the identification of at-risk children (Facoetti et al., 2010a). This result therefore also offers a new approach for the early identification of DD.

The SAS hypothesis (Hari & Renvall, 2001) proposes that there is a specific deficit in DD for rapid and automatic attentional orienting and engagement onto auditory and visual objects (Facoetti et al., 2010b; Lallier et al., 2010) which is argued to have an impact on reading acquisition based on orthographic–phonological binding (Blomert, 2011). The proposed multisensory SAS also has implications for efficient functioning of the perceptual noise exclusion mechanism (Sperling et al., 2005; Geiger et al., 2008; Ziegler et al., 2009). Testing theories about the aetiology of DD require developmental designs (Goswami, 2003), and recent work from different research groups, using both at-risk and longitudinal studies, suggests that reading acquisition is based not only on speech segmentation (Goswami et al., 2011), but also on visual MD-based serial attentional orienting onto letter strings (e.g. Plaza & Cohen, 2006; Boets et al., 2008; Ferretti et al., 2008; Kevan & Pammer, 2008, 2009; Facoetti et al., 2010a; Franceschini et al., 2010; 2012). I propose that the core neural deficit underlying DD is the fundamental multimodal attentional mechanism that mediates efficient orthographic-phonological binding. This proposal has the ultimate aim of improving the efficacy of neuroscience-based educational interventions in DD. Indeed, some intervention studies have clearly shown that both auditory and visual orienting of attention can be improved by training in children with both DD and/or SLI (e.g. Geiger et al., 1994; Facoetti et al., 2003; Stevens et al., 2008). In particular, these studies consistently demonstrate that the inhibitory aspects of attention—that are crucial for perceptual noise exclusion—can be remediated by appropriate rehabilitation programmes (Geiger et al., 1994; Facoetti et al., 2003; Stevens et al., 2008). Our data demonstrate that a pure visual spatial treatment (based on rapid letter string presentation) not only improved phonological decoding, but also improved the inhibitory attentional mechanisms required for left-to-right serial searching of letter strings (Facoetti & Lorusso, unpublished data; see Vidyasagar & Pammer, 2010 for discussion). In fact, even the 'pure' phonologically-based treatment programmes that are typically used to rehabilitate DD, have to make use of fundamental auditory attentional mechanisms.

It is intriguing to note that playing action video games significantly improves visual attentional orienting and engagement (for a recent review see Dye et al., 2009). Critically, this increase in rapid attentional orienting generalizes to various tasks beyond game situations. Thus action video game play improves general attentional resources, allowing gamers to better allocate their attention across both space and time (Dye et al., 2009). Video gaming might, therefore, provide an efficient attentional training regimen to induce reading improvement in DD children as well as in pre-reading children at risk of DD. Overall, the findings reported here offer the possibility of developing new, more efficient, treatments of DD through the use of intensive training to improve multisensory orienting of spatial attention in pre-reading children at risk of reading failure.

Acknowledgements

This chapter is dedicated to Giulio, Camilla and Tiziana. A.F. is supported by grants from the Italian Ministry of University and Scientific Research ('PRIN2007'), CARIPARO Foundation ('Borse di Dottorato CARIPARO 2009'), and the University of Padova ('Assegni di Ricerca 2009' and 'Progetto di Ateneo 2009'). I sincerely thank Milena Ruffino, Anna Noemi Trussardi, Simone Gori, and Sandro Franceschini for helpful discussions.

References

American Psychiatric Association (1994). *Diagnostic and statistical manual of mental disorders 4th edition* [DSM-IV]. Washington, DC: APA.

Amitay, S., Ben-Yehudah, G., Banai, K., & Ahissar, M. (2002). Disabled readers suffer from visual and auditory impairments but not from a specific magnocellular deficit. *Brain*, 125, 2272–85.

Ans, B., Carbonnel, S., & Valdois, S. (1998). A connectionist multiple-trace memory model for polysyllabic word reading. *Psychological Review*, 105, 678–723.

Asbjørnsen, A.E., & Bryden, M.P. (1998). Auditory attentional shifts in reading-disabled students: quantification of attentional effectiveness by the Attentional Shift Index. *Neuropsychologia*, 36, 143–8.

Auclair, L., & Sieroff, E. (2002). Attentional cueing effect in the identification of words and pseudowords of different length. *Quarterly Journal of Experimental Psychology*, 55, 445–63.

Blomert, L. (2011). The neural signature of orthographic-phonological binding in successful and failing reading development. *Neuroimage*, 57, 695–703.

Boden, C., & Giaschi, D. (2007). M-stream deficits and reading-related visual processes in developmental dyslexia. *Psychological Bulletin*, 133, 346–66.

Boets, B., Wouters, J., van Wieringen, A., De Smedt, B., & Ghesquière, P. (2008). Modelling relations between sensory processing, speech perception, orthographic and phonological ability, and literacy achievement. *Brain and Language*, 106, 29–40.

Bosse, M.L., & Valodis, S. (2009). Influence of the visual attention span on child reading performance: a cross-sectional study. *Journal of Research in Reading*, 32, 230–53.

Bosse, M.L., Tainturier, M.J., & Valdois, S. (2007). Developmental dyslexia: The visual attention span deficit hypothesis. *Cognition*, 104, 198–230.

Bouma, H. (1970). Interaction effects in parafoveal letter recognition. *Nature*, 226, 177–8.

Buchholz, J., & McKone, E. (2004). Adults with dyslexia show deficits on spatial frequency doubling and visual attention tasks. *Dyslexia*, 10, 24–43.

Carrasco, M.,Williams, P., & Yeshurum, Y. (2002). Covert attention increases spatial resolution with or without masks: Support for signal enhancement. *Journal of Vision*, 2, 467–79.

Castles, A., & Coltheart, M. (2004). Is there a causal link from phonological awareness to success in learning to read? *Cognition*, 91, 77–111.

Cestnick, L., & Coltheart, M. (1999). The relationship between language-processing and visual processing deficit in developmental dyslexia. *Cognition*, 71, 231–55.

Cohen, L., & Dehaene, S. (2009). Ventral and dorsal contributions to word reading. In: M.S. Gazzaniga (Ed.) *The Cognitive Neuroscience* (4th edn.), pp. 789–804. Cambridge, MA: The MIT Press.

Corbetta, M., & Shulman, G.L. (2002). Control of goal-directed and stimulus-driven attention in the brain. *Nature Review Neuroscience*, 3, 201–15.

Cornelissen, P., Richardson, A., Mason, A., Fowler, S., & Stein, J. (1995). Contrast sensitivity and coherent motion detection measured at photopic luminance levels in dyslexics and controls. *Vision Research*, 35, 1483–94.

DeFries, J.C. (1985). Colorado reading project. In: D.B. Gray & J.F. Kavanagh (Eds.) *Biobehavioral measures of dyslexia*, pp. 107–122. Parkton, MD: York Press.

Démonet, J.F. & Reilhac, C. (2012). A Neurological Account of Dyslexia. In:J. Stein & Z. Kapoula (Eds.) *Visual Aspects of Dyslexia*, pp. 1–14. Oxford: Oxford University Press.

Dosher, B.N., & Lu, Z. (2000). Noise exclusion in spatial attention. *Psychological Science*, 11, 139–46.

Dye, M.W., Green, C.S., & Bavelier, D. (2009). Increasing speed of processing with action video games. *Current Direction in Psychological Science*, 18, 321–6.

Eden, G.F., & Zeffiro, T.A. (1998). Neural systems affected in developmental dyslexia revealed by functional neuroimaging. *Neuron*, 21, 279–82.

Enns, J.T., & Di Lollo, V. (2000). What's new in visual masking? *Trends in Cognitive Science*, 4, 345–52.

Facoetti, A., Lorusso, M. L., Paganoni, P., Umiltà, C., & Mascetti, G.G. (2003). The role of visuospatial attention in developmental dyslexia: evidence from a rehabilitation study. *Cognitive Brain Research*, 15, 154–64.

Facoetti, A., Ruffino, M., Peru, A., Paganoni, P., & Chelazzi, L. (2008). Sluggish engagement and disengagement of non-spatial attention in dyslexic children. *Cortex*, 44, 1221–33.

Facoetti, A., Gori, S., Bigoni, A., Ruffino, M., Molteni, M., & Cecchini, P. (2009). Magnocellular-dorsal pathway and sub-lexical route in developmental dyslexia. *Perception* 38, 103.

Facoetti, A., Corradi, N., Ruffino, M., Gori, S., & Zorzi, M. (2010a). Visual spatial attention and speech segmentation are both impaired in preschoolers at familial risk for developmental dyslexia. *Dyslexia*, 16, 226–39.

Facoetti, A., Trussardi, A.N., Ruffino, M., Lorusso, M.L., Cattaneo, C., Galli, R., *et al.* (2010b). Multisensory spatial attention deficits are predictive of phonological decoding skills in development dyslexia. *Journal of Cognitive Neuroscience*, 22, 1011–25.

Facoetti, A., Ruffino, M., Gori, S., Bigoni, A., Benassi, M., Bolzani, R., *et al.* (2010c). On the relationship between magnocellular pathway and automatic attentional orienting: evidences from developmental dyslexia. *Journal of Vision*, 10, 281.

Ferretti, G., Mazzotti, S., & Brizzolara, D. (2008). Visual scanning and reading ability in normal and dyslexic children. *Behavioral Neurology*, 19, 87–92.

Fisher, J.H. (1905). Case of congenital word blindness (Inability to learn to read). *Ophthalmological Review*, 24, 315–18.

Franceschini, S., Gori, S., Ruffino, M., Pedrolli, K., & Facoetti, A. (2012). A causal link between visual spatial attention and reading acquisition. *Current Biology*, 22, 1–6.

Franceschini, S., Corradi, N., Ruffino, M., Gori, S., Gianesini, T., & Facoetti, A. (2010). Atypical local perception precedence in preschooler poor readers. *Perception*, 39, 79.

Fritz, J.B., Elhilali, M., David, S.V., & Shamma, S.A. (2007). Auditory attention focusing the searchlight on sound. *Current Opinion in Neurobiology*, 17, 437–55.

Gabrieli, J.D. (2009). Dyslexia: a new synergy between education and cognitive neuroscience. *Science*, 325, 280–3.

Gayán, J., & Olson, R.K. (2001). Genetic and environmental influences on orthographic and phonological skills in children with reading disabilities. *Developmental Neuropsychology*, 20, 483–507.

Geiger, G., Lettvin, J.Y., & Fanhle, M. (1994). Dyslexic children learn a new visual strategy for reading: a controlled experiment. *Vision Research*, 34, 1223–33.

Geiger, G., Cattaneo, C., Galli, R., Pozzoli, U., Lorusso, M.L., Facoetti, A., *et al.* (2008). Wide and diffuse perceptual modes characterized dyslexics in vision and audition. *Perception*, 37, 1745–64.

Gormley Jr, W.T., Philips, D., & Gayer, T. (2008). Preschool programs can boost school readiness. *Science*, 320, 1723–24.

Goswami, U. (2003). Why theories about developmental dyslexia require developmental designs? *Trends in Cognitive Science*, 7, 534–40.

Goswami, U., Thomson, J., Richardson, U., Stainthorp, R., Hughes, D., Rosen, S., *et al.* (2002). Amplitude envelope onsets and developmental dyslexia: A new hypothesis. *Proceedings of the National Academy of Sciences of the United States of America*, 99, 10911–16.

Goswami, U., Wang, H.L., Cruz, A., Fosker, T., Mead, N., & Huss, M. (2011). Language-universal sensory deficits in developmental dyslexia: English, Spanish, and Chinese. *Journal of Cognitive Neuroscience*, 23, 325–37

Grünling, C., Ligges, M., Huonker, R., Klingert, M., Mentzel, H.J., Rzanny, R., *et al.* (2004). Dyslexia: the possible benefit of multimodal integration of fMRI- and EEG-data. *Journal of Neural Transmission*, 111, 951–69.

Habib, M. (2000). The neurological basis of developmental dyslexia an overview and working hypothesis. *Brain*, 123, 2373–99.

Hallgren, B. (1950). Specific dyslexia (congenital word-blindness); a clinical and genetic study. *Acta Psychiatrica and Neurology Supplement*, 65, 1–287.

Hari, R., & Renvall, H. (2001). Impaired processing of rapid stimulus sequences in dyslexia. *Trends in Cognitive Science*, 5, 525–32.

Hari, R., Renvall, H., & Tanskanen, T. (2001). Left minineglect in dyslexic adults. *Brain*, 124, 1373–80.

Harm, M.W., & Seidenberg, M.S. (1999). Phonology, reading acquisition, and dyslexia: insights from connectionist models. *Psychological Review*, 106, 491–528.

Hawelka, S., & Wimmer, H. (2005). Impaired visual processing of multi-element arrays is associated with increased number of eye movements in dyslexic reading. *Vision Research*, 45, 855–63.

Hawelka, S., Huber, C., & Wimmer, H. (2006). Impaired visual processing of letter and digit strings in adult dyslexic readers. *Vision Research*, 46, 718–23.

Hoeft, F., Hernandez, A., McMillon, G., Taylor-Hill, H., Martindale, J.L., Meyel, A., *et al.* (2006). Neural basis of dyslexia: a comparison between dyslexic and nondyslexic children equated for reading ability. *Journal of Neuroscience*, 26, 10700–8.

Jones, M.W., Branigan, H.P., & Kelly, M.L. (2008). Visual deficits in developmental dyslexia: relationships between non-linguistic visual tasks and their contribution to components of reading. *Dyslexia*, 14, 95–115.

Kevan, A., & Pammer, K. (2008). Visual deficits in pre-readears at familial risk for dyslexia. *Vision Research*, 48, 2835–9.

Kevan, A., & Pammer, K. (2009). Predicting early reading skills from pre-reading measures of dorsal stream functioning. *Neuropsychologia*, 47, 3174–81.

Kinsey, K., Rose, M., Hansen, P., Richardson, A., & Stein, J. (2004). Magnocellular mediated visual-spatial attention and reading ability. *Neuroreport*, 15, 2215–18.

Ladavas, E., Umiltà, C., & Mapelli, D. (1997). Lexical and semantic processing in the absence of word reading: Evidence from neglect dyslexia. *Neuropsychologia*, 35, 1075–85.

Lallier, M., Tainturier, M.J., Dering, B., Donnadieu, S., Valdois, S., Thierry, G. (2010). Behavioral and ERP evidence for amodal sluggish attentional shifting in developmental dyslexia. *Neuropsychologia*, 48, 4125–35.

Livingstone, M.S., Rosen, G.D., Drislane, F.W., & Galaburda, A.M. (1991). Physiological and anatomical evidence for a magnocellular defect in developmental dyslexia. *Proceedings of the National Academy of Sciences of United States of America*, 88, 7943–7.

Martelli, M., Di Filippo, G., Spinelli, D., & Zoccolotti, P. (2009). Crowding, reading, and developmental dyslexia. *Journal of Vision*, 9, 1–18.

McCandliss, B.D., Cohen, L., & Dehaene, S. (2003). The visual word form area: expertise for reading in the fusiform gyrus. *Trends in Cognitive Science*, 7, 293–9.

Menghini, D., Finzi, A., Benassi, M., Bolzani, R., Facoetti, A., Giovagnoli, S., *et al.* (2010). Different underlying neurocognitive deficits in developmental dyslexia: a comparative study. *Neuropsychologia*, 48, 863–72.

Montani, V., Facoetti, A., & Zorzi, M. (2010). Crowding effect in lexical and sublexical recognition. *Perception*, 39, 148.

Pammer, K., Lavis, R., Hansen, P., & Cornelissen, P.L. (2004). Symbol-string sensitivity and children's reading. *Brain & Language*, 89, 601–10.

Pelli, D.G. (2008). Crowding: A cortical constraint on object recognition. *Current Opinion in Neurobiology*, 18, 445–51.

Pennington, B.F. (2006). From single to multiple deficit models of developmental disorders. *Cognition*, 101, 385–413.

Pernet, C., Anderssn, J., Paulesu, E., & Demonet, J.F. (2009). When all hypotheses are right: a multifocal accounf of dyslexia. *Human Brain Mapping*, 30, 2278–92.

Perry, C., Ziegler, J.C., & Zorzi, M. (2007). Nested incremental modeling in the development of computational theories: The CDP+ model of reading aloud. *Psychological Review*, 114, 273–315.

Plaza, M., & Cohen, E. (2006). The contribution of phonological awareness and visual attention in early reading and spelling. *Dyslexia*, 13, 67–76.

Potter, M.C., Staub, A., & O'Connor, D.H. (2002). The time course of competition for attention: Attention is initially labile. *Journal of Experimental Psychology: Human Perception and Performance*, 28, 1149–62.

Pugh, K.R., Mencl, W.E., Jenner, A.R., Kats, L., Frost, S.J., Lee, J.R., *et al.* (2000) Functional neuroimaging studies of reading and reading disability (developmental dyslexia). *Mental Retardation and Developmental Disabilities Research Reviews*, 6, 207–13.

Ramus, F. (2003). Developmental dyslexia: specific phonological deficit or general sensorimotor dysfunction? *Current Opinion in Neurobiology*, 13, 212–18.

Renvall, H., & Hari, R. (2002). Auditory cortical responses to speech-like stimuli in dyslexic adults. *Journal of Cognitive Neuroscience*, 14, 757–68.

Reynolds, J.H., & Heeger, D.J. (2009). The normalization model of attention. *Neuron*, 61, 168–85.

Roach, N.W., & Hogben, J.H. (2007). Impaired filtering of behaviourally irrelevant visual information in dyslexia. *Brain*, 130, 771–85.

Ruffino, M., Trussardi, A.N., Gori, S., Finzi, A., Giovagnoli, S., Menghini, D., *et al.* (2010a). Attentional engagement deficits in dyslexic children. *Neuropsychologia*, 48, 3793–801.

Ruffino, M., Gori, S., Franceschini, S., & Facoetti, A. (2010b). Developmental dyslexia: Perceptual noise exclusion deficit or spatial attention dysfunction? *Perception*, 39, 80.

Shamma, S.A., & Micheyl, C. (2010). Behind the scenes of auditory perception. *Current Opinion Neurobiology*, 20, 361–6.

Share, D.L. (1995). Phonological recoding and self-teaching: Sine qua non of reading acquisition. *Cognition*, 55, 151–218.

Shaywitz, S.E., & Shaywitz, B.A. (2005). Dyslexia specific reading disability. *Biological Psychiatry*, 57, 1301–9.

Sieroff, E., Pollatsek, A., & Posner, M. (1988). Recognition of visual letter strings following injury to the posterior visual spatial attention system. *Cognitive Neuropsychology*, 5, 427–49.

Sperling, A.J., Lu, Z.L., Manis, F.R., & Seidenberg, M.S. (2005). Deficits in perceptual noise exclusion in developmental dyslexia. *Nature Neuroscience*, 8, 862–3.

Stein, J., & Walsh, V. (1997). To see but not to read: The magnocellular theory of dyslexia. *Trends in Neuroscience*, 20, 147–52.

Stevens, C., Fanning, J., Coch, D., Sanders, L., & Neville, H. (2008). Neural mechanisms of selective auditory attentional enhanced by computerized training: Electrophysiological evidence from language-impaired and typically developing children. *Brain Research*, 1205, 55–69.

Stevens, C., Sanders, L., & Neville, H. (2006). Neurophysiological evidence for selective auditory attention deficits in children with specific language impairment. *Brain Research*, 1111, 143–52.

Tallal, P. (2004). Improving language and literacy is a matter of time. *Nature Review Neuroscience*, 5, 721–8.

Thomas, C.J. (1905). Congenital word blindness and its treatment. *Ophthalmoscope*, 3, 380–5.

Turkeltaub, P.E., Gareau, L., Flowers, D.L., Zeffiro, T.A., & Eden, G.F. (2003). Development of neural mechanisms for reading. *Nature Neuroscience*, 6, 767–73.

Valdois, S., Bosse, M.L., & Tainturier, M.J. (2004). The cognitive deficits responsible for developmental dyslexia: review of evidence for a selective visual attentional disorder. *Dyslexia*, 10, 339–63.

Valdois, S., Carbonnel, S.,Juphard, A., Baciu, M., Ans, B., Peyrin, C., *et al.* (2006). Polysyllabic pseudo-word processing in reading and lexical decision: Converging evidencefrom behavioral data, connectionist simulations and functional MRI. *Brain Research*, 1085, 149–62.

Van der Lubbe, R.H., & Keuss, P.J. (2001). Focused attention reduces the effect of lateral interference in multi-element arrays, *Psychological Research*, 65, 107–18.

Vellutino, F.R., Fletcher, J.M., Snowling, M.J., & Scanlon, D.M. (2004). Specific reading disability (dyslexia): What have we learned in the past four decades? *Journal of Child Psychology and Psychiatry*, 45, 2–40.

Vidyasagar, T.R., & Pammer, K. (2010). Dyslexia: a deficit in visuo-spatial attention, not in phonological processing. *Trends in Cognitive Science*, 14, 57–63.

Whitney, C., & Cornelissen, P. (2005). Letter position encoding and dyslexia. *Journal of Research in Reading*, 28, 274–301.

Wright, B.A., Bowen, R.W., & Zecker, S.G. (2000). Nonlinguistic perceptual deficits associated with reading and language disorders. *Current Opinion in Neurobiology*, 10, 482–6.

Ziegler, J.C., & Goswami, U. (2005). Reading acquisition, developmental dyslexia and skilled reading across languages: A psycholinguistic grain size theory. *Psychological Bulletin*, 131, 3–29.

Ziegler, J.C., Perry, C., Wyatt, A.M., Ladner, D., & Schülte-Korne, G. (2003). Developmental dyslexia in different languages: Language-specific or universal? *Journal of Experimental Child Psychology*, 86, 169–93.

Ziegler, J.C., Pech-Georgel, C., George, F., Alario, F.X., Lorenzi, C. (2005). Deficits in speech perception predict language learning impairment. *Proceedings of the National Academy of Sciences of the United States of America*, 27, 14110–15.

Ziegler, J.C., Pech-Georgel, C., George, F., & Lorenzi, C. (2009). Speech perception in noise deficits in dyslexia. *Developmental Science*, 12, 732–45.

Zorzi, M. (2005). Computational models of reading. In: G. Houghton (Ed.) *Connectionist models in cognitive psychology*, pp. 403–44. London: Psychology Press.

Zorzi, M., Barbiero, C., Facoetti, A., Lonciari, I., Carrozzi, M., Montico M., Bravar, L., George, F., Pech-Georgel C., & Ziegler, J. (2012). Extra-Large Letter Spacing Improves Reading in Dyslexia. *Proceedings of the National Academy of Sciences of the United States of America*, in press.

Chapter 9

The Role of the Dorsal Pathway in Word Recognition

Kristen Pammer

It is well accepted that reading is a learned skill that requires the precise synthesis of visual and verbal information. In order to read successfully, we must have a visual system that is sufficiently tuned to recognizing contrast borders in the form of edges, curves, lines, corners, and dots. The visual system must then put these features in the correct spatial positions to form identifiable letters, phonemes, morphemes, and words. This latter form of identification, requires input from higher cognitive processes such as memory and language centres, because up until this point in time in the reading network (approximately 150 ms in), the visual system is only sensitive to the fact that the pattern of contrasts on the page are words as opposed to a picture of a vase of flowers. Therefore, the visual system has recognized contrast boundaries, identified their locations, coded them into a neural signal reflecting the relative positions of the lines, edges, corners, and curves, has started sending the signals to higher cortical areas, received feedback from the higher cortical areas to facilitate the recognition of the pattern as letters and words, put the letters and words in the correct locations, and—if we are reading a line or page of text as normal—programmed the next saccadic jump to do it all again. The amazing thing, is that the visual system is extracting all of this during a single fixation and saccade in order to be ready for the subsequent fixation—in about 200 ms (Starr & Rayner, 2001), depending on the difficulty of the text that is being read. The complexity of the whole cortical reading network in terms of engagement of cognitive resources such as attention, verbal working memory, long-term memory, language, phonological processing, and a multitude of other components, is staggering. However, the feat achieved by the visual system just within the first 200 ms of seeing a word, deserves its own little round of applause.

Existing as it does at the front end of the reading network, early visual coding has a unique role in the integrity of the overall network. Like a spark-plug that fails to fire when the car is started, if these initial early visual signals are delayed or degraded, it can have serious knock-on effects throughout the system as a whole. Thus while a huge amount of scientific research has shown poor reading to be related to poor skills in high-level cognition, such as working memory (e.g. Beneventi et al., 2010), executive functioning (Poljac et al., 2010) and phonological coding (e.g. Snowling, 2000), a serious amount of research has also shown that the efficiency of early visual coding strongly affects reading (e.g. Cornelissen et al., 1998; Au & Lovegrove, 2001; Pammer et al., 2005; Levi et al., 2010), poor reading (e.g. Cornelissen et al., 1995; Talcott et al., 1998; Pammer & Wheatley, 2001), and reading acquisition (Kevan & Pammer, 2009). If the reader of this chapter has read any other chapters in this book, then they will probably already be familiar with the concept of the dorsal and ventral (sometimes called the magnocellular and parvocellular) visual pathways. However, to set the context of the current discussion: there are two primary neural pathways that carry visual information from the eye to the brain (actually, there are three, the koniocellular is the third (Hendry & Reid, 2000) but for the sake of parsimony, I am going to acknowledge its presence, but ignore it from this point on). Each of the pathways are responsible for transmitting different types of visual information (Maunsell et al., 1990); the dorsal pathway transmits information quickly and is responsible for coding qualities such as motion, spatial location, and low contrast, while the ventral pathway is slower and responsible for transmitting information about things like colour, detail, and high contrast. About 30 years ago, it was demonstrated (Lovegrove et al., 1980) that dyslexic children were poorer compared to normal reading children at processing visual information that was handled by the dorsal pathway. But they were perfectly normal in processing visual information handled by the ventral pathway. This started a veritable avalanche of research investigating the role of the dorsal pathway in reading, with a current literature count standing well over 300 articles. In most cases the research is more-or-less united in the finding that dyslexic readers are poorer at detecting visual stimuli that is transmitted by the dorsal visual pathway (Livingstone et al., 1991; Stein & Walsh, 1997; Stein, 2001; Vidyasagar & Pammer, 2010), that dorsal sensitivity predicts reading ability, that dorsal visual deficits exist in children at risk for dyslexia even before they learn to read (Kevan & Pammer, 2008), and dorsal processing predicts subsequent reading acquisition 2 years later (Kevan & Pammer, 2009). These findings have been replicated in many different labs over the world, using many different methodologies, in different countries and languages, and in both children and adults. However, like all good scientific analysis, the findings are by no means universal, and there is considerable dissension from other researchers (e.g. Skottun, 2000; Skottun & Skoyles, 2010). Nevertheless, there is substantial evidence to suggest that the dorsal visual pathway may in some way be involved in reading and word recognition. At first this seems counterintuitive; physiologically the dorsal stream is activated most strongly when processing visual information that is moving and colourless. Hence it is not immediately obvious how the dorsal stream may be so important in reading. Therefore, in order to get some sense of how the dorsal pathway may have a role in reading and word recognition, we need to start by looking more closely at the role that the dorsal pathway has in vision in general.

The dorsal visual pathway in vision

As already mentioned, the dorsal pathway is responsible for transmitting specific types of visual information such as motion, low contrast, and spatial coding (Van Essen, 1985; Livingstone & Hubel, 1988; Merigan & Maunsell, 1993; Logothetis & Sheinberg, 1996). It is primarily made up of magnocellular cells which are large cells that transmit information quickly (Laycock et al., 2007), primarily to the posterior parietal cortex (PPC)—the area of the brain considered to be responsible for processing spatial information

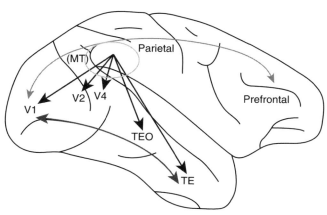

Fig. 9.1 (Also see Colour plate 1.) A model of interactions between different components of the visual cortex. The PPc is indicated by the yellow circle. Reprinted from *Brain Research Reviews*, 30(1), Trichur Raman Vidyasagar, A neuronal model of attentional spotlight: parietal guiding the temporal, pp. 69, Copyright (1990), with permission from Elsevier.

(Coby & Goldberg, 1999; Corbetta & Shulman, 2002), see Fig. 9.1. A large amount of research has described the different ways in which the PPC and the dorsal pathway is responsible for different aspects of spatial coding, such as orienting, covert attention, sustained attention, and visual search. However, for our purposes, it is the specific role that the dorsal pathway and PPC has in very early, preattentive, spatial coding of visual information that is of the most interest.

It is reasonably well accepted now that visual coding of information does not proceed purely in a feedforward, hierarchical flow of information, coding general features through to specific detail. Rather, early visual coding is highly interactive with much higher parts of the network, coding different elements of the visual object and feeding information both forward and back through the system (Lamme & Roelfsema 2000; Bullier, 2001; Bar et al., 2006; Lauritzen et al., 2009; Noudoost et al., 2010). When we direct our attention to an object in a visual scene we increase our responsivity to the object by increasing acuity and reducing reaction time (Posner, 1980; Posner & Peterson, 1990). Thus mechanisms within the visual system conduct a very fast analysis of the visual scene, coding information such as the spatial location of objects, and feeding this information back to other visual centres for more detailed analysis of the attended object. It has been suggested that the cortical mechanism responsible for this fast allocation of spatial attention is the dorsal pathway via the PPC (Shomstein & Behrmann, 2006; Saalman et al., 2007; Bressler et al., 2008). A comprehensive model of visual coding (Vidyasagar 1998, 1999) involves the integration of information over the two different visual pathways; the ventral stream, important for identification of objects via the occipital temporal cortex (OTC), and the dorsal stream via the PPC, crucial for the identification of spatial relations between objects (Merigan & Maunsell, 1993). Feedback loops between the PPC, the primary visual cortex, and associated lateral connections to the OTC provide a neurophysiological framework for a model of visual attention in which the dorsal pathway produces a fast analysis of spatial, global form information. This information is then used to extract and bind more detailed, local components of the visual scene which would occur by the ventral pathway in the OTC and visual cortex. The model is dependent upon very fast feedforward and feedback connections between the dorsal and ventral pathways, and the visual cortex. Therefore, the evidence thus far suggests that the rapid dorsal pathway may have a role in reading, by virtue of its role in early visual-spatial encoding. What then is the evidence that the dorsal stream may be involved in the visual-spatial aspects of reading words?

Visual-spatial encoding in word recognition

Behaviourally, we know that disrupting the visual-spatial qualities of text makes it more difficult to read—hAvInG iNcOnSisTeNt FoNt can severely disrupt reading speed and decoding, even having ALL UPPERCASE FONT WILL DECREASE READING SPEED, and although the 'Cambridge Effect' shows us that the 'lteters can be a taotl mses and you can sitll raed wothiut a porbelm', this is not strictly true. Yes, as adult, good readers we can decode the words—eventually—but reading speed slows down dramatically, our eye stops on each word for much longer than in normal reading and the eye jumps backwards far more frequently. However, the question of interest here is whether these word decoding difficulties occur because the dorsal stream is—perhaps—working harder to conduct its natural function, which is to sample the spatial qualities of the words, thus delaying the feedforward/feedback signal through the ventral system that would trigger detailed coding and recognition of the word?

Mayall, Humphreys, Mechelli, Olson and Price (2001) demonstrated that disrupting spatial allocation over text, e.g. with inconsistent fonts, engages the PPC. They conducted a positron emission tomography (PET) study presenting words in mixed font or normal font. They demonstrated a significant activation in the PPC (see Fig. 9.2) when the font was mixed for long and short words, presented at low or high contrast. Later, Braet and Humphreys (2006) disrupted processing of words and mixed-font words in the area identified by Mayall et al. by using transcranial magnetic stimulation (TMS). Consistent with the idea that the PPC is involved in word recognition, particularly when font is disrupted, they found that TMS increased reaction time (RT) for word recognition compared to no-TMS and control-TMS conditions. Moreover, RT for word naming increased even further for the mixed-font words.

We conducted a neuroimaging study, using magnetoencephalographic (MEG) neuroimaging to look at whether the dorsal pathway is at least involved when we spatially distort text (Pammer et al., 2006). MEG neuroimaging measures the tiny magnetic field patterns that are generated by the brain when large populations of cells fire (refer to Hämäläinen et al. (1993) for a review of MEG neuroimaging). We made an assumption that if the dorsal stream is involved when we read words, then the PPC should be active. Moreover, if the dorsal stream is involved by virtue of its specialization for early spatial encoding, then activity in the PPC should occur early in the sequence of events—so as to give sufficient time to send the information to the ventral stream—and, such activity

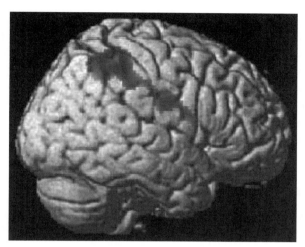

Fig. 9.2 Using a PET study, Mayall et al. (2001) demonstrated activation here in the PPc for words of mixed font compared to words presented normally. Adapted from Kate Mayall, Glyn W. Humphreys, Andrea Mechelli, Andrew Olson, and Cathy J. Price, 'The Effects of Case Mixing on Word Recognition: Evidence from a PET Study', *Journal of Cognitive Neuroscience*, 13:6 (August 15, 2001), pp. 844–53. © 2001 by the Massachusetts Institute of Technology.

should be stronger when we distort the spatial qualities of text, because the dorsal stream is being 'pushed' and has to work harder to do its job properly, thus maximizing the cortical response (Pulvermüller et al., 1997). We presented participants with words flashed on the screen for 100 ms, the words were either presented as normal such as 'HOUSE', or they were presented with the individual letters shifted relative to each other, such as 'H^OU^SE'. There were also words in which the letters were rearranged to form non-words such as 'HUOSE'. It was a lexical decision task such that with each word presentation the participant had to identify if the letter string was a word or not. The neuroimaging signals demonstrated that there was indeed a clear signal in the PPC early in the processing stream, and that this signal was stronger in the Shifted Words condition (Fig. 9.3).

It was apparent then from this study that the dorsal pathway is involved in word recognition, and when we push the system to work harder by disrupting the automatic spatial

Shifted words ROI
100–300 ms, 35–40 Hz

Shifted words vs. Words ROI
100–300 ms, 35–40 Hz

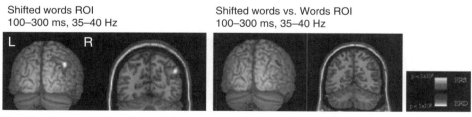

Fig. 9.3 (Also see Colour plate 2.) The MEG signal in the PPc is much stronger in the Shifted Words condition as represented in the left figure. The right figure is the contrast between the 'Normal' and the 'Shifted' words conditions. The signals were high frequency at 35–40 Hz, and was maximal within 300 ms of the presentation of the word.

encoding of familiar words, we get increased activation in the dorsal pathway—as indicated by increased activation in the PPC, suggesting that one of the roles the dorsal pathway may have in word recognition is in the spatial encoding of letter features.

The cumulative evidence from these studies is that when the spatial qualities of words are disrupted, there is activation in the part of the brain that receives major input from the dorsal visual pathway. As demonstrated in the figures, the consistency of these findings is compelling and suggests that the PPC, and putatively the dorsal pathway, is involved in processing the spatial qualities of text, and this occurs early in the processing sequence.

The unique contribution of the right PPC?

Thus far the evidence points to a unique role for the right PPC in the coding of spatial information in word recognition. However, the neuropsychological evidence to support this conclusion is not quite so clear-cut.

Braet and Humphreys (2006) describe two patients; G.K. and F.L. (see also Hall et al. (2001) for a full description of G.K.'s impairment) who demonstrate reading impairments that are consistent with what one would expect with right-PPC impairment. Compared to another patient with occipital but not parietal lesions, G.K and F.L. demonstrated clear difficulties in reading words particularly when presented in mixed case. This was independent of their ability to read words of low contrast, indicating that it was not the physical degradation of the word representation that was the problem, but the unusual spatial displacement of the letters. However, both G.K and F.L had brain lesions that extended bilaterally into the PPC regions. Patients with 'neglect dyslexia' have lesions in the right PPC and the manifestation of their reading difficulty is in terms of 'neglecting' or substituting the left side of presented words (Lee et al., 2009), this neglect often extends to the visual world in general, demonstrating a 'spatial neglect' (Ellis et al., 1993). Conversely, patients with left-hemisphere lesions may demonstrate neglect or substitution for the right ends of words, but the neglect often does not extend to the visual world in general (Greenwald & Berndt, 1999). Other patients have demonstrated reading impairments that are more consistent with impaired spatial coding; Patent D.E.S (Petrich, et al., 2007) demonstrated extremely poor, to almost non-existent, non-word reading, and positional errors and/or substitutions at the start of words (to the left). Patients B.S and P.Y. (Friedmann & Gvion, 2001) demonstrated letter-position dyslexia where their reading errors represented swaps or substitutions of letters within words. However, all these patients demonstrate left-hemisphere lesions. Similarly, F.M and P.T. also with left-hemisphere lesions (Shallice & Warrington, 1977) demonstrated an inability to recognize letters when presented within words, with otherwise preserved letter and word recognition.

How can these findings be resolved? Mesulam (1999) has suggested that the left and right frontoparietal networks, which includes the PPC areas that we have been discussing and the frontal eye fields, may have different representations of hemifield space. Specifically they suggest that the left frontoparietal network processes information from the contralateral visual hemifield, while the right frontoparietal network processes visual information from both the left and right visual space. If this were to be the case, then

words presented foveally will engage the right PPC as a consequence of spatial information to be processed from the left and right hemifields. However, only word information
from the right hemifield will engage the left PPC. However, Sommer et al. (2008) demonstrated that this heuristic was different depending on the spatial requirements; spatial
orienting resulted in a pattern of results consistent with those predicted by Mesulam such
that the right hemisphere appeared to process an equal representation of the left and right
hemifield, while the left hemisphere processed primarily right hemisphere information.
Visual search on the other hand, revealed the opposite pattern of results with specific
contralateral sensitivity shown by the right hemisphere, and non-specific hemifield sensitivity shown by the left hemisphere. What these results suggest regarding the role of the
dorsal stream in spatial encoding and reading is that it is likely that the left and right PPC
are engaged in different aspects of spatial encoding in reading. Mesulam's model would
explain why it is predominately right-PPC activity that is seen when we engage the spatial
mechanisms when reading because spatial information is coded from the left and right
visual fields. However, just the right PPC alone is not sufficient for spatial encoding when
reading and it is possible that the left PPC has a necessary—albeit more subtle—role in
spatial coding. Ultimately, carefully designed research teasing out the different spatial
requirements of word recognition can test this possibility.

Training the dorsal stream?

Anybody who works in the area of reading and dyslexia research is routinely asked the
question 'So what can we do about the problem?'. As discussed, there is good evidence
linking the dorsal stream to reading and dyslexia. Moreover, if the dorsal stream is intrinsically related to reading, then we should be able to demonstrate that training the dorsal
stream independently of reading increases reading speed and/or accuracy. However, little
research has actually been done in this area.

Lorusso et al. (2006) and Solan et al. (2004) demonstrated increased sensitivity with
dyslexic children on reading measures such as reading speed and word-attack. However,
in both studies it is unclear if the visual training was uniquely responsible for the better
reading scores. For example, in Lorusso et al.'s study, the children were trained on fast
attentional shifting, but the stimuli to be detected were words that 'became increasingly
difficult in terms of word length and complexity of spelling' (p. 201).Thus it is difficult to
disentangle whether it was the effect of practice in attentional shifting, or exposure to
increasingly more difficult words, that increased reading speed and accuracy.

Conlon et al. (2009) demonstrated that coherent motion thresholds improved for dyslexic readers after a single practice trial. The same practice did not significantly improve
the sensitivity of the control readers and despite the improvement in motion threshold in
the dyslexic readers they remained significantly less sensitive than the normal readers. The
improvement in only one practice session is remarkable, and begs the question whether
sensitivity in the dyslexic readers would have normalized with further practice. Similarly,
Fischer and Harnegg (2000) trained children for 3 weeks on a saccadic control task. After
the training period the children's saccadic control measures normalized to those of the
control children. However, while these studies demonstrated that it is possible to improve

visual sensitivity in dyslexic readers, there is no indication as to whether or not this translates into improved reading or word decoding. Moreover, it could be possible that training the dorsal stream in a way that would translate into increased word decoding skills, may need to be more targeted, and commensurate with the role that the dorsal stream is suggested to play in word decoding and reading. In other words, if the dorsal stream is involved in word decoding by virtue of its physiological role in preattentive coding and synthesizing the spatial qualities of text, then it may be exactly this aspect of dorsal processing that needs to be trained in order to translate into improved reading skills. Candidates for such training might be *visual search*, *attentional blink*, and *change detection*.

Change detection is a task in which two visual scenes are presented quickly one after the other with a short blank period in between. From scene one to scene two a change occurs; the colour of the bus, the presence of a tree, for example. The object is to identify what, if anything, changed from scene one to scene two. *Attentional blink* is the observation that when required to detect two targets in a stream of items (target 1 and target 2), the second target (T2) is harder to detect if it is presented between 300–500 ms after T1, resulting in what has been called an 'attentional blink' (Raymond et al., 1992). In *visual search* a number of objects are presented on the screen and the object is to search the display for the target object—the red circle within a random search array of blue circles and red squares—for example.

For our purposes, the critical element in these tasks is the requirement for fast spatial coding of a cluttered visual scene—a requirement that is explicitly the domain of the dorsal pathway. Indeed neurophysiological studies have implicated the dorsal pathway in change detection (Beck et al., 2001, 2006; Tseng et al., 2010), attentional blink (Shapiro, 2009), and visual search (refer to Behrmann et al. (2004) for a review), refer to Fig. 9.4 for

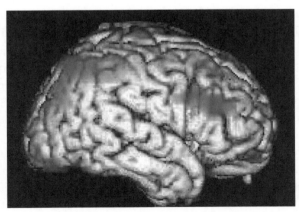

Fig. 9.4 (Also see Colour plate 3.) Brain activity in a change blindnesss task when participants detected the change from scene 1 to scene 2. Once again, note the engagement of the PPc consistent with the activation that occurs when decoding single words that have had their internal configuration spatially disrupted. Reprinted by permission from Macmillan Publishers Ltd: *Nature Neuroscience*, 4(6), Diane M. Beck, Geraint Rees, Christopher D. Frith, and Nilli Lavie, Neural correlates of change detection and change blindness, p. 464, copyright (2001).

an example. Moreover, visual search is impaired in dyslexic readers (e.g. Vidyasagar & Pammer, 1999), as is change detection (Rutkowski et al., 2003) and attentional blink (McLean et al., 2009).

Therefore, the evidence suggests that the dorsal pathway is intrinsically involved in word decoding by virtue of its role in the sequential analysis of the spatial components of word and word elements. Therefore acquiring good reading skills should be dependent upon the development of good visuo-spatial coding skills. Subsequently, it is not unreasonable to predict that visuo-perceptual training in non-linguistic tasks that draw heavily on the same spatial coding of symbols required for reading—such as change blindness and visual search—should translate into better reading and/or word decoding skills. However, this possibility is still speculative and currently under investigation in our laboratory.

Conclusions

Like most of the chapters here, this section is designed to characterize in some way the significance of the cognitive-perceptual processing that occurs in the very early stages of reading. While enormous scientific effort has been dedicated to examining the 'higher-order' components of the reading network, relatively little is known about the functioning and significance of the early stages (see Fig. 9.5) and in many cases an assumption is

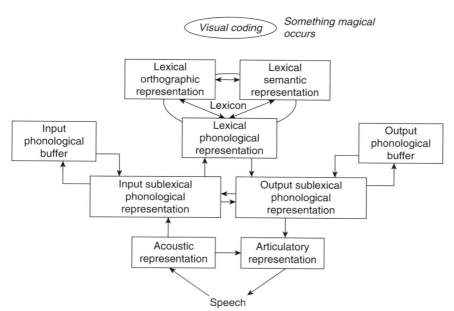

Fig. 9.5 Adapted from Ramus and Szenkovits' excellent review of phonological coding on reading. I have facetiously added the top 'box' in which visual coding occurs. Adapted from What phonological deficit? Franck Ramus and Gayaneh Szenkovits, *Quarterly Journal of Experimental Psychology*, © 2008 Taylor & Francis, reprinted by permission of the publisher (Taylor & Francis Ltd, http://www.tandf.co.uk/journals).

made that information gets from the page to the higher cortical centres, but the significance of such mechanisms remains elusive.

The evidence presented here and elsewhere is that there is no magical process that transmits visual information from the page to the cortical reading network. It is a highly sophisticated neural exchange with a dynamic transfer of information between the visual centres. Word recognition—identifying common words, decoding unfamiliar words, and recognizing orthographically similar words such as 'form' and 'from' is dependent upon fast spatial coding which is the domain of the dorsal visual pathway. It is likely that disruption to this process could cause a significant 'knock-on' effect throughout the network resulting in poor word decoding and reading skills. Thus, the evaluation of dorsally-mediated spatial tasks as a viable training tool in reading is a sensible step forward in this area.

References

Au, A., & Lovegrove, B. (2001). Temporal processing ability in above average and average readers. *Perception and Psychophysics*, 63, 148–55.

Bar, M., Kassam, K., Ghuman, A., Boshyan, J., Schmid, A., Dale, A.M., *et al.* (2006). Top-down facilitation of visual recognition. *Proceedings of the National Academy of Sciences of the United States of America*, 103, 449–54

Beck, D.M., Rees, G., Frith, C.D., & Lavie, N. (2001). Neural correlates of change detection and change blindness. *Nature Neuroscience*, 4, 645–50.

Beck, D.M., Muggleton, N., Walsh, V., & Lavie, N. (2006). Right parietal cortex plays a critical role in change blindness. *Cerebral Cortex*, 16, 712–17.

Behrmann, M., Geng, J.J., & Shomstein, S. (2004). Parietal cortex and attention. *Current Opinion in Neurobiology*, 14, 212–17.

Beneventi, H., Tonnessen, F., Ersland, L., & Hugdahl, K. (2010). Executive working memory processes in dyslexia; Behavioral and fMRI evidence. *Scandinavian Journal of Psychology*, 51, 192–202.

Braet, W., & Humphreys, G. (2006). Case mixing and the right parietal cortex: evidence from rTMS. *Experimental Brain Research*, 168, 265–71.

Bressler, S., Tang, W., Sylvester, C., Shulman, G., & Corbetta, M. (2008). Top-down control of human visual cortex by frontal and parietal cortex in anticipatory visual spatial attention. *Journal of Neuroscience*, 28, 10056–61.

Bullier, J. (2001). Integrated model of visual processing. *Brain Research Reviews*, 36, 96–107.

Colby, C., & Goldberg, M. (1999). Space and attention in parietal cortex. *Annual Review of Neuroscience*, 22, 319–49.

Conlon, E., Sanders, M., & Wright, C. (2009). Relationships between global motion and global form processing, practice, cognitive and visual processing in adults with dyslexia or visual discomfort. *Neuropsychologia*, 47, 907–15.

Corbetta, M., & Shulman, G. (2002). Control of goal-directed and stimulus-driven attention in the brain. *Nature Reviews; Neuroscience*, 3, 201–15.

Cornelissen, P., Richardson, A., Mason, A., Fowler, S., & Stein, J. (1995) Contrast sensitivity and coherent motion detection measured at photopic luminance levels in dyslexics and controls. *Vision Research* 35, 1483–94.

Cornelissen, P., Hansen, P., Gilchrist, I., Cormack, F., Essex J., & Frankish, C. (1998). Coherent motion detection and letter position encoding. *Vision Research*, 38, 2181–91.

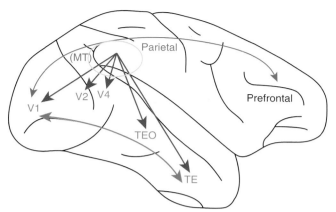

Colour plate 1 (Also see Fig. 9.1.) A model of interactions between different components of the visual cortex. The PPc is indicated by the yellow circle. Reprinted from *Brain Research Reviews*, 30(1), Trichur Raman Vidyasagar, A neuronal model of attentional spotlight: parietal guiding the temporal, pp. 69, Copyright (1990), with permission from Elsevier.

Shifted words ROI
100–300 ms, 35–40 Hz

Shifted words vs. Words ROI
100–300 ms, 35–40 Hz

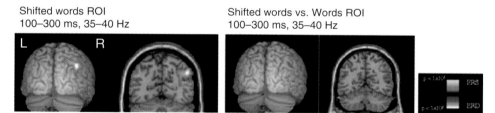

Colour plate 2 (Also see Fig. 9.3.) The MEG signal in the PPc is much stronger in the Shifted Words condition as represented in the left figure. The right figure is the contrast between the 'Normal' and the 'Shifted' words conditions. The signals were high frequency at 35–40 Hz, and was maximal within 300 ms of the presentation of the word.

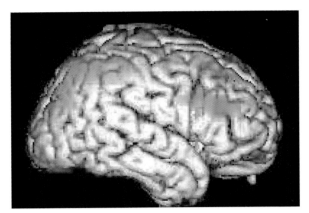

Colour plate 3 (Also see Fig. 9.4.) Brain activity in a change blindnesss task when participants detected the change from scene 1 to scene 2. Once again, note the engagement of the PPc consistent with the activation that occurs when decoding single words that have had their internal configuration spatially disrupted. Reprinted by permission from Macmillan Publishers Ltd: *Nature Neuroscience*, 4(6), Diane M. Beck, Geraint Rees, Christopher D. Frith, and Nilli Lavie, Neural correlates of change detection and change blindness, p. 464, copyright (2001).

Ellis, A., Young, A., & Flude, B. (1993). Neglect and visual language. In: I.H. Robinson & J.C. Marshall (Eds.) *Unilateral Neglect: Clinical and Experimental Studies*, pp. 233–55. Hillsdale, NJ: Lawrence Erlbaum Associates Inc.

Fischer, B., & Hartnegg, K. (2000). Effects of visual training on saccade and control in dyslexia. *Perception*, 29, 531–42.

Friedmann, N., & Gvion, A. (2001). Letter position dyslexia. *Cognitive Neuropsychology*, 18, 673–96.

Greenwald, M., & Berndt, R. (1999). Impaired encoding of abstract letter order: Severe alexia in a mildly aphasic patient. *Cognitive Neuropsychology*, 16, 513–56.

Hall, D., Humphreys, G., & Cooper, A.(2001). Neuropsychological evidence for case-specific reading: Multiletter units in visual word recognition. *Quarterly Journal of Experimental Psychology*, 54A, 439–67.

Hämäläinen, M., Hari, R., Ilmoniemi, R., Knuutila, J., & Lounasmaa, O. (1993). Magnetoencephalography—theory, instrumentation, and applications to noninvasive studies of the working human brain. *Reviews of Modern Physics*, 65, 413–97.

Hendry, S., & Reid, C. (2000). The koniocellular pathway in primate vision. *Annual Review of Neuroscience*, 23, 127–53.

Kevan, A., & Pammer, K. (2008). Visual deficits in in pre-readers at familial risk for dyslexia. *Vision Research*, 48, 2835–9.

Kevan, A., & Pammer, A. (2009). Predicting early reading skills from pre-reading measures of dorsal stream functioning. *Neuropsychologia*, 47, 3174–81.

Lamme, V.A., & Roelfsema, P.R. (2000). The distinct modes of vision offered by feedforward and recurrent processing. *Trends in Neuroscience*, 23, 571–9.

Lauritzen, T., D'Esposito, M., Heeger, D., & Silver, M. (2009). Top-down flow of visual spatial attention signals from parietal to occipital cortex. *Journal of Vision*, 9, 1–14.

Laycock, R., Crewther, D., Fitzgerald, P.B., & Crewther, S. (2007). Evidence for fast signals and later processing in human V1/V2 and V5/MT+: A TMS study of motion perception. *Journal of Neurophysiology*, 98, 1253–62.

Lee, B., Suh, M., Kim, E-J., Seo, S., Choi, K., Kim, G-M., *et al.* (2009). Neglect dyslexia: Frequency, association with other hemispatial neglects, and lesion localization. *Neuropsychologia*, 47, 704–10.

Levi, T., Walsh, V., & Lavidor, M. (2010). Dorsal stream modulation of visual word recognition in skilled readers. *Vision Research*, 50, 883–8.

Livingstone, M., & Hubel, D. (1988). Segregation of form, colour, movement and depth: anatomy, physiology and perception. *Science*, 240, 740–9.

Livingstone, M., Rosen, G., Drislane, F., & Galaburda, A. (1991). Physiological and anatomical evidence for a magnocellular defect in developmental dyslexia, *Proceedings of the National Academy of Sciences of the United States of America*, 88, 7943–7.

Logothetis, N., & Sheinberg, D. (1996). Visual object recognition. *Annual Review of Neuroscience*, 19, 577–621.

Lorusso, M.L., Facoetti, A., Paganoni, P., Pezzani, M., & Molteni, M. (2006) Effects of visual hemisphere-specific stimulation versus reading-focused training in dyslexic children. *Neuropsychological Rehabilitation*, 16, 194–212.

Lovegrove, W.J., Bowling, A., Badcock, B., & Blackwood, M. (1980). Specific reading disability: differences in contrast sensitivity as a function of spatial frequency. *Science*, 210, 439–440.

Mayall, K., Humphreys, G., Mechelli, A., Olson, A., & Price, C. (2001). The effects of case mixing on word recognition: Evidence from a PET study. *Journal of Cognitive Neuroscience*, 13, 844–53.

McLean, G.M.T., Stuart, G.W., Visser, T.A.W., & Castles, A. (2009). The attentional blink in developing readers. *Scientific Studies of Reading*, 13, 334–57.

Maunsell, J., Nealey, T., & DePriest, D. (1990). Magnocellular and parvocellular contributions to responses in the middle temporal visual area (MT) of the macaque monkey. *Journal of Neuroscience*, 10, 3323–34.

Merigan, W., & Maunsell, J. (1993). How parallel are the primate visual pathways? *Annual Review of Neuroscience*, 16, 369–402.

Mesulam, M. (1999) Spatial attention and neglect: parietal, frontal and cingulate contributions to the mental representation and attentional targeting of salient extrapersonal events. *Philosophical Transactions of the Royal Society of London B Biological Sciences*, 354, 1325–46.

Noudoost, B., Chang, M., Steinmetz, N., & Moore, T. (2010). Top-down control of visual attention. *Current Opinion in Neurobiology*, 20, 183–90.

Pammer, K., & Wheatley, C. (2001). Isolating the M(y)-cell response in dyslexia using the spatial frequency doubling illusion. *Vision Research*, 41, 2139–47.

Pammer, K., Lavis, R., Cooper, C., Hansen, P., & Cornelissen, P. (2005). Symbol-string sensitivity and adult performance in lexical decision. *Brain and Language*, 94, 278–96.

Pammer, K., Hansen, P., Holliday, I., & Cornelissen, P. (2006). Attentional shifting and the role of the dorsal pathway in visual word recognition. *Neuropsychologia*, 44, 2926–36.

Petrich, J., Greenwald, M., & Berndt, R. (2007). An investigation of attentional contributions to visual errors in right 'neglect dyslexia'. *Cortex*, 43, 1036–46.

Poljac, E., Simon, S., Ringlever, L., Kalcik, D., Groen, W., Buitelaar, J., *et al.* (2010). Impaired task switching performance in children with dyslexia but not children with autism. *Quarterly Journal of Experimental Psychology*, 63, 401–16.

Posner, M.I. (1980). Orienting of attention. *Quarterly Journal of Experimental Psychology*, 32, 3–25.

Posner, M.I., & Petersen, S.E. (1990). The attention system of the human brain. *Annual Reviews Neuroscience*, 13, 25–42.

Pulvermüller, F., Birbaumer, N., Lutzenberger, W., & Mohr, B. (1997). High-frequency brain activity: Its possible role in attention, perception and language processing. *Progress in Neurobiology*, 52, 427–45.

Ramus, F., & Szenkovits, G. (2008). What phonological deficit? *The Quarterly Journal of Experimental Psychology*, 61, 129–41.

Raymond, J., Shapiro, K., & Arnell, K. (1992). Temporary suppression of visual processing in an RSVP task: An attentional blink? *Journal of Experimental Psychology: Human Perception and Performance*, 18, 849–60.

Rutkowski, J., Crewther, D., & Crewther, S. (2003). Change detection in impaired in children with dyslexia. *Journal of Vision*, 3, 95–105.

Saalman, Y., Pigarev, I., & Vidyasagar, T. (2007). Neural mechanisms of visual attention: How top-down feedback highlights relevant locations. *Science*, 316, 1612–15.

Shapiro, K. (2009). The functional architecture of divided visual attention. *Progress in Brain Research*, 176, 101–21.

Shallice, T., & Warrington, E. (1977). The possible role of selective attention in acquired dyslexia. *Neuropsychologia*, 15, 31–41.

Shomstein, S., & Behrmann, M. (2006). Objects modulate competition in human parietal and extrastriate cortices. *Proceedings of the National Academy of Sciences of the United States of America*, 103, 11387–92.

Skottun, B. (2000). The magnocellular deficit theory of dyslexia: the evidence from contrast sensitivity. *Vision Research*, 40, 111–27.

Skottun, B., & Skoyles, J. (2010). L-and M-cone ratios and magnocellular sensitivity in reading. *International Journal of Neuroscience*, 120, 241–4.

Snowling, M. (2000). *Dyslexia* (2nd edn). Oxford: Blackwell.

Solan, H., Shelley-Tremblay, J., Hansen, P., Silverman, M., Larson, S., & Ficarra, A. (2004) M-cell deficit and reading disability: a preliminary study of the effects of temporal vision-processing therapy. *Optometry*, 75, 640–50.

Sommer, W., Kraft, A., Schmidt, S., Olma, M., & Brandt, S. (2008). Dynamic spatial coding within the dorsal fronto-parietal network during a visual search task. *PLoS ONE*, 3, 1–10.

Starr, M., & Rayner, K. (2001). Eye movements during reading; Some current controversies. *Trends in Cognitive Sciences*, 5, 156–63.

Stein, J. (2001). The magnocellular theory of developmental dyslexia. *Dyslexia*, 7, 12–36.

Stein, J., & Walsh, V. (1997). To see but not to read; the magnocellular theory of dyslexia. *Trends in Neurosciences*, 20, 147–52.

Talcott, J., Hansen, P., Willis-Owen, C., McKinnell, I., Richardson, A., & Stein, J. (1998). Visual magnocellular impairment in adult developmental dyslexics. *Neuro-ophthalomology*, 60, 187–201.

Tseng, P., Hsu, T.Y., Muggleton, N.G., Tzeng, O.J., Hung, D.L., & Juan, C.H. (2010). Posterior parietal cortex mediates encoding and maintenance processes in change blindness. *Neuropsychologia*, 48, 1063–70.

Van Essen, D. (1985). Functional organisation of primate visual cortex. In: J.E. Peters (Ed.) *Cerebral Cortex*, Vol 3, pp. 259–329. New York: Plenum.

Vidyasagar, T.R. (1998). Gating of neuronal responses in macaque primary visual cortex by an attentional spotlight. *Neuroreport*, 9, 1947–52.

Vidyasagar, T.R. (1999). A neuronal model of attentional spotlight: parietal guiding the temporal *Brain Research Reviews*, 30, 66–76.

Vidyasagar, T.R., & Pammer, K. (1999). Impaired visual search in dyslexia relates to the role of the magnocellular pathway in attention. *NeuroReport*, 10, 1283–7.

Vidyasagar, T.R., & Pammer, K. (2010). Dyslexia: A deficit in visuo-spatial attention, not phonological processing. *Trends in Cognitive Sciences*, 14, 57–63.

Chapter 10

Aetiology of Dyslexia: A Visual Perspective on a Phonological Marker

Trichur R. Vidyasagar

Over the last many decades, a number of theories have been proposed as the basic cause of dyslexia, but the most dominant of them has been the idea that it is caused by a phonological deficit (reviewed in Goswami & Bryant, 1990; Shaywitz & Shaywitz, 2005; Goswami, 2011). This concept has received most of its support from the profound deficits in phonological awareness commonly seen in most children with developmental dyslexia (reviewed in Ramus, 2003). Furthermore, many of these children also show deficits in auditory processing (Tallal, 1980), especially for rapidly presented stimuli. These experiments have been taken as supporting the thesis that dyslexia is fundamentally a problem within the stream that processes auditory signals to extract the phonological building blocks, with no causative factor within the visual system.

However, there are good reasons to doubt that this idea of a phonological aetiology is the whole story. While there is a strong correlation between phonological deficits and reading disabilities, no causal link has yet been established (Castles & Coltheart, 2004). Not all those with dyslexia have phonological difficulties and there are also those with significant phonological deficits but no accompanying reading impairment (Castles & Coltheart, 1993, 2004; Broom & Doctor, 1995; Hanley & Gard, 1995; Valdois et al., 2003; Tree & Kay, 2006). Furthermore, in the hierarchy of neural stages involved in reading, vision occurs before grapheme–phoneme correspondence and so it is important to exclude upstream deficits in visual or orthographic processing that could lead to impaired reading and even poor development of phonological skills before attributing the core deficit to a downstream process.

This chapter makes a case that even if we are to exclude cases of 'surface dyslexia' which exhibit no phonological deficits, developmental dyslexia should still be considered as arising primarily in the visual system, with deficits in phonological processing being either a consequence of impairments in orthographic processing or at best an independent contributory factor in a multifactorial disorder that primarily arises from a defect within the visual pathways.

Spatiotemporal parsing of the visual input—an essential step in reading

Reading and writing are very recent developments in the history of our species and it is unlikely that the underlying mechanisms that enable them evolved specifically for this purpose. It is far more likely that humans are using neural systems that had originally evolved for some other purpose. Stanislas Dehaene (2005) has coined the term 'neuronal recycling' to describe how culture has exploited evolutionarily long-established neuronal systems to enable functions such as reading and arithmetic. He reviews the case for specific areas in the human brain that evolved for other purposes, but are nevertheless well suited for reading, such as parts of the left occipitotemporal cortex and more specifically, the visual word form area (VWFA) or the 'letterbox' area (Dehaene, 2009). The human occipitotemporal cortex has been shown to be involved in object recognition, with subdivisions of it being specialized for different categories such as places, houses, faces, words, and objects (Puce et al., 1996; Kanwisher et al., 1997; Ishai et al., 1999; Haxby et al., 2001; Malach et al., 2002). These studies show that there is a gradient across these areas that goes from analysis of fine form laterally to large forms such as landscapes and houses medially. The VWFA is possibly just an area among these modules which deals with representations of objects of a particular spatial scale (Dehaene, 2009). The human cortical region for object identification has also its homologue in the inferotemporal cortex of the macaque brain as revealed in the many studies of the activity of single neurons in the awake, trained macaque (Sary et al., 1993; Logothetis et al., 1995; Tanaka, 1996; Tamura & Tanaka, 2001; Vogels & Biederman, 2002).

Having a cortical area that is specialized for recognizing the forms of letters that go to make up words is by itself far from sufficient to recognize the words. There is another fundamental issue in pattern recognition that goes hand in hand with having an area that has stored representations for letters. The electrophysiological studies previously cited have not only shown that neurons in these areas respond specifically for complex shapes, faces, letters, etc., but that they also show remarkable invariance across many dimensions, such as position, illumination, size, rotation, contrast, etc. Such invariance permits us to identify, for example, a letter whatever its font-size, font-type, rotation, location in the visual field, or perspective. However, such object identification is associated with a problem—because of loss of information about specific variants. Thus, for example, when information on location is lost (as in the large receptive fields of inferotemporal neurons), it can be problematic in tasks where such position information of the identified object is necessary for meaningful perception, as in reading text. Furthermore, since different attributes of an object such as colour, form, depth, etc. are processed in separate cortical areas (Zeki, 1978; Ungerleider & Mishkin, 1982; Livingstone & Hubel, 1988; Merigan & Maunsell, 1993; Logothetis & Scheinberg, 1996), there emerges also the binding problem (Treisman, 1996) of how the attributes of each object can be correctly recombined and perceived. This is a particularly challenging issue when we consider the natural world which is usually a clutter of innumerable objects.

The solution that the visual system might have developed to solve this conundrum is what is proposed here as the primary neuronal process that is also 'recycled' to enable reading; its derangement may underlie dyslexia (Vidyasagar, 1999, 2001). As a solution to the binding problem, one set of models (Treisman & Gelade, 1980; Wolfe, 1994; Vidyasagar, 1999) has proposed that a 'spotlight of attention' acting at a relatively early stage in the visual pathways selects just one location or object to be processed at any one time. Thus, say, when one is looking for a face in a crowd, a serial search is executed across the items until the face one is looking for is identified. Since each object is processed sequentially, though it takes more time as set size increases, the system is able to process and combine the attributes of each item correctly. It has been proposed (Vidyasagar, 1999) that the same mechanism of visual search is 'recycled' for reading, allocating attentional resources to one or two letters at a time. This process, as explained later, requires a complex interplay between different submodalities of the afferent visual pathway and between different cortical areas.

The visual signals from the eyes are carried in three parallel submodalities—magnocellular, parvocellular, and koniocellular—up to V1, from where two streams carry these further, one along a dorsal route into the parietal cortex and the other along a ventral route into the temporal neocortex (e.g. Livingstone & Hubel, 1988). The dorsal stream that is also dominated by the fast magnocellular pathway is concerned more with the spatial locations and relations of objects and mediates associated perceptual functions such as motion and depth perception that are essential for action. On the other hand, the ventral stream, which gets most of the parvocellular inputs, is largely concerned with identification of objects, such as letters in a written script (Ungerleider & Mishkin, 1982; Livingstone & Hubel, 1988; Goodale & Milner, 1992). Thus spatial locations of objects are well coded in the dorsal stream, whereas the features themselves are only crudely processed there, but in fine detail in the ventral stream. It has been proposed that the dorsal stream, which gets a dominant magnocellular input, may use the spatial map of the locations of objects to direct a spotlight of attention to gate responses in area V1 or areas along the ventral stream (Vidyasagar, 1999). That the receptive fields of neurons along the ventral stream get larger and larger from V1 to the subsequent pattern processing areas also means that the site along this line of cortical areas where the spotlight of attention is targeted may depend upon the degree of clutter and the size of objects in the visual scene. The gating at a small spatial scale that feedback to area V1 may enable, needs to happen only when there is a lot of clutter with a large number of small-sized objects. In the presence of many distracters, gating on a fine-grain retinotopic map is necessary to facilitate processing of the each restricted portion of the visual field to the exclusion of the rest. In situations where not much clutter is present and there are only one or two objects present in the visual field, as indeed in many highly controlled, classical visual physiology experiments, the attentional gating does not need the involvement of the fine-grain map of area V1. This may be the reason why in early experiments that looked for attentional effects in macaque V1, little top-down influences were observed (Mohler & Wurtz, 1977), whereas in later experiments in macaques (Motter, 1993; Vidyasagar, 1998) and humans (Brefzynski & DeYoe, 1999; Somers et al., 1999), which introduced clutter in the visual scene, significant attentional gating was clearly demonstrated.

The neural substrate that underlies such a gating process is likely to be the synchronized neuronal oscillations that have recently received much attention. It is now being increasingly appreciated that temporal coding by way of synchronized oscillations plays an important role in brain function. Electrophysiological studies in macaques have shown that neuronal activity entrained in specific oscillatory frequencies mediate both synchronized activity within cortical areas (Eckhorn et al., 1988; Gray et al., 1989; Womelsdorf et al., 2007) and between cortical areas (Buschman & Miller, 2007; Saalmann et al., 2007; Gregoriou et al., 2009). In a study on macaques (Saalmann et al., 2007), spatial attention within the lateral intraparietal area (LIP) was shown to be carried by oscillations in the frequency range of 20–45 Hz and this activity led to synchrony with the retinotopically corresponding region in an earlier visual area, namely area MT (middle temporal). Such top-down modulation of activity in area MT was instrumental in mediating facilitation of responses in area MT at the attended location and suppression of responses in unattended locations. Such feedback further down to even earlier visual areas, such as area V1 (primary visual cortex) has been postulated (Vidyasagar, 1999, 2001) to underlie the attention-related responses seen in area V1, both in single-unit studies (Motter, 1993; Vidyasagar, 1998; McAdams & Reid, 2005; Vidyasagar & Pigarev, 2007) and in human brain imaging (Brefzynski & DeYoe, 1999; Gandhi et al., 2001; Simola et al., 2009). The main purpose of such a feedback may be to select at the level of V1, neuronal representations of specific objects for further detailed processing along the ventral stream.

I suggest that such spatiotemporal parsing of the visual input that originally evolved to solve the problem of visual search in a cluttered environment and also to solve the binding problem in perception, has been exploited in recent human history to enable reading (Vidyasagar, 1999, 2001; Vidyasagar & Pammer, 1999). In processing a text, such as the one you are reading now, one usually fixates at a point for about 250 ms, taking in seven or eight letters and then one makes a saccade to a new fixation point along the line. In doing so, if the brain were to process these letters in parallel during any of the fixation periods, the high density of the many small visual patterns forming the letters would make it impossible for a pattern recognition system with position invariance to order the letters in their proper spatial sequence. On the other hand, a serial, sequential processing of the letters could enable the ventral stream to process just one or two letters at a time. The magnocellular inputs to the dorsal stream probably only have the spatial resolution to resolve the presence of letters and thus code their locations, but not to resolve the fine detail that would enable recognizing them. Nevertheless these signals that code the locations of the letters could help in gating the stream of letters into the ventral stream in a temporal sequence, so that the letters can be recognized individually (or in pairs or triplets). The temporal sequence of this process automatically provides the spatial sequence of the letters, which would otherwise be lost in a pattern recognition system with position invariance. A somewhat similar suggestion, that a serial left-to right allocation of attention is needed for reading non-words was also made by Cestnick and Coltheart (1999). Accuracy in letter-position encoding is predicted by performance in a (magno-mediated) coherent motion detection task (Cornelissen et al., 1998), indicating that a gating feedback function by the dorsal stream may be critical for reading.

Most probably, a similar process happening in the auditory system is what enables communication by spoken language. There is now considerable evidence that the human auditory system not only has a spectrum of channels each sensitive to a relatively narrow range of sound frequencies, but that it is also sensitive to amplitude modulation occurring across these frequency channels and on different timescales (for review, see Joris et al., 2004).

In decoding speech, it uses such amplitude modulation at different timescales as a way of sampling syllables and phonemes (Luo & Poeppel, 2007; Schroeder et al., 2008; Kerlin et al., 2010). While such temporal sampling may be a ubiquitous way of attention select-ing parcels of sensory inputs for detailed processing in each sensory modality, it acquires a unique status in the case of reading, involving temporal sampling in two different modalities. During early language training, when the child is only exposed to spoken words, temporal sampling in the auditory domain is essential for segmenting words into syllables and phonemes, creating onset/rime and in developing phonological awareness (reviewed in Goswami, 2011). The auditory lexicon so developed is admittedly the one used by the child to access the meanings of known words when it begins to read. However, it is important to note that as the child learns to read and even after many months when s/he has learnt to recognize letters, only short words with big letters and with little crowd-ing are presented to the child. While children easily learn many spoken words in a day, why is actual reading so difficult, even for those children who will eventually become good readers? Is it simply the learning of the correspondence between a visual object and its corresponding sound (in the case of reading, the grapheme–phoneme correspond-ence) that is difficult? That is unlikely, since children are generally very good at learning their auditory counterparts, i.e. spoken names, of new objects that are shown to them.

In the case of reading, the real difficulty, I believe, is in the processing within the visual system. As the child is exposed to the first written letters and words and 'taught to read', visual attentional mechanisms are put on great demand to focus attention on one letter at a time and to parse the letter stream in the right order at the appropriate locations and in the right direction—say, right to left in English around the fixation point. If the same attentional mechanisms used for serial visual search are used in this process, one particu-lar difficulty to be gotten over is the fact that the visual search mechanism that evolution has given us is a relatively random process which does not usually have to perform a sys-tematic search. It does not keep a meticulous memory of where it has been to avoid these locations, but performs a nearly random run of the items until the target is found (Horowitz & Wolfe, 1998). For reading, however, this neural network needs to learn to move the spotlight of attention, not randomly across the items in a text, but sequentially and in a particular direction. This probably takes years to perfect and may explain how slowly most children learn to read, compared to so many other areas in life where chil-dren learn the task very much faster. It is commonplace that, even though the visual acu-ity of children entering primary school is adequate to resolve small print, their books have large letters, fewer words, and avoid word clutter. Even then, the processing of the graph-emes is at a much slower pace than the rate of phonemes and syllables in spoken language with which they are already familiar. With the spoken words that they easily comprehend, the phonemes and syllables already occur at a much faster rate. Thus slowness in learning to read may have little to do with phonological difficulties. Over the years, as they get better and better at reading, the speed of reading eventually gets much faster than speech. That speaking words in all languages is slower than the average speed of adult reading may be simply due to the fact that speech is a social act and so the speed has to be limited by the necessity to cater to everyone, including the slower members of the social group.

On the other hand, reading to oneself does not have that restriction and can get developed to a very fast speed. All these considerations point to the fact that the temporal sampling that occurs in the visual pathways during reading, parallel to that in the auditory system when we listen to speech, can be an independent and possibly the main rate-limiting step in reading. However, it eventually achieves in most people a higher temporal efficiency than spoken language.

Dyslexia as a disorder of visuo-spatial attention

Against the backdrop described so far regarding the neural processes possibly involved in reading, it would not be unreasonable to speculate that a disorder affecting the operation of the spatiotemporal parsing of the text could lead to impaired reading (Vidyasagar, 1999, 2001; Vidyasagar & Pammer, 2010). The basic defect could be anywhere along the visual pathway from the retina to the VWFA that compromises the speed and accuracy with which individual letters or graphemes are recognized before the information is transmitted for performing the grapheme–phoneme correspondence. Among the studies of essential visual perceptual functions such as visual acuity, none have suggested a specific deficit in the parvocellular pathways, but there are many which have found magnocellular impairments (e.g. Lovegrove et al., 1980, 1986; Livingstone et al., 1991; Cornelissen et al., 1995; Eden et al., 1996; Stein & Walsh, 1997; Pammer & Wheatley, 2001; Solan et al., 2004). While some studies have failed to find an association between developmental dyslexia and a magnocellular deficit (Williams et al., 2003; Heim et al., 2010), it should be noted that the crucial magnocellular deficit need only be in a very restricted portion of the visual field near the centre of the fovea or the deficit could be further in dorsal stream cortical areas or even with the top-down spatiotemporal parsing of the parvocellular input going into the ventral stream. However, a common outcome for any of these lesions would be impaired attentional gating at the spatiotemporal scale required for normal reading and thus a poorer and/or slower letter stream entering the VWFA (Vidyasagar, 1999).

In support of this suggestion, there is now an impressive list of studies that have shown poorer visuo-spatial attention among dyslexic children (Casco et al., 1996; Hari et al., 1999, 2001; Vidyasagar & Pammer, 1999; Facoetti et al., 2000, 2008, 2009, 2010; Facoetii & Molteni, 2001; Rutkowski et al., 2003; Bednarek et al., 2004; Kinsey et al., 2004; Pammer et al., 2004; Schulte-Körne et al., 2004; Valdois et al., 2004; Strasburger, 2005; Thomson et al., 2005; Valdois et al., 2006; Bosse et al., 2007; Dubois et al., 2007; Roach & Hogben, 2007; Solan et al., 2007; Dhar et al., 2008; Kevan & Pammer, 2008; Jones et al., 2008; Bosse & Valdois, 2009; Ruffino et al., 2010). Apart from these studies which have shown direct deficits in some aspect or other of visual attention itself, many other studies have shown deficits at one or other level of the visual pathway that can potentially compromise the ability to perform efficient spatiotemporal parsing of the letter stream. This includes not only impairments that could be attributed to the early magnocellular pathways themselves, but also to any of the dorsal stream functions such as directional motion contrast sensitivity (Slaghuis & Ryan, 2006), visual motion sensitivity (Cornelissen et al., 1995;

Eden et al., 1996), visual sensitivity measured by the magno-mediated frequency doubling illusion (Pammer & Kevan, 2007), motion onset visual-evoked potentials (Schulte-Körne et al., 2004), Ternus apparent motion task (Cestnick & Coltheart, 1999; Davis et al., 2001), etc. For a comprehensive review of possible dorsal stream contributions to developmental disorders including dyslexia, see Grinter et al. (2010).

By now, as cited earlier, there are a large number of studies that are consistent with a possible causal link between attentional deficits and dyslexia, but few that have come up with a negative result with the possible exception of just one study (Ziegler et al., 2010). The main challenge to this view does not derive from experimental findings, but rather from the commentaries of Skoyles and Skottun (e.g. Skoyles & Skottun, 2004) that there is an inherent 'control group fallacy' in all the experimental work linking either attentional or magnocellular deficits to dyslexia. Their claim goes like this: since dyslexics form only a small proportion in the population (4–15%) even if this group have a higher proportion of subjects with magnocellular deficits, the numbers of those with magnocellular disorders who are not dyslexic will be higher than those with dyslexia. Using the figures published by Lovegrove et al. (1986), Skoyles & Skottun (2004) calculate that at a dyslexia prevalence of 4% in the population and a prevalence rate of magnocellular deficits in the dyslexic population of 75% and in the control population of 8%, there would be 2.56 times as many people with magnocellular deficits who will not have a reading problem, than those with dyslexia. They also point out that only at a dyslexia prevalence rate of 9.64 would the chances of those with magnocellular deficits also having dyslexia reach 50%.

However, this argument is misleading. While their argument is flawless to the point described earlier, they fail to continue their line of thought to the next step. If one does, their major argument gets turned on its head: while it is true that if you have a magnocellular deficit your chance of also being a dyslexic may be only 28% at a dyslexia prevalence rate of 4%, if you do *not* have a magnocellular deficit, your chance of being a dyslexic is far less. I calculate this to be 1.1%, using the same data that Skoyles and Skottun used. Thus, having a magnocellular deficit 'increases' the likelihood of having dyslexia 25 times! As in countless other relationships in clinical medicine (such as smoking and cancer or saturated fats and coronary artery disease), it appears that a child having a magnocellular deficit has a higher likelihood of having a reading disability as well. This argument applies also to the calculations that Skoyles and Skottun use elsewhere with regard to the visual attention data of Bosse et al. (2007) and Facoetti et al. (2010). Their argument is akin to questioning the relationship of smoking to cancer by pointing out that the majority of smokers do not develop lung cancer.

However, a more pertinent value of their line of argument would have been to raise the issue of (1) whether dyslexia could be a multifactorial disorder, with a visuo-spatial attentional deficit just being one of the main contributing factors (Bosse et al., 2007; Menghini et al., 2010) or (2) whether there is just one subset among the many types of attention that can potentially provide a perfect, diagnostic metric, explaining the full variance in reading skills. At present, the experimental evidence cannot make an unequivocal distinction between these two possibilities.

Phonological deficits—cause or symptom?

While there has been accumulating evidence in favour of a visual contribution to developmental dyslexia, the claim that poor phonological development is the main cause has become weaker. Firstly, the correlation between phonological deficits and developmental dyslexia has been found to be wanting in many cases (Castles & Coltheart, 1993, 2004; Broom & Doctor, 1995; Hanley & Gard, 1995; Valdois et al., 2003; Tree & Kay, 2006). Second, phonological representations themselves have been shown to be normal in dyslexic children, but it is the access to these representations that exhibit task-specific deficits (Ramus & Szenkovits, 2008).

Third, phonological training has not been shown to improve dyslexics' reading skills very much. Even in the earliest study that claimed a causal connection between sound categorization and reading and spelling abilities (Bradley & Bryant, 1983), the only group that improved significantly in reading and spelling was the group that received *both* visual spelling and auditory/phonological categorization training; they improved much more than those who received training only in auditory categorization. A number of other studies have shown that auditory training at different timescales may improve auditory skills, but it rarely generalizes to improve either phonological or reading skills (McAnally et al., 1997; Strehlow et al., 2006) More recently, an acoustic remediation programme (commercially available as FastForWord) was reported to improve language and reading skills (Tallal et al., 1996; Temple et al., 2003), but attempts to replicate the results by other groups that incorporated more rigorous controls, have not been successful (Hook et al., 2001; Pokorni et al., 2004; McArthur et al., 2008). Though the programme was effective in improving auditory processing skills, there were no comparable improvements in reading performance. In fact, in one study (Hook et al., 2001), reading scores did not improve with FastForWord, but they did with Orton–Gillingham training. It is noteworthy that the latter is an elaborate and highly structured multimodal training programme that combines visual, auditory, and kinaesthetic stimuli. Thus the improvements could partly or even all be due to the visual component of the training. The idea that temporal processing within the auditory system could be related to phonological skills (e.g. Tallal, 1980; Rey et al., 2002) has itself been questioned by other studies (e.g. Paul et al., 2006). Interestingly, Paula Tallal herself hinted at the possibility that auditory processing deficits are not the main cause of reading impairments (Tallal & Stark, 1982). They found that auditory processing deficits were not associated with reading impairments unless there were also impairments in spoken language.

Fourth, in contrast, orthographic training has actually been shown to improve phonological skills, leading to suggestions that the poorer phonological processing and phonemic awareness seen in dyslexics could be due to a deficit in the visual pathways. An early study by Ehri (1989) had already shown that phonological deficits tend to be seen mainly when children are not taught to read and spell. More recently, when literate and illiterate Portuguese-speaking women were compared in a well-controlled study, it was found that the illiterates had poorer phonemic awareness, especially as seen in their reproduction of pseudowords, but this improved after orthographic training (Reis & Castro-Caldas, 1997;

Castro-Caldas et al., 1998). Furthermore, there were even significant morphological changes in the brain that seemed to be related to acquisition of visual literacy. Significantly higher levels of activations were seen in a number of brain regions of literate subjects when they repeated pseudowords than in illiterates (Castro-Caldas et al., 1998, 1999; Petersson et al., 2007; Dehaene et al., 2010), indicating that the reading years of a child may actually help develop a parallel neural system. A study by Mann and Wimmer (2002) used the pedagogical differences in the way American and German kindergartners were taught reading to investigate the development of phonemic awareness and concluded that the awareness of phonemes develops primarily as a result of literacy training rather than spontaneously from listening to spoken words.

A good test for causality is a longitudinal design that can show that a deficit precedes and predicts reading skills and that appropriate training to ameliorate the deficit reduces the reading disability. Pre-school performance in coherent motion perception (Boets et al., 2006), visual contrast sensitivity (Kevan & Pammer, 2009) and temporal order judgement (Hood & Conlon, 2004) all predict reading skills in primary school. Though phonological skills may also predict reading skills, an upstream deficit in the visual system can potentially cause a reading impairment as well as cause or at least aggravate a phonological deficit, explaining the strong association between phonological deficits and reading difficulties.

As noted earlier, the effects of training in auditory processing on development of reading skills are equivocal, though it may improve phonological awareness. This is entirely consistent with the idea that the process of grapheme–phoneme correspondence is a quasi-independent process not necessarily helped by specific auditory training. If there is any improvement at all, it may be only in those cases where the auditory impairment is so severe that the original development of a phonemic memory itself had been affected.

Remediation studies using visual tasks are in their early days and more controlled studies are needed to establish their usefulness. However, the studies conducted so far, employing saccade control (Fischer & Hartnegg, 2000) visual-perceptual training (Solan et al., 2004), and visual attentional training (Lorusso et al., 2005) have all shown some promise. Furthermore, different subtypes of dyslexia are likely to respond to different training programmes as early studies seem to suggest (Lorusso et al., 2011).

Dyslexia as a deficit in the temporal sampling framework?—Yes, but where?

As a neural mechanism supporting the phonological theory, one influential suggestion has been that the deficit arises possibly out of a temporal processing disorder that would explain the deficits in rapid auditory processing and in the phonological awareness commonly seen in dyslexics (Tallal, 1980). In providing a detailed neural framework for such an aetiology, Usha Goswami (2011) argues that a deficit in temporal sampling at the rates that help in segmenting syllables within spoken words is the core deficit in dyslexia. This framework (with the acronym, TSF) proposes that the deficit is primarily in coding low frequency amplitude modulations and explains many features seen with auditory processing in dyslexics (McAnally & Stein, 1997; Witton et al., 1998; Lorenzi et al., 2000; Talcott etal. 2000; Abrams et al., 2009).

On the other hand, the temporal sampling deficit may be a generalized deficit affecting other sensory modalities as well, especially vision, or one affecting mainly the visual system. Goswami regards the visual system as doing a spatial sampling of the sensory input, while the auditory system is performing a temporal sampling of its acoustic input. However, even for static visual stimuli, when the target is embedded in a cluttered field, the visual system needs to perform both spatial and temporal sampling of the visual input, as described in an earlier section of this chapter. This rapid spatiotemporal parsing of information that is necessary to string letters in proper sequence into a word will be affected if there is a generalized deficit in temporal sampling and the rate at which the graphemic sequence is prepared for the next stage of grapheme–phoneme correspondence would then be slower. In that case, an accompanying deficit in auditory processing may not only independently affect auditory processing of syllables and other acoustic inputs as shown by many studies on dyslexic individuals, but it can potentially augment the reading difficulty caused by the visual deficit. On the other hand, since reading text silently is usually much faster than reading it out loud or normal speech, the rate-limiting step in reading may actually be the visual, rather than the phonological, component. The auditory deficit in dyslexics may just be incidental, but it might be expected to show a certain degree of robust correlation with the reading impairment due to the simple fact that children may have a generalized temporal sampling deficit and that successful reading itself improves phonemic awareness.

In line with the studies cited earlier, I would actually go one step further and propose the following: the orthographic training that is done during the early years of reading helps in the development of grapheme–phoneme correspondence and phonemic awareness since, in normal readers, the internal, mental process of 'sounding out' the words in a written text is eventually faster than the rate at which the same words are spoken in real life. It is a commonplace observation that, when watching a foreign-language film, normal readers would have read the subtitles long before they are spoken by the actors. Thus the neural networks subserving grapheme–phoneme correspondence and stringing together the phonemes of a word can deal with a much faster rate of sampling coming from the visual system than the usual rate at which phonemes are heard in normal speech. The sounding out of the phonemes in a written text and stringing them together in the correct sequence may well be a parallel process to that which strings the phonemes together from the spoken train and may gain very little from the latter, slower process, though both may ultimately access the same auditory word lexicon. The impressive success of 'phonics' in primary schools (Goswami & Bryant, 1990) may be attributed to the specific training given to the process of identification of graphemes and developing the grapheme–phoneme correspondence, not to any independent development of phonological processing skills.

As children learn to read and by the age of 7 or 8, as they 'take to reading' and learn many new words at a remarkable rate, they don't really know whether they are regular or irregular words, because there are no corresponding listings in their auditory lexicon for them. There are also no syllable segmentation, syllable stress, or onset/rime corresponding to these words that had been 'acoustically' learnt from listening to speech to guide the reader to a specific target in the lexicon. Thus phonological processing and prior auditory training are of little use in learning to read new irregular words and little help in developing grapheme–phoneme correspondence. In fact, as the children try to 'sound out' these words, they simply apply the rules that they have already learnt and this very process, whether they get the pronunciation and accent right or not, is likely to strengthen their phonemic awareness. This is very apparent in the speech of many people from non-English speaking countries who are well-read in English and who may have excellent vocabulary and writing skills in English, but who often pronounce words 'incorrectly' though they try to follow the phonological rules precisely for uncommon words that they hardly hear in their daily lives. Extensive reading by itself helps one to rehearse the 'sounds' of letters and words and can improve phonological processing.

In the early stages of reading, all levels of phonological ability—awareness of syllable, onset/rime and phoneme, corresponding to different rates of temporal sampling—'seem' to contribute to reading skills, whereas subsequently, only phoneme-level ability is correlated with development of reading skills. This is usually cited in support of the phonological theory of dyslexia (Goswami, 2011). However, the development of phonemic awareness and reading capacity may be determined by the temporal sampling upstream in the visual domain and any parallel developmental defects in temporal sampling in the auditory domain may lead to just an incidental correlation with reading skills, rather than a causal one. The visual attentional mechanisms proposed here as orchestrating the sequential processing of the letter stream may use a dynamic spatiotemporal scale, parsing the letter stream at a frequency and spatial extent depending upon a variety of factors such as letter size, word length, and prior expectation arising from preceding words and syllables. There is ample evidence that visual search mechanisms are flexible in terms of the size of the window (Belopolsky et al., 2007), the speed of the attentional scan (Kröse & Julesz, 1989) and even the number of spotlights of attention that can be handled simultaneously (McMains & Somers, 2004). Thus depending upon task demands, top-down mechanisms of the frontoparietal network can execute the spatiotemporal allocation of attention at the required temporal sampling rates. Therefore, the temporal sampling deficits that Goswami (2011) prefers to localize to the auditory system in developmental dyslexia could well be happening in the visual system.

A parsimonious, temporal sampling deficit hypothesis regarding dyslexia may be one that localizes the core deficit in temporal sampling in the visual system, since being an upstream process in the hierarchy of perceptual and cognitive functions in reading, an impairment in the visuospatial attentional mechanisms will have a flow-on effect on subsequent processes such as grapheme–phoneme correspondence and phonemic awareness, whereas a purely auditory sampling deficit might not lead to a serious reading handicap. This is consistent with the reports of lack of correlation in many cases between non-word reading and phonological skills (Castles & Coltheart, 2004).

Some of the impairment in temporal sampling in dyslexia is seen in rhythmic entrainment of sounds; this can be at the relatively low temporal frequency of around 2 Hz

(Wolff et al., 2002; Thomson & Goswami, 2008, 2010). This is close to the rate at which syllables are segmented and has been taken as support for a phonological aetiology for dyslexia (Goswami, 2011). However, temporal sampling deficits at a comparable rate in the visual system would also seriously affect the spatiotemporal parsing of letters into graphemes and syllables by the visual attentional system. In fact parsing at this slower rate is also crucial for directing shifts of fixation along the letter stream.

In many cases, the phonological processing difficulties may partly arise from the orthographic difficulties due to visual attentional problems. However, if the basic phonological processing itself is also severely impaired due to a temporal sampling deficit in the auditory domain with consequently poorer phonological representations prior to the start of reading, it is then likely to affect reading acquisition even without any visual deficit occurring upstream. However, I believe that this effect is likely to be transitory if there are no deficits in the speed and accuracy with which the visual system and the attentional networks process the visual signals.

Merav Ahissar (2007), in questioning the pure phonological and the auditory temporal processing deficit models, has suggested that the core deficit in dyslexia may be in working memory capacity. In an elegant variation of the classical Tallal experiment, she has shown that it is not an ability to process rapidly presented tones per se that is affected in dyslexic individuals, but rather the ability to keep individual tones long enough in working memory. While an inefficient short-term memory may be an explanation of the experimental results, it is unlikely, since poorer general working memory would lead to many other cognitive deficits that would show up in intelligence scores; this is not the case in developmental dyslexia. On the other hand, a normal capacity working memory will be overloaded if an impaired attentional system is not able to process the packets of sensory information (tones or phonemes in the auditory domain and graphemes in the visual) fast enough. This explains both the 2-tone/3-tone and the reference/no-reference experimental results of Ahissar (figs 1 and 2 in Ahissar, 2007). In fact, Ahissar goes on to show that in visual equivalents of the auditory task, similar deficits are found (fig. 3 of Ahissar, 2007) and also admits that her anchoring-deficit hypothesis can actually be considered as a type of impaired-attention hypothesis.

Most of those (e.g. Stuart et al., 2001; Skoyles & Skottun, 2004; Ram-Tsur et al., 2006; McLean et al., 2010; Goswami, 2011) who have questioned the magnocellular or visual attentional models of developmental dyslexia have failed to appreciate that the crucial deficit is likely to be in the 'spatiotemporal' parsing of the letter stream by the visual system, not in pure temporal sampling. Thus unless the task requires parsing *both in space and time* and at the *specific foveal region* of the visual field, there may be only weak if any correlation between spatiotemporal processing abilities and reading skills. Few studies have addressed this issue specifically. Furthermore, the critical deficit could occur anywhere in the visual pathway that affects the magnocellular submodality or the dorsal stream attention-related structures. All of these would lead to poorer parsing of the letter stream and thus reading difficulty. This may explain the finding (Solan et al., 2007) that performance in a magnocellular processing test could correctly categorize 78.3% of poor readers, while an attention test could correctly categorize as many as 95.7% of poor readers.

Site of the visual deficit: visuo-spatial attentional network or the VWFA?

If the deficit in developmental dyslexia is in the visual pathways, is it in the VWFA or at a site prior to it that ultimately compromises the rate at which attentional mechanisms parse the letter stream for processing by the VWFA? I have argued above and in earlier work (Vidyasagar, 1999; Vidyasagar & Pammer, 2010) that the core deficit in dyslexia is in visuo-spatial processing upstream from VWFA, but there is also more recent evidence in support. Dehaene et al. (2010) studied the functional magnetic resonance imaging activation of different brain areas between illiterate, literate, and ex-literate (i.e. people who learnt to read as adults) groups. They imaged the occipital areas as well as the ventral visual cortex, which has a series of compartments specialized for recognizing a variety of visual objects such as places, houses, tools, faces, and letters. Apart from the finding that literacy enhanced phonological activation to speech sounds in the planum temporale, they also showed an impressive plasticity of the ventral visual cortex. They found that literacy training in childhood leads to an expansion of the VWFA compared with other areas. If the ventral visual cortex is capable of such plasticity, unless the deficit is one that affects the whole ventral visual cortex which would then be apparent as poor visual object recognition in general (something never reported in developmental dyslexia), the core deficit in dyslexia is likely to be happening in the way that the letter stream arrives at the VWFA rather than in the VWFA itself.

Furthermore, if in dyslexia, as proposed earlier, the attentional feedback to the primary visual cortex (V1) necessary for sequential facilitation of the letter string is affected, one would also expect that activation of area V1 during reading should be poorer in dyslexics. This can be clearly seen in the published data of many studies (e.g. Demb et al., 1998; Blau et al., 2010). The study by Dehaene et al. (2010) also shows that the degree of activation of early visual areas is higher in literates compared to the illiterates. If reading involves using the attentional system to sequentially gate the visual inputs as they arrive in V1, this process should be highly developed in literates, thus explaining the greater V1 activation.

Summary

In conclusion, the fundamental deficit in developmental dyslexia may be one in spatio-temporal attentional sampling of the visual input which can lead not only to poor reading ability, but potentially also to poorer phonological skills. While a generalized temporal sampling deficit could also contribute to phonological impairment due to impaired sampling in the auditory domain, the phonological deficit per se may play only a minor part in causing the reading disability, despite its strong correlation with reading skills that is commonly seen within the dyslexic population.

Acknowledgements

The author's experimental work cited in this chapter was supported by grants from the Australian National Health and Medical Research Council and the Australian Research Council.

References

Abrams, D.A., Nicol, T., Zecker, S., & Kraus, N. (2009). Abnormal cortical processing of the syllable rate of speech in poor readers. *Journal of Neuroscience*, 29, 7686–93.

Agnew, J.A., Dorn, C., & Eden, G.F. (2004). Effect of intensive training on auditory processing and reading skills. *Brain and Language*, 88, 21–5.

Ahissar, M. (2007). Dyslexia and the anchoring hypothesis. *Trends in Cognitive Sciences*, 11, 458–65.

Bednarek, D.B., Saldana, D., Quintero-Gallego, E., Garcia, I., Grabowska, A., & Gomez, C.M. (2004). Attentional deficit in dyslexia: a general or specific impairment? *NeuroReport*, 15, 1787–90.

Belopolsky, A.V., Zwaan, L., Theeuwes, J., & Kramer, A.F. (2007). The size of an attentional window modulates attentional capture by color singletons. *Psychonomic Bulletin & Review*, 14, 934–8.

Blau, V., Reithler, J., van Atteveldt, N., Seitz, J., Gerretsen, P., Goebel, R., *et al.* (2010). Deviant processing of letters and speech sounds as proximate cause of reading failure: a functional magnetic resonance imaging study of dyslexic children. *Brain*, 133, 868–79.

Boets, B., Wouters, J., van Wieringen, A., & Ghesquière, P. (2006). Coherent motion detection in preschool children at family risk for dyslexia. *Vision Research*, 46, 527–35.

Bosse, M.L., & Valdois, S. (2009). Influence of the visual attention span on child reading performance: a cross-sectional study. *Journal of Research in Reading*, 32, 230–53.

Bosse, M.L., Tainturier, M.J., & Vadois, S. (2007). Developmental dyslexia: the visual attention span deficit hypothesis. *Cognition*, 104, 198–230.

Boussaoud, D., Desimone, R., & Ungerleider, L.G. (1991). Visual topography of area TEO in the macaque, *Journal of Comparative Neurology*, 306, 554–75.

Bradley, L., & Bryant, P.E. (1983). Categorizing sounds and learning to read: A causal connection. *Nature*, 301, 419–21.

Brefzynski, J.A., & DeYoe, E.A. (1999). A physiological correate of the 'spotlight' of visual attention. *Nature Neurosciences*, 2, 370–4.

Broom, Y.M., & Doctor, E.A. (1995). Devleopmental surface dyslexia: a case study of the efficacy of a remediation programme. *Cognitive Neuropsychology*, 12, 69–110.

Buschman, T.J., & Miller, E.K. (2007). Top-down and bottom-up control of attention in the prefrontal and posterior parietal cortices, *Science*, 315, 1860–2.

Casco, C., & Prunetti, E. (1996). Visual search of good and poor readers: effects with targets having single and combined features. *Perceptual and Motor Skills*, 82, 1155–67.

Castles, A., & Coltheart, M. (1993). Varieties of developmental dyslexia. *Cognition*, 47, 149–80.

Castles, A., & Coltheart, M. (2004). Is there a causal link from phonological awareness to success in learning to read? *Cognition*, 91, 77–111.

Castro-Caldas, A., Petersson, K.M., Reis, A., Stone-Elander, S., & Ingvar, M. (1998). The illiterate brain: Learning to read and write during childhood influences the functional organization of the adult brain. *Brain*, 121, 1053–63.

Castro-Caldas, A., Miranda, P.C., Carmo, I., Reis, A., Loete, F., Ribeiro, C., *et al.* (1999). Influernece of learning to read and write on the morphology of the corpus callosum. *European Journal of Neurology*, 6, 23–8.

Cestnick, L., & Coltheart, M. (1999). The relatinship between language-processing and visual-processing deficits in developmental dyslexia. *Cognition*, 71, 231–55.

Cornelissen, P., Hansen, P., Gilchrist, I., Cormack, F., Essex, J., & Frankish, C. (1998). Coherent motion detection and letter position encoding. *Vision Research*, 38, 2181–91.

Cornelissen, P., Richardson, A., Mason, A., Fowler, S., & Stein, J. (1995). Contrast sensitivity and coherent motion detection measured at photopic luminance levels in dyslexics and controls, *Vision Research*, 35, 1483–94.

Davis, C., Castles, A., McAnally, K., & Gray, J. (2001). lapses of concentration and dyslexic performance on the Ternus task. *Cognition*, 81, B21–31.

Dehaene, S. (2005). Evolution of human cortical circuits for reading and arithmetic: The 'neuronal recycling' hypothesis. In: S. Dehaene, J.R. Duhamel, M. Hauser, & G. Rizzolatti (Eds.) *From Monkey Brain to Human Brain*, pp. 133–57. Cambridge, MA: MIT Press.

Dehaene, S. (2009). *Reading in the Brain: The science and evolution of a human invention*. New York: Viking.

Dehaene, S., Pegado, F., Barga, L.W., Ventura, P., Nunes Filho, G., Jobert, A., *et al.* (2010). How learning to read changes the cortical networks for vision and language. *Science*, 330, 1359–64.

Demb, J.B., Boynton, G.M., & Heeger, D.J. (1998). Functional magnetic resonance imaging of early visual pathways in dyslexia. *Journal of Neuroscience*, 18, 6939–51.

Dhar, M., Been, P.H., Minderaa, R.B., & Althaus, M. (2008). Distinct information processing charactristics in dyslexia and ADHD during a covert orienting task: An event-related potential study. *Clinical Neurophysiology*, 119, 2011–25.

Dubois, M., Micheau, P.F., Noel, M.-P., & Valdois, S. (2007). Preorthographic constraints on visual word recognition: Evidence from a case study of developmental surface dyslexia. *Cognitive Nueropsychology*, 24, 623–60.

Eckhorn, R., Bauer, R., Jordan, W., Brosch, M., Kruse, M., Munk, M., *et al.* (1988). Coherent oscillations: a mechanism of feature linking in the visual cortex? Multiple electrode and correlation analyses in the cat. *Biological Cybernetics*, 60, 121–30.

Eden, G.F., VanMeter, J.W., Rumsey, J.M., Maisog, J.M., Woods, R.P., & Zeffiro, T.A. (1996). Abnormal processing of visual motion in dyslexia revealed by functional brain imaging, *Nature*, 382, 66–9.

Ehri, L. (1989). The development of spelling knowledge and its role in reading acquisition and reading disability. *Journal of Learning Disabilities*, 22, 356–65.

Facoetti, A., & Molteni, M. (2001). The gradient of visual attention in developmental dyslexia. *Neuropsychologia*, 39, 352–7.

Facoetti, A., Paganoni, P., Turatto, M., Marzola, V., & Mascetti, G.G. (2000). Visual-spatial attention in developmental dyslexia, *Cortex*, 36, 109–23.

Facoetti, A., Ruffino, M., Peru, A., Paganoni, P., & Chelazzi, L. (2008). Sluggish engagement and disengagement of non-spatial attention in dyslexic children. *Cortex*, 44, 1221–33.

Facoetti, A., Trussardi, A.N., Ruffino, M., Lorusso, M.L., Cattaneo, C., Galli, R., *et al.* (2009). Multisensory spatial attention deficits are predictive of phonological decoding skills in developmental dyslexia. *Journal of Cognitive Neuroscience*, 22, 1011–25.

Facoetti, A., Corradi, N., Ruffino, M., Gori, S., & Zorzi, M. (2010). Visual attention and speech segmentation are both impaired in preschoolers at familial risk for developmental dyslexia. *Dyslexia*, 16, 226–39.

Fischer, B., & Hartnegg, K. (2000). Effects of visual training on saccade control in dyslexia. *Perception*, 29, 531–42.

Gandhi, S.P., Heeger, D.J., & Boynton, G.M. (2001). Spatial attention affects brain activity in human primary visual cortex. *Proceedings of the National Academy of Sciences of the United States of America*, 96, 3314–19.

Goodale, M.A., & Milner, A.D. (1992). Separate visual pathways for perception and action. *Trends in Neuroscience*, 15, 20–5.

Goswami, U. (2011). A temporal sampling framework for developmental dyslexia. *Trends in Cognitive Science*, 15, 3–10.

Goswami, U., & Bryant, P. (1990). *Phonological skills and learning to read*. Hove: Erlbaum.

Gray, C.M., Konig, P., Engel, A.K., & Singer, W. (1989). Oscillatory responses in cat visual cortex exhibit inter-columnar synchronization which reflects global stimulus properties. *Nature*, 338, 334–7.

Gregoriou, G.G., Gotts, S.J., Zhou, H., & Desimone, R. (2009). High-frequency, long-range coupling between prefrontal and visual cortex during attention. *Science,* 324, 1207–10.

Grinter, E.J., Maybery, M.T., & Badcock, D.R. (2010). Vision in developmental disorders: Is there a dorsal stream deficit? *Brain Research Bulletin,* 82, 147–60.

Hanley, J.R., & Gard, F. (1995). A dissociation between developmental surface and phonological dyslexia in two undergraduate students. *Neuropsychologia,* 13, 909–14.

Hari, R., Valta, M., & Uutela, K. (1999). Prolonged attentional dwell time in dyslexic adults. *Neuroscience Letters,* 271, 202–4.

Hari, R., Renvall, H., & Tanskanen, T. (2001). Left mininegelct in dyslexic adults. *Brain,* 124, 1373–80.

Haxby, J.V., Gobbini, M.I., Furey, M.L., Ishai, A., Schouten, J.L., & Pietrini, P. (2001). Distributed and overlapping representations of faces and objects in ventral temporal cortex. *Science,* 293, 2425–30.

Heim, S., Grande, M., Pape-Neumann, J., von Ermingen, M., Meffert, E., Grabowska, A., *et al.* (2010). Interaction of phonological awareness and 'magnocellular processing during normal and dyslexic reading: Behavioural and fMRI investigations. *Dyslexia,* 16, 258–82.

Hood, M., & Conlon, E. (2004). Visual and auditory temporal processing and early reading development. *Dyslexia,* 10, 234–52.

Hook, P.E., Macaruso, P., & Jones, S. (2001). Efficacy of Fast ForWord training on facilitating acquisition of reading skills by children with reading difficulties—A longitudinal study. *Annals of Dyslexia,* 51, 75–96.

Horowitz, T.S., & Wolfe, J.M. (1998). Visual search has no memory, *Nature* 394, 575–7.

Ishai, A., Ungertleder, L.G., Martin, A., Schouten, J.L., & Haxby, J.V. (1999). Distributed representation of objects in human ventral visual pathway. *Proceedings of the National Academy of Sciences of the United States of America,* 96, 9379–84.

Jones, M.W., Branigan, H.P., & Kelly, M.L. (2008). Visual deficits in developmental dyslexia: relationships between non-linguistic visual tasks and their contribution to components of reading. *Dyslexia,* 14, 95–115.

Joris, P.X., Schrienr, C.E., & Rees, A. (2004). Neural processing of amplitude-modulated sounds. *Physiological Review,* 84, 541–77.

Kanwisher, N., McDermott, J., & Chun, M.M. (1997). The fusiform face area: A module in human extrastriate cortex specialized for face perception. *Journal of Neuroscience,* 17, 4302–11.

Kerlin, J.R., Shahin, A.J., & Miller, L.M. (2010). Attentional gain control of ongoing cortical speech representations in a 'Cocktail Party'. *Journal of Neuroscience,* 30, 620–8.

Kevan, A., & Pammer, K. (2008). Visual processing deficits in preliterate children at familial risk for dyslexia. *Vision Research,* 48, 2835–39.

Kevan, A., & Pammer, K. (2009). Predicting early reading skills from pre-reading measures of dorsal stream functioning. *Neuropsychologia,* 47, 3174–81.

Kinsey, K., Rose, M., Hansen, P., Richrdson, A., & Stein, J. (2004). Magnocellular mediated visual-spatial attention and reading ability. *NeuroReport,* 15, 2215–18.

Kröse, B.J., & Julesz, B. (1989). The control and speed of shifts of attention. *Vision Research,* 29, 1607–19.

Livingstone, M.S., & Hubel, D.H. (1988). Segregation of form, color, movement and depth: anatomy, physiology and perception. *Science,* 240, 740–9.

Livingstone, M.S., Rosen, G.D., Drislane, F.W., & Galaburda, A.M. (1991). Physiological and anatomical evidence for a magnocellular defect in developmental dyslexia. *Proceedings of the National Academy of Sciences of the United States of America,* 88, 7943–7.

Logothetis, N.K., & Scheinberg, D.L. (1996). Visual object recognition. *Annual Review of Neuroscience,* 19, 577–621.

Logothetis, N.K., Pauls, J., & Poggio, T. (1995). Shape representation in the inferior temporal cortex of monkeys. *Current Biology,* 5, 552–63.

Lorenzi, C., Dumont, A., & Füllgrabe, C. (2000). Use of temporal envelope cues by children with developmental dyslexia. *Journal of Speech, Language, and Hearing Research* 43, 1367–79.

Lorusso, M.L., Facoetti, A., Toraldo, A., & Molteni, M. (2005). Tachistoscopic treatment of dyslexia changes the distribution of visual-spatial attention. *Brain and Cognition,* 57, 135–42.

Lorusso, M.L., Facoetti, A., & Bekker, D.J. (2011). Neuropsychological treatment of dyslexia: Does type of treatment matter? *Journal of Learning Disabilities,* 44, 136–49.

Lovegrove, W.J., Bowling, A., Badcock, D., & Blackwood, M. (1980). Specific reading disability: differences in contrast sensitivity as a function of spatial frequency, *Science* 210, 439–40.

Lovegrove, W.J., Martin, F., & Slaghuis, W.L. (1986). A theoretical and experimental case for a visual deficit in specific reading disability. *Cognitive Neuropsychology,* 3, 225–67.

Luo, H., & Poepppel, D. (2007). Phase patterns of neuronal responses reliably discriminate speech in human auditory cortex. *Neuron,* 54, 1001–10.

Malach, R., Levy, I., & Hasson, U. (2002). The topography of high-order human object areas. *Trends in Cognitive Science,* 6, 176–84.

Mann, V.A., & Wimmer, H. (2002). Phoneme awareness and pathways to literacy: a comparison of German and American children. *Reading and Writing,* 15, 653–82.

McAdams, C.J., & Reid, R.C. (2005). Attention modulates the responses of simple cells in monkey primary visual cortex. *Journal of Neuroscience,* 25, 11023–33.

McAnally, K.I., Hansen, P.C., Cornelissen, P.L., & Stein, J.F. (1997). Effect of time and frequency manipulation on syllable perception in developmental dyslexics. *Journal of Speech, Language, and Hearing Research,* 40, 912–24.

McAnally, K.I., & Stein, J.F. (1997). Scalp potentials evoked by amplitude modulated tones in dyslexia. *Journal of Speech, Language, and Hearing Research* 40, 939–45.

McArthur, G.M., Ellis, D., Atkinson, C.M., & Coltheart, M. (2008). Auditory processing deficits in children with reading and language impairments: Can they (and should they) be treated? *Cognition,* 107, 946–77.

McMains, S.A., & Somers, D.C. (2004). Multiple spotlights of attentional selection in human visual cortex. *Neuron,* 42, 677–86.

McLean, G.M.T., Casstles, A., Coltheart, V., & Stuart, G.W. (2010). No evidence for a prolonged attentional blink in developmental dyslexia. *Cortex,* 46, 1317–29.

Menghini, D., Finzi, A., Benassi, M., Bolzani, R., Facoetti, A., Giovagnoli, S., et al. (2010). Different underlying neurocognitive deficits in developmental dyslexia: a comparative study. *Neuropsychologia,* 48, 863–72.

Merigan, W.H., & Maunsell, J.H.R. (1993). How parallel are the primate visual pathways? *Annual Review of Neuroscience,* 16, 369–402.

Mohler, C.W., & Wurtz, R.H. (1977). Role of striate cortex and superior colliculus in visual guidance of saccadic eye movements in monkeys. *Journal of Neurophysiology,* 40, 74–94.

Morais, J., Cary, L., Alegria, J., & Bertelson, P. (1979). Does awareness of speech as a sequence of phones arise spontaneously? *Cognition,* 7, 323–31.

Motter, B.C. (1993). Focal attention produces spatially selective processing in visual cortical areas V1, V2 and V4 in the presence of competing stimuli. *Journal of Neurophysiology,* 70, 909–19.

Pammer, K., & Kevan, A. (2007). The contribution of visual sensitivity, phonological processing and nonverbal IQ to children's reading. *Scientific Studies of Reading,* 11, 33–53.

Pammer, K., & Wheatley, C. (2001). Isolating the M(y)-cell response in dyslexia using the spatial frequency doubling illusion. *Vision Research,* 41, 2139–47.

Pammer, K., Lavis, R., Hansen, P., & Cornelissen, P.L. (2004). Symbol-string sensitivity and children's reading. *Brain and Language,* 89, 601–10.

Paul, I., Bott, C., Heim, S., Wienbruch, C., & Elbert, T.R. (2006). Phonological but not auditory discrimination is impaired in dyslexia. *European Journal of Neuroscience,* 24, 2945–53.

Petersson, K.M., Silva, C., Castro-Caldas, A., Ingvar, M., & Reis, A. (2007). Literacy: A cultural influence on functional left-right differences in the inferior parietal cortex. *European Journal of Neuroscience*, 26, 791–9.

Pokorni, J.L., Worthington, C., & Jamison, P. (2004). Phonological awareness intervention: Comparison of Fast ForWord, Earobics, and LiPS. *Journal of Educational Research*, 97, 147–57.

Puce, A., Allison, T., Asgari, M., Gore, J.C., & McCarthy, G. (1996). Differential sensitivity of human visual cortex to faces, letterstrings and textures: A functional magnetic resonance imaging study. *Journal of Neuroscience*, 16, 5205–15.

Ram-Tsur, R., Faust, M., & Zivotofsky, A.Z. (2006). Sequential processing deficits of reading disabled persons is independent of stimulus interval. *Vision Research*, 46, 3949–60.

Ramus, F. (2003). Developmental dyslexia: specific phonological deficit or general sensorimotor dysfunction. *Current Opinion in Neurobiology*, 13, 212–18.

Ramus, F., & Szenkovits, G. (2008). What phonological deficit? *Quarterly Journal of Experimental Psychology*, 61, 129–41.

Resi, A., & Castro-Caldas, A. (1997). Illiteracy: a cause for based cognitive development. *Journal of the International Neuropsychological Society*, 3, 444–50.

Rey, V., De Martino, S., Espesser, R., & Habib, M. (2002). Temporal processing and phonological impairment in dyslexia: effect of phoneme lengthening on order judgment of two consonants. *Brain and Language*, 80, 576–91.

Roach, N.W., & Hogben, J.H. (2007). Impaired filtering of behaviourally irrelevant visual information in dyslexia. *Brain*, 130, 771–85.

Ruffino, A., Trussardi, A.N., Gori, S., Finzi, A., Giovagnoli, S., Menghini, D., *et al.* (2010). Attentional engagement deficits in dyslexic children. *Neuropsychologia*, 48, 3793–801.

Rutkowski, J.S., Crewther, D.P., & Crewther, S.G. (2003). Change detection is impaired in children with dyslexia. *Journal of Vision*, 3, 95–105.

Saalmann, Y.B., Pigarev, I.N., & Vidyasagar, T.R. (2007). Neural mechanisms of visual attention: How top-down feedback highlights relevant locations. *Science*, 316, 1612–15.

Sary, G., Vogels, R., & Orban, G.A. (1993). Cue-invariant shape selectivity of macaque inferior temporal neurons. *Science*, 260, 995–7.

Schroeder, C.E., Lakatos, P., Kajikawa, Y., Partan, S., & Puce, A. (2008). Neuronal oscillations and visual amplification of speech. *Trends in Cognitive Sciences*, 12, 106–13.

Schulte-Körne, G., Bartling, J., Deimel, W., & Remschmidt, H. (2004). Motion-onset VEPs in dyslexia: Evidence for visual perceptual deficit. *NeuroReport*, 15, 1075–8.

Shaywitz, S.E., & Shaywitz, B.A. (2005). Dyslexia (specific reading disability). *Biological Psychiatry*, 57, 926–33.

Simola, J., Stenbacka, L., & Vanni, S. (2009). Topography of attention in the primary visual cortex. *European Journal of Neuroscience*, 29, 188–96.

Skoyles, J., & Skottun, B.C. (2004). On the prevalence of magnocellular deficits in the visual system of non-dyslexic individuals. *Brain and Language*, 88, 79–82.

Slaghuis, W.L., & Ryan, J.F. (2006). Directional motion contrast sensitivity in developmental dyslexia. *Vision Research*, 46, 3291–303.

Snowling, M.J. (2001). From language to reading and dyslexia. *Dyslexia*, 7, 37–46.

Solan, H.A., Shelley-Tremblay, J., Hansen, P.C., Silverman, M.E., Larson, S., & Ficarra, A. (2004). M-cell deficit and reading disability: a preliminary study of the effects of temporal vision-processing therapy. *Optometry*, 75, 640–50.

Solan, H.A., Shelley-Tremblay, J., Hansen, P.C., & Larson, S. (2007). Is there a common linkage among reading comprehension, visual attention and magnocellular processing? *Journal of Learning Disabilities*, 40, 270–8.

Somers, D.C., Dale, A.M., Seiffert, A.E., & Tootell, R.B.H. (1999). Functional MRI reveals spatially specific attentional modulation in human primary visual cortex. *Proceedings of the National Academy of Sciences of the United States of America*, 96, 1663–8.

Stein, J.F., & Walsh, V. (1997). To see but not to read: the magnocellular theory of dyslexia, *Trends in Neurosciences* 20, 147–52.

Strasburger, H. (2005). Unfocussed spatial attention underlies the crowding effect in indirect form vision. *Journal of Vision*, 5, 1024–37.

Strehlow, U., Haffner, J., Bischof, J., Grtazka, V., Parzer, P., & Resch, F. (2006). Does successful training of temporal processing of sound and phoneme stimuli improve reading and spelling? *European Child & Adolescent Psychology*, 15, 19–29.

Stuart, G.W., McAnally, K.I., & Castles, A. (2001). Can contrast sensitivity functions in dyslexia be explained by inattention rather than a magnocellular deficit? *Vision Research*, 41, 325–11.

Talcott, J.B., Witton, C., McLean, M.F., Hansen, P.C., Rees, A., Green, G.G., *et al.* (2000). Dynamic sensory sensitivity and children's word decoding skills. *Proceedings of the National Academy of Sciences of the United States of America*, 14, 2952–7.

Tallal, P. (1980). Auditory temporal perception, phonics, and reading disabilities in children, *Brain and Language*, 9, 182–98.

Tallal, P., & Stark, R.E. (1982). Perceptual/motor profiles of reading impaired children with or without concomitant oral language deficits. *Annals of Dyslexia*, 32, 163–76.

Tallal, P., Miller, S.L., Bedi, G., Byma, G., Wang, X., Nagarajan, S.S., *et al.* (1996). Language comprehension in language earning impaired children improved with acoustically modified speech. *Science*, 271, 81–4.

Tamura, H., & Tanaka, K. (2001). Visual response properties of cells in the ventral and dorsal parts of the macaque inferotemporal cortex. *Cerebral Cortex*, 11, 384–99.

Tanaka, K. (1996). Inferotemporal cortex and object vision. *Annual Review of Neuroscience*, 19, 109–39.

Temple, E., Deutsch, G.K., Poldrack, R.A., Miller, S.A., Tallal, P., Merzenich, M.M., *et al.* (2003). Neural deficits in children with dyslexia ameliorated by behavioral remediation: evidence from functional MRI. *Proceedings of the National Academy of Sciences of the United States of America*, 100, 2860–5.

Thomson, J.B., Chenault, B., Abbott, R.D., Raskind, W.H., Richards, T., Aylward, E., *et al.* (2005). Converging evidence for attentional influences on the orthographic word form in child dyslexics. *Journal of Neurolinguistics*, 18, 93–126.

Thomson, J.M., & Goswami, U. (2008). Rhythmic processing in children with developmental dyslexia: auditory and motor rhythms link to reading and spelling. *Journal of Physiology Paris*, 102, 120–9.

Thomson, J.M., & Goswami, U. (2010). Learning novel phonological representations in developmental dyslexia: associations with basic auditory processing of rise time and phonological awareness, *Reading and Writing*, 23, 453–69.

Tree, J.J., & Kay, J. (2006). Phonological dyslexia and phonological impairment: an exception to the rule? *Neuropsychologia*, 44, 2861–73.

Treisman, A.M. (1988). Features and objects: the fourteenth Bartlett memorial lecture. *Quarterly Journal of Experimental Psychology*, 40, 201–37.

Treisman, A.M. (1996). The binding problem. *Current Opinion in Neurobiology*, 6, 171–8.

Treisman, A.M., & Gelade, G. (1980). A eature integration theory of attention. *Cognitive Psychology*, 12, 97–136.

Ungerleider, L.G., & Mishkin, M. (1982). Two cortical visual systems. In: D.J. Ingle, M.A. Goodalem, & R.J. Mansfield (Eds) *Analysis of visual behavior*, PP. 549–86. Cambridge MA: MIT Press.

Valdois, S., Bosse, M.-L., Ans, B., Carbonnel, S., Zorman, M., David, D., *et al.* (2003). Phonological and visual processing deficits can dissociate in developmental dyslexia: evidence from two case studies. *Reading and Writing*, 16, 541–72.

Valdois, S., Bosse, M.-L., & Tainturier, M.-J. (2004). The cognitive deficits responsible for developmental dyslexia: Review of evidence for a selective visual attentional disorder. *Dyslexia*, 10, 339–63.

Valdois, S., Carbonnel, S., Juphard, A., Baciu, M., Ans, B., Peyrin, C., *et al.* (2006). Polysyllabic pseudo-word processing in reading and lexical decision: converging evidence from behavioral data, connectionist simulations and functional MRI. *Brain Research*, 1085, 149–62.

Vidyasagar, T.R. (1998). Gating of neuronal responses in macaque primary visual cortex by an attentional spotlight. *NeuroReport*, 9, 1947–52.

Vidyasagar, T.R. (1999). A neuronal model of attentional spotlight: parietal guiding the temporal. *Brain Research Reviews*, 30, 66–76.

Vidyasagar, T.R. (2001). From attentional gating in macaque primary visual cortex to dyslexia in humans. *Progress in Brain Research*, 134, 297–312.

Vidyasagar, T.R., & Pammer, K. (1999). Impaired visual search in dyslexia relates to the role of the magnocellular pathway in attention. *NeuroReport*, 10, 1283–7.

Vidyasagar, T.R., & Pammer, K. (2010). Dyslexia: a deficit in visuo-spatial attention, not in phonological processing. *Trends in Cognitive Sciences*, 14, 57–63.

Vidyasagar, T.R., & Pigarev, I.N. (2007). Modulation of neuronal responses in macaque primary visual cortex in a memory task. *European Journal of Neuroscience*, 25, 2547–57.

Vogels, R., & Biederman, I. (2002). Effects of illumination intensity and direction on object coding in macaque inferior temporal cortex. *Cerebral Cortex*, 12, 756–66.

Williams, M.J., Stuart, G.W., Castles, A., & McAnally, K.I. (2003). Contrast sensitivity in subgroups of developmental dyslexia. *Vision Research*, 43, 467–77.

Witton, C., Talcott, J.B., Hansen, P.C., Richardson, A.J., Griffiths, T.D., Rees, A., *et al.* (1998). Sensitivity to dynamic auditory and visual stimuli predicts nonword reading ability in both dyslexic and normal readers. *Current Biology*, 8, 791–7.

Wolfe, J.M. (1994). Guided search 2.0: a revised model of visual search. *Psychonomic Bulletin & Review*, 1, 202–38.

Wolff, P.H. (2002). Timing precision and rhythm in developmental dyslexia. *Reading and Writing*, 15, 179–206.

Womelsdorf, T., Schoffelen, J.M., Oostenveld, R., Singer, W., Desione, R., Engel, A.K., *et al.* (2007). Modulation of neuronal interactions through neuronal synchronization. *Science*, 316, 1609–12.

Zeki, S. (1978), Functional specialization in the visual cortex of the rhesus monkey. *Nature*, 274, 423–8.

Ziegler, J.C., Pech-Georgel, C., Dufau, S., & Grainger, J. (2010). Rapid processing of letters, digits and symbols: what purely visual-attentional deficit in developmental dyslexia? *Developmental Science*, 13, F8–F14.

Chapter 11

Visual Contributions to Reading Difficulties: The Magnocellular Theory

John Stein

Introduction

Many children who have unusual difficulty learning to read complain of visual perceptual anomalies, such as the letters appearing to blur, move around, or split into two. Naturally these interfere with their ability to identify the letters and their order, and reduce the accuracy with which they can lay down reliable representations of the visual form of words in their sight vocabularies ('visual lexicon'). Since, despite some views, the visual system provides the most important processing for reading, such problems very severely impede these children's acquisition of both orthographic and phonological skills.

You might think that this is obvious. It is obvious that blind people cannot read print at all; so lesser degrees of visual impairment would probably impair reading as well. But the idea that children's reading difficulties are ever due to visual deficiencies is highly controversial, despite the clear descriptions of visual symptoms that so many children give. The current consensus is that reading problems are mainly due to failure to acquire phonological skills, and that the visual system usually does its job perfectly well in dyslexics.

Visual reading pathways

Nevertheless most people agree that visual processing is important for reading. There are two main routes to understanding written material: sublexical (phonological) and lexical (whole word). Just how separate these routes are is not wholly clear; there are clearly interactions between them, so that both are activated during normal reading (Manis et al., 1997). Nevertheless, the two routes exist.

Beginning readers have very few words in their sight vocabulary; so they mainly rely on the sublexical, phonological route. First they have to visually identify individual letters and their order and then translate them into the sounds they stand for. Then these are melded into the word's complete sound and associated with its meaning. All these stages mean that this route is relatively slow and only used for unfamiliar words.

However, practised readers already have many words which they can recognize by sight in their visual lexicon. So they can use the lexical or 'visual semantic' route for these which is much faster. They merely have to identify the whole word visually to rapidly gain its meaning.

Visual requirements of reading

Both these routes rely first and foremost on visual analysis: in the sublexical route the letters first have to be visually identified and ordered properly; in the lexical route the whole word is recognized visually. Thus a very large proportion of the information processing required for reading is indeed visual.

What are the specific visual requirements of reading? Retinal ganglion cells gather signals from the photoreceptors, bipolar, horizontal, and amacrine cells, and relay them to the lateral geniculate nucleus (LGN) in the thalamus, thence to the cerebral cortex—to the primary visual, 'striate' or 'calcarine', cortex (V1) which is situated at the back of the occipital lobe. Ten per cent of these retinal ganglion cells are much larger than the others—hence they are called magnocellular—magnus is Latin for large; they provide rapid information about timing and movement, for the control of attention and eye movements. The other 90% are known as parvocellular (parvus, P—Latin for small) and koniocellular (even smaller—konio—Greek for dust); these provide information about fine detail and colour for object identification ('what' information). From the primary visual cortex two main visual pathways then project forwards, the ventral, 'what', and the dorsal, 'where', routes.

Obviously letters have to be identified correctly; so it is often assumed that the most important pathway employed for reading is the ventral 'what' route since this specializes in object identification. It passes from V1 ventrally via V2–V4 and culminates in the visual word form area (VWFA) which lies in the anterior part of the left fusiform gyrus on the under surface of the left occipitotemporal junction (Cohen & Dehaene, 2004) and it clearly plays an important role in reading. But probably just as important is the more rapid dorsal stream that can also identify words rapidly because it controls the focus of attention.

In addition to identifying letters we need to see them in the correct order. In fact dyslexics are more inaccurate and slow at attending to the sequence of letters than they are at identifying each individually. Correct sequencing depends on being able to focus attention, integrate, and memorize information about what the fovea was seeing with where the eyes were pointing at the time, since what is centred on the fovea is dependent on how the eyes have just moved. This integration depends on the properties of the other forward route from the primary visual cortex—the dorsal 'where' route that passes dorsally via V2–V5 and culminates in the posterior parietal cortex (PPC). This dorsal stream is primarily devoted to determining *where* objects are for the visual guidance of attention and of eye and limb movements (Ungerleider & Mishkin, 1982; Goodale & Milner, 1992).

Visual magnocellular neurons

The visual input to this 'where' route is mainly provided by the magnocellular neurons. Their axons project to the magnocellular layers of the LGN and also to the superior colliculus to help control eye movements (Maunsell, 1992). These axons are heavily myelinated so that the signals they project to the visual cortex arrive there *c.*10 ms before the smaller, slower P cells. Also their dendritic fields are 20–50 times the size of those of the

P cells. At the reading distance this means that M cells respond best to large images— around 0.5 cm in size; this is about half the average size of a word. Despite their large size they can probably still resolve images 10 times smaller than optimal, so that they can easily contribute to identifying the shapes of letters, which in small print subtend only about 1 mm. But they probably cannot detect small letter features, such as serifs, 0.1 mm in size. Thus they can rapidly indicate the positions of each letter and begin their identification. They have high sensitivity to low contrasts and rapid temporal frequencies, but lower spatial frequency sensitivity; thus they are specialized for indicating letter shape, position, change, flicker, and motion, even at very low light levels and contrasts. But although they are most sensitive to the longer wavelengths, such as yellow, they do not contribute to colour vision.

This combination of features makes their function not only to detect letter position and shape, but also in conjunction with motor signals to track self-movements, in particular of the eyes. Knowing where the eyes are pointing in relation to your head and body enables you to locate and attend to objects in relation to your egocentre independently of their retinal positions (Stein, 1992). Hence the M system is important both for correctly determining the order of letters in a word, and for identifying them.

Visual stabilization

Because M cells detect any unwanted image motion, they also provide crucial input to the systems that stabilize visual perception. Our eyes move around constantly, hence images swish across the retina much of the time. Yet we do not usually see the world appear to move—because the predicted visual consequences of each eye movement are subtracted from the image motion it causes to yield a stable percept. The prediction is carried out by the cerebellum and integrated with M-dominated motion signals in the PPC.

This compensation therefore also depends on the integrity of the visual magnocellular system. This picks up the motion of images across the retina caused by eye movements and projects these to the dorsal visual pathway culminating in the PPC. This is the area whose main function is to determine where things are in relation to the body's egocentre. At the same time a copy of the motor signals triggering the muscles to move the eyes is also sent to the PPC via the cerebellum, to forewarn how the eyes will move. After the movement, eye muscle proprioceptors also signal to the PPC their new lengths. All these signals are used by the PPC to calculate how far the eyes will move, then how far they did in fact move. In this way they help to determine where each visual object is in relation to the body (Stein, 1992). Although crucial for attention and eye control, the motion of these images across the retina never reaches consciousness, so the world remains perceptually stationary.

Between saccades from one object to the next, the eyes are kept fixated to inspect each one by a negative feedback servocontrol system. The eyes make small movements all the time; this is essential to prevent too much bleaching of the retinal pigments (Yarbus, 1965). But these miniature eye movements would cause unwanted image motion. This is detected by the retinal magno cells, and fed back via the superior colliculus to the oculomotor servosystem. This then brings the eyes back on target. So the integrity of the M system is crucial not only for tracking eye movements to help indicate where the eyes are pointing, but also for keeping them fixated on a single letter when required.

Even this servomechanism does not manage to keep the eyes absolutely stationary, however; images are always 'jittering' on the retina. This jitter would cause images to appear to blur if there were no mechanism to compensate for it. But most of us perceive a clear image most of the time. Murakami & Cavanagh (1998) proposed that normally the visual system removes jitter by estimating the minimal 'baseline' amount of retinal movement that is caused by miniature eye movements. This is signalled by the M-ganglion cells. The retinal area showing the least motion then corresponds to features in the visual scene which are actually stationary. Hence if this 'motion minimum' is subtracted from the motion signals coming from all over the retina, then any motion surviving this subtraction will denote real object motion in the outside world. This will correct for the small eye movements and allow a stable percept of truly stationary objects during fixation.

Thus the magnocellular system plays crucial roles not only in sequencing small objects such as letters, but also in achieving stable visual perception. If it is deficient in any way these operations will be less precise and the subject will neither know precisely where his eyes are pointing, nor achieve a stable percept. He will not have accurate knowledge of where letters are positioned and his eyes will move around more than they should during fixation. Being unintended and uncontrolled these movements will not be accompanied by motor efference signals to indicate how large they were, so the image movements they cause will be treated as real movements of the external target. Hence, letters will appear to move around and will be mislocated after each eye movement.

These problems will be exacerbated when the eyes need to converge for reading small print. For example, if at one moment the right eye is looking at the d in the word dog and then a moment later this eye shifts to point at the g, the g will appear to have moved into the position previously occupied by the d. At the same time the other eye might be doing the opposite and so letters can appear to cross over each other, blur, go double, or move in and out of the page.

Visual symptoms

These are exactly the kinds of 'visual stress' symptom of which many children with reading difficulties complain (Singleton & Henderson, 2007; Singleton, Chapter 6; Wilkins, Chapter 4, this volume). 'The letters blur'; 'they move over each other, so I can't tell what order they're meant to be in.' Many of the children that we see at our clinics for those with reading problems report such symptoms. But in adults such overt problems with clearly seeing text seem to be less common, and the dominant symptom in compensated adults is very poor spelling. These inaccurate spellings probably reveal the deficiencies in how their visual representations of words were laid down in their sight vocabulary during childhood. Thus such spelling errors are probably visual in origin and not 'phonological'.

Nevertheless, at the moment the prevailing opinion among experts is that reading problems are mainly phonological, and not visual. Even though everyone agrees that at least some children have visual problems with reading, many put their prevalence very low, at less than 10% of all dyslexics (Snowling, 2000). On the contrary, however, we find that over 50% of the children we see in our clinics have significant visual problems and that these often contribute to their phonological ones (Stein & Fowler, 2005).

These estimates depend on what is counted as visual. If someone says that letters and words appear to move around, that is clearly a visual problem. But many children are so used to the motion that they don't realize that it is abnormal, unless they are specifically asked. In adults apparent letter motion is much less common. But their visual word representations for spelling are often very poor as noted earlier. Even without having symptoms of letters appearing to move around, not having a clear idea of the order of letters is also likely to have a visual origin.

Normally before you move your eyes something has attracted your attention. It grabs your attention; then you move your eyes. Accordingly the visual magnocellular system is engaged before any eye movements, to control the focus of your attention. Shifting attention accurately from one letter to another is therefore equally important for determining letter order. The visual dorsal route dominated by M-cell input shifts attention to each letter or word and this brings the ventral route to bear on identifying it (Cheng et al., 2004).

Developmental dyslexia

So far we have referred mainly to reading problems in general rather than to dyslexia specifically. Since most of the research to be reviewed here has studied developmental dyslexics we now need briefly to define what we mean by developmental dyslexia, since there is controversy even about its definition. Having regard to the strong evidence for a genetic, hence neurobiological, basis for this condition we distinguish dyslexia from other causes of poor reading, such as absent parental support and poor schooling, which do not have a genetic basis. Dyslexia is a distinct entity because of its specificity for reading and spelling, hence its other name, 'specific reading disability'. Therefore we subscribe to the 'discrepancy definition' of dyslexia, namely reading and spelling significantly behind what would be expected from the person's general intelligence.

Since dyslexia has been shown to be associated with differences in brain structure and connectivity we see it as a more general neurological syndrome despite its specificity for literacy; so we expect to see many of the other characteristic features of a dyslexic such as a family history of literacy difficulties and often of immunological problems such as allergies, eczema, asthma, and autoimmune disease; overlap with other neurodevelopmental conditions such as developmental dysphasia (also known as specific language impairment), developmental dyspraxia (developmental coordination disorder), attention deficit hyperactivity disorder (ADHD), central auditory processing disorder, even autistic spectrum disorders. We also expect to find poor sequencing in all domains, not just of letters in a word, but also of the order of sounds in a word (phonology), the alphabet, days of the week, months of the year, arithmetic tables, remembering telephone numbers, digit recall, motor sequencing, (hence clumsiness is characteristic), poor punctuality, poor ordering of his own life!

Visual magnocellular impairments in dyslexia

Strictly speaking, visual magno cells can only be defined in the subcortical visual system because they are only anatomically separated from the parvo cells in the retina, LGN, and layer 4c of the primary visual cortex. Thereafter M and P inputs converge and interact strongly. Hence the best way to test for deficits is to use stimuli that are selectively processed by the subcortical magnocellular areas. In fact there is evidence of M abnormalities in dyslexics at all levels: in the retina and LGN, and also in the primary visual cortex, and later in the cortical dorsal where pathway from the primary visual cortex to MT/V5, PPC, and the ultimate goal of both magno and parvo routes, the prefrontal cortex.

Retina

One of the most important features of M cells is their non-linear character. They fire transiently not only when a light is switched on in their receptive field centre but also when it is switched off (rectification), so that if a grating is moved across the field they will fire at twice the temporal and spatial frequency of the grating. Since they are much more sensitive to low contrasts than parvocells are, as contrast is increased from zero they are the cells that begin to respond much earlier than the P cells. Since they signal at twice the frequency of the stimulus this is interpreted perceptually as the grating having twice the number of bars. This is called the spatial frequency doubling effect; it provides a selective test of magnocellular sensitivity in the retina (Maddess et al., 1999). Pammer & Wheatley (2001) showed that dyslexics tend to have a higher contrast threshold for perceiving such low spatial, high temporal frequency gratings than good readers, confirming that their M system is mildly impaired (Pammer, Chapter 9, this volume).

The same non-linearity can be seen in the visual evoked potential recorded from the primary visual cortex. If an oscillating grating or chequer board is used as a stimulus, the M cells fire twice each time a bar crosses their receptive field, first when it enters its receptive field, then when it exits i.e. they fire at the second harmonic of the stimulus frequency. Since parvocells fire to the entry of the bar only and are inhibited by its exit they mainly respond just to the fundamental rather than the second harmonic. So by recording over the occipital pole the ratio of the second harmonic to the fundamental frequency we can index the sensitivity of an individual's M system relative to his P system. We have found that this ratio is very much lower in dyslexics; and this has turned out to be a sensitive technique for detecting magnocellular impairment.

As discussed earlier, another effect mediated by retinal M cells is the 'jitter illusion'. When patterns imaged onto one part of the retina are jittered for several seconds by a small amount equivalent to the size of miniature eye movements, the M cells there adapt and so give a falsely low estimate of the amplitude of the motion. Hence after the jitter is stopped images on unadapted adjacent parts of the retina will now appear to jitter. The duration of this illusion therefore gives a measure of the sensitivity of retinal M cells. The more sensitive they are, the more adapted they will become, so the longer they will take to return to normal after the jitter stimulus, and the longer the subsequent jitter illusion will be (Murakami & Cavanagh, 1998). We have recently shown that in many adult dyslexics this illusory percept is much shorter, and its duration correlates not only with another measure of M cell function, visual motion sensitivity, but also with the dyslexics' reading accuracy and speed. These findings again support the view that dyslexics have deficits in visual magnocellular processing.

Lateral geniculate nucleus

This is the main thalamic relay of visual information between the eye and the visual cortex. Here the M-retinal ganglion cells terminate in their own M-cell layers, separately from the parvocell layers, one for each eye. Although the properties of the peripheral M system have been mainly worked out by recording from the M layers in the LGN in monkeys, we have as yet no non-invasive way of recording responses in the LGN directly in intact humans. But perhaps the best evidence for a magnocellular deficit came from Galaburda's postmortem studies of five dyslexic human brains from the Orton brain bank. He found that the M layers in the LGN in these brains were selectively impaired. Not only were the cells c.25% smaller in the dyslexic compared with the control brains, but also they were not confined to their proper M layers—many had mismigrated into the adjacent konio and parvo layers of the LGN (Livingstone et al., 1991).

Such mismigration was also seen in the cerebral cortex in dyslexic brains. Neurons, particularly large ones, were found to have migrated beyond the outer limiting membrane to form little blebs on the cortical surface: these are known as ectopias (Galaburda et al., 1985). It was highly exciting therefore to find, as we shall see later, that at least three of the genes that have been associated with reading problems are involved in controlling neuronal migration early in brain development (Galaburda et al., 2006).

Grating contrast sensitivity—Primary visual cortex

Sensitivity to the contrast of black and white gratings is thought to be mediated mainly by the primary visual cortex (VI). Since Lovegrove's first report (Lovegrove et al., 1980) there have been several studies that have confirmed that the contrast sensitivity (CS) of many dyslexics is lower than that of controls, particularly at the low spatial and high temporal frequencies mediated by the M system (Cornelissen et al., 1995; Bednarek & Grabowska, 2002). Other tests of M function involving the primary visual cortex in dyslexics that have been reported are: abnormal temporal gap detection for low contrast and low spatial frequency stimuli (Badcock & Lovegrove, 1981), reduced critical flicker frequency (Chase & Jenner, 1993) and decreased low spatial frequency contrast sensitivity for flickering and moving stimuli (Martin & Lovegrove, 1984, 1987; Mason et al. 1993; Felmingham & Jakobson, 1995; Edwards et al., 2004).

However, some studies have failed to confirm these differences. On the basis of his study over 25 years ago with Gross-Glen of 18 adult dyslexics (Gross-Glen et al., 1995) together with over two dozen reviews of others' work, Skottun has repeatedly criticized the hypothesis that dyslexics have specifically impaired M-stream processing, even though he seems to accept that many dyslexics do indeed have visual problems. The reading of Gross-Glen's sample of dyslexics was actually better than normal for their age, but behind that expected from their IQ. Although they found that the dyslexics did have CS deficits when compared with good readers, these were not so marked at the low spatial frequencies that were expected to stimulate the magno system best. Instead they were more impaired at higher ones. Two points should be noted here. First M cells can respond to much higher spatial frequencies than Skottun seems to be aware of. Second Gross-Glen et al. used very brief stimuli lasting only 17 or 34 ms (equivalent to temporal frequencies of 59 and 29 Hz respectively), frequencies that would in fact preferentially stimulate the M system. Thus their results actually confirmed others' findings that if gratings are flickered at high temporal frequencies, dyslexics show lower CS than controls even at high spatial frequencies, hence that dyslexics often show M weakness.

Williams et al. (2003) also failed to find any significant differences between dyslexics and controls at either low or high spatial frequencies. However, they studied only a small number of subjects, and they chose to stimulate the M system using a high contrast grating at a temporal frequency of only 8 Hz. The P system is not completely silenced at this high contrast and rate and can still respond, so large differences would not be expected, especially with such a small number of subjects.

Sperling and collagues have suggested that dyslexics' visual problems are not the result of a magnocellular impairment, but of a failure to filter out 'visual noise' (Sperling et al., 2005). Clearly the source of such noise is crucial. Probably the impaired M system in dyslexics spatially undersamples the visual world (Talcott et al., 2000a). This would leave response gaps between retinal M cells that would clearly add noise to any visual processing, just as Sperling et al. found.

Like Gross-Glen et al. (1995) they failed to find lower contrast sensitivity in dyslexics at the low than higher spatial frequencies which they had expected of a M impairment. But they used stationary gratings; whereas for stationary gratings contrast sensitivity is not mediated by the M system alone, even at low spatial frequencies (Merigan & Maunsell, 1990). Hence their dyslexics' surviving sensitivity to low spatial frequencies was probably mediated by the parvo system because this can signal even low spatial frequency gratings if they are stationary. A flickering light is equivalent to a very low spatial and high temporal frequency stimulus, and almost all those who have measured dyslexics' flicker sensitivity have found it to be slightly reduced (Talcott, 2003).

In summary, the great majority of studies (c.90%) that have specifically looked for subcortical visual M-cell deficits in dyslexics have shown that many do suffer from mild M impairments, particularly displayed in tests employing low contrasts, high temporal, and low spatial frequencies.

Dorsal stream areas

The magnocellular system provides the main visual input to the dorsal 'where' corticofugal stream, so that tests focusing on these higher cortical areas can also provide evidence about M impairments. However, one always has to bear in mind that higher dorsal stream tasks depend on the whole dorsal stream. Although 90% of its visual input is provided by the M system, 10% is provided by P and K sources. Therefore higher area visual tasks provide only circumstantial evidence for deficits in the subcortical visual magnocellular system.

Nevertheless there is enough direct evidence from studying the subcortical visual M stream specifically, together with the more circumstantial evidence from higher areas that receive large M-cell input, to conclude that many dyslexics do indeed have impaired M-cell function.

Visual motion sensitivity

The best way of assessing the M sensitivity of neurons in individuals at a crucial stage of the dorsal stream, the middle temporal visual motion area (MT/V5), is to measure their responses to visual motion in 'random dot kinematograms'. Clouds of dots moving in the same direction, 'coherently', are progressively diluted with noise dots moving in random directions until the subject can no longer detect any coherent motion in the display. This threshold therefore defines the sensitivity of that individual's visual dorsal stream system for the detection of motion. Several researchers have shown that this is reduced in many dyslexics (Cornelissen et al., 1995; Talcott et al., 2000b; Hill & Raymond, 2002; Downie et al., 2003; Samar & Parasnis, 2005). Over the whole range of reading abilities from good readers to dyslexics, the lower a person's motion sensitivity the worse is his reading (Talcott et al., 2000b). Other work has shown reduced velocity discrimination (Eden et al., 1996; Demb et al., 1998a) and elevated speed thresholds for motion-defined form (Felmingham & Jakobson, 1995) in dyslexics.

Furthermore Fischer (Chapter 2, this volume) demonstrated that many visual and optomotor tasks which are dependent for their speed and accuracy upon M-cell input, are weak in dyslexics at the age of 7 and become progressively more deficient compared with those of good readers as the children grow older. Indeed cohort studies have shown that children's motion sensitivity measured before they start reading predicts their reading progress by the time they are 8 years old (Boets et al., 2011). Thus it is clear that M-cell function plays an important, though not exclusive, role in the acquisition of reading skills.

Nevertheless some people with low motion sensitivity can still be good readers (Skoyles & Skottun, 2004), since visual motion sensitivity is by no means the only influence on their reading. Yet individual differences in motion sensitivity explain over 25% of the variance in reading ability over a whole population (Talcott et al., 2000b). In other words individuals' dorsal stream performance dominated by M-cell input probably does help to determine how well their visual reading skills develop, and this is true of everybody, not just dyslexics.

Higher-level dorsal stream tasks

The PPC receives its main visual input from V5/MT; this input plays a crucial role in its functions of guiding visual attention, eye, and limb movements (Vidyasagar, 2004, Chapter 10, this volume). Dyslexics have been found to be worse than good readers at cueing visual attention (Facoetti et al., 2001; Kinsey et al., 2004, Facoetti, Chapter 8, this volume), visual search (Facoetti et al., 2000; Iles et al., 2000), visual short-term 'retain and compare' memory (Ben-Yehudah et al., 2001) and attentional grouping in the Ternus test

(Cestnick & Coltheart, 1999), visual attention span (Valdois, Chapter 10, this volume). These findings again suggest that dorsal stream function tends to be impaired in dyslexics.

Since none of these tests stimulates the peripheral magnocellular system entirely selectively, these results do not unequivocally prove that impaired magnocellular function is entirely responsible, as Skottun repeatedly reminds us (Skottun & Skoyles, 2011). Nevertheless, as the visual input to the dorsal stream is dominated by the M system, its contribution is clearly important.

Moreover many of the studies mentioned earlier incorporated control tests for P function, such as measuring visual acuity or colour discrimination; dyslexics usually proved to be as good or better at these P-dominated tasks (Hansen et al., 2001). This suggests that their poor performance can be mainly attributed to M-system weakness even in the presence of robust parvocellular function (Fukushima et al., 2005).

Eye movement control by the dorsal stream

Normally the dorsal stream not only directs visual attention to a target but also directs the eyes towards it. Hence numerous studies have found not only that the direction of visual attention is disturbed in dyslexics (Vidyasagar, 2004, Chapter 10, this volume), but also that their eye control during reading is abnormal. This is generally accepted. But these abnormalities are often ascribed to the subject not understanding the text, rather than themselves causing the reading problems. Yet poor eye control has also been demonstrated in several non-reading situations, by tests in children of fixation stability (Fischer & Hartnegg, 2000, Fischer, Chapter 2, this volume), smooth pursuit, and saccadic control (Stein & Fowler, 1982; Crawford & Higham, 2001). In one study, however, although the dyslexics did display abnormal eye movements, these were not significantly associated with worse dorsal stream function as measured by coherent motion detection; but the number of dyslexics studied was very small (Hawelka & Wimmer, 2005).

Event-related potentials

Recording averaged electroencephalogram potentials in response to a moving, low-contrast visual target provides a more objective measure of cortical dorsal stream processing than psychophysical techniques. Of recent visual event-related potential (ERP) studies in dyslexics, the great majority have either confirmed the original observation of Livingstone et al. (1991) that dyslexics have weaker responses to moving, low-contrast, targets than good readers (Kuba et al., 2001), or they have found that dyslexics show slower, smaller, and spatially abnormal, focused visual attentional ERP responses in line with the psychophysical results. Only one study with small numbers found no sensory or attentional abnormalities (Robichon et al., 2002).

Visual treatments

The main purpose of trying to understand the mechanisms causing dyslexics to have reading problems is to help develop effective means of overcoming them. Although evidence that a particular technique works does not by itself prove that the theory underlying it is correct, it provides strong evidence in its favour. Although there is a plethora of claims about visual treatments that help dyslexics to learn to read better, very few have been rigorously designed on the basis of modern understanding of the information processing stages of reading.

Often also they were not properly controlled for placebo effects. The very fact that somebody is taking notice of their reading problems is often sufficient for a child to try harder, to focus his attention more effectively, and to feel better about himself (Hawthorne effect). So reading may improve even if the treatment has no specific effect at all. Such placebo effects should not be denigrated, however; whatever their cause, any improvements should be welcomed. But if they are placebos, they do not justify charging large sums for the treatment, as is often the case. To be plausible also they need to have a clear rationale.

Here, therefore, I will only consider a few techniques that have a rationale that is relevant to the magnocellular theory and that have been subjected to appropriate controls. In 1985 we published the results of a double-blind randomized controlled trial of monocular occlusion when reading (Stein & Fowler, 1985). We studied children with significant reading difficulties who also had unstable binocular control measured using a standard orthoptic test. Randomly selected, we gave them either spectacles with the left lens occluded with opaque tape or placebo clear plano spectacles. We found that those who received the occlusion were more likely to achieve stable binocular control. If they did so, their reading improved significantly more than those receiving placebo who did not achieve stable control (p <0.005). In 2000 we repeated this study using pale yellow spectacles as a better placebo and obtained similar results (Stein et al., 2000). We argued that dyslexics' binocular instability was due to a significant visual magnocellular deficit, and that occluding the left eye when reading helped the ocular motor control system to overcome this deficit to achieve more stable fixation.

We noted that the placebo response to pale yellow filters in 2000 was considerably greater than that to plano clear lenses in 1985. By then we had also found that we could improve amblyopia in some children using deep yellow filters (Fowler et al., 1991). We argued that these effects were because yellow light actually stimulates the magnocellular system specifically. M-ganglion cells do not contribute to conscious colour vision; but they receive mainly from both the long (red) and medium wavelength (green) cones; hence they are optimally activated by yellow light. Therefore we tested whether deep yellow filters designed to maximally activate M cells, might be even more effective at improving M-cell function and reading in children with visual reading difficulties. In a double-blind randomized controlled trial we showed that this was indeed the case for some children (Ray et al., 2005). We gave to randomly selected children who had found that yellow made small print look clearer, either yellow filters or placebo to use for all close work for 3 months. The placebo was a card with a slit to place over text to restrict reading to a single word at a time, as suggested by (Geiger & Lettvin, 1987). Those who received the yellow filters increased their sensitivity to visual motion in random dot kinematograms, i.e. their M responses improved, and this was accompanied by significantly greater progress in single word reading and spelling than with the placebo (p <0.05). We have since confirmed that the yellow filters actually do increase the amount of long wavelength light falling on the retina, hence stimulating M cells more, because they cause the pupil to dilate.

Serendipitously we also observed that some children benefited more from wearing deep blue filters than yellow. Probably the Oxford blue filters selectively activate intrinsically photosensitive retinal ganglion cells (IPRGCs) which contain the blue sensitive pigment melanopsin (Hankins et al., 2008). These cells project, not to the conscious, image signalling, retinogeniculate visual system, but to the hypothalamus. Their function there is to entrain the body's internal clock in the hypothalamic suprachiasmatic nucleus (SCN) to seasonally varying day length. We wake up earlier in the summer because the IPRGCs signal the amount of blue light entering the eye, which is maximal in the morning. This arousal is mediated by the SCN which specifically activates the dorsal M-dominated 'where' visual pathway. Hence when we give children blue filters we facilitate the dorsal visual stream and this seems to help the children to focus their attention and eye movements more reliably. Accordingly we have recently shown in another randomized control trial that giving most children with visual reading problems blue filters increases their single word reading accuracy more than giving them yellow.

Improving the synchronization of diurnal rhythms has other benefits as well. Many children with visual reading difficulties have disturbed sleep patterns. Their parents are often surprised that the blue filters seem to improve their child's sleeping as well as his reading.

Likewise many such children complain of headaches when they try to read. Migraine headaches are known to be accompanied by disturbed sleep rhythms. Hence we now have many anecdotal reports that successful treatment of reading difficulties with blue filters is also accompanied by fewer headaches, and we are now following this up more systematically.

Multicoloured filters

There are many commercial companies selling ranges of coloured filters for reading problems with the claim that each person needs an individually prescribed colour for best effect; thus using only yellow and blue would fail to meet individual requirements. In one study (Wilkins et al., 1994), 68 children viewed text illuminated by coloured light in an apparatus that allowed the separate manipulation of hue (colour) and saturation (depth of colour), at constant luminance, in order to find the colour that would help them most. A pair of plastic spectacle lenses was then dyed so as to provide the appropriate chromaticity under conventional white (F3) fluorescent light for each child. A placebo pair was also made that looked a similar colour but had a chromaticity outside the range which they had previously found to improve their visual symptoms. Each pair was worn for 1 month. Neither the children, nor the examiner, knew who had received correct or placebo colour.

Almost half the children dropped out of the study altogether, presumably because the glasses did not help them. Of those who did complete it slightly more did indeed report a reduction in their symptoms of eye strain and headache when the filter had the chromaticity that they had chosen, which was different for each individual. Significantly from our point of view, however, most of these chromaticities clustered around yellow or blue (Wilkins et al., 1994). The children kept diaries recording their symptoms; but only 36 (53%) of these were completed. Symptoms were slightly less frequent during the month that the correct lenses had been worn; but the difference was small and there is no evidence that simple yellow and blue would not have been equally or more efficacious.

Thus the evidence for requiring a large range of filter colours is not strong; the individual colours chosen usually cluster around yellow and blue and if the M theory outlined here is correct, yellow and blue alone should suffice. In an as yet unpublished head-to-head study comparing our Oxford blue and yellow filters with another company's much wider range of colours, our Oxford filters actually achieved superior results.

In summary there are now a fair number of clinical trials showing that visual treatments derived from the visual magnocellular theory of reading problems have produced worthwhile improvements in children's reading. These will remain controversial until many more and larger, properly controlled, trials have been carried out. But they are at least consistent with the M theory.

Opposition to the magnocellular theory

The great critic of the view that impaired visual magnocellular development may contribute to visual dyslexic problems is Brent Skottun (Gross-Glen, 1995; Skottun, 2010). In nearly 50 papers so far, mainly criticizing others' work, he points out that it is difficult selectively to activate only visual magno cells, and it is impossible to record responses either psychophysiologically or physiologically in the cortex which are not to some extent contaminated by parvocellular input. However parvo influence can be made very small because dorsal 'where' pathway responses are dominated by their visual magnocellular input. Skottun claims that of the papers that use selective magnocellular stimuli to test dyslexics' M sensitivity, there are more that fail to find such a selective deficit than show it. Nevertheless of the experimental studies in which stimuli have been used that mainly excite M cells, 90% have shown some degree of impairment in dyslexics.

Note that even Skottun is not claiming that dyslexics do not suffer a visual deficit, merely that it has not been clearly shown to be dependent upon impaired peripheral visual magnocellular processing. He suggests that the visual deficit can affect both parvocellular and magnocellular systems and that it may be attributed to deficiencies in visual attention. However, since the evidence is now overwhelming that the magnocellular system dominates both bottom-up capture of visual attention and dorsal stream-mediated top-down voluntary orientation of visual attention (Vidyasagar, Chapter 10, this volume), this still leaves the major visual deficit in dyslexia attributable to a magnocellular deficit.

An extended magnocellular system for temporal processing?

Large nerve cells with rapid temporal processing, 'transient', sensitivity are not confined to the peripheral visual system but are found throughout the whole of the rest of the nervous system, in the auditory and cutaneous sensory systems, and in memory and motor systems, such as the cerebellum (Hockfield & Sur, 1990). These large cells are probably all related through development, because they all express similar surface antigens, recognized by antibodies such as CAT 301. These surface signature molecules enable them to make preferential functional connections with each other.

Shatz and her colleagues have shown that the development of these magno cells and their connections, at least in the visual system and the hippocampus, is regulated by the major histocompatibility complex (MHC) cell recognition and immune regulation gene system (Corriveau et al., 1998). Most of the 150 known MHC genes reside on the short arm of chromosome 6. When M cells start information processing, MHC class 1 proteins begin to be expressed on their surfaces, probably to help them find other M cells to interact with. This is why CAT 301 staining can be used to identify magnocellular neurons throughout the nervous system.

If neurons do not make useful connections during development they are eliminated by the process of apoptosis, summed up in the epithet 'use it or lose it'. Ninety per cent of all the neurons generated in the germinal zones are eliminated in this way during the assembly of functional processing networks during development. The 10% of M cells that survive form an extended network specialized for rapid temporal processing, particularly for the direction of attention.

The surface signatures on neurons are not only important to recognize each other and make such connections, but also to label them as 'self' so that microglial scavenging cells recognize them and do not to attempt to destroy them as foreign invaders. But magno cells seem to be particularly vulnerable to genetic, immunological, and other general environmental influences. They are selectively damaged in prematurity, birth hypoxia, malnutrition, autoimmune diseases, and in the many overlapping neurodevelopmental conditions described earlier, not only dyslexia, but also dyspraxia, dysphasia, dyscalculia, ADHD, and autistic spectrum disorders.

Auditory transient processing

Although we do it without thinking, identifying and ordering the sequences of sounds that make up speech is hardly less difficult than sequencing letters. All doctors in training know this when they try to identify whether a heart murmur is systolic or diastolic. Whether the murmur comes before or after the second heart sound is often very difficult to decide; yet cardiac events are far slower than in average speech. This serial analysis depends on being able to accurately detect changes in sound frequency and amplitude, such as those that convey information in speech, and to memorize their order. Like the visual M system this tracking of auditory transients in real time is mediated by a set of large neurons specialized for rapid temporal processing. These contrast with the smaller neurons that identify different mixtures of frequencies, such as chords, by their spectral composition. These neurons work less rapidly and may be likened to visual parvo cells. Thus in the auditory system there are equivalents to the M and P systems, though at no stage are they entirely separate; so they are not named as in the visual system. Also there are auditory equivalents to the dorsal and ventral streams (Rauschecker & Tian, 2000).

We therefore began testing children's ability to detect simple amplitude or frequency changes to see whether dyslexics might have impaired amplitude and frequency transient sensitivity (McAnally & Stein, 1996). Indeed the dyslexics did display lower sensitivity to amplitude (AM) or frequency modulations (FM) of a 500-Hz carrier, up to modulation frequencies of 40 Hz. Above this rate there were no significant differences between dyslexics and controls, probably because the auditory system can no longer follow these high rates in real time. Instead the percept becomes qualitatively different; rather than individual modulations we hear a single chord. Analysis of this is mediated by the smaller neurons which identify the whole spectrum generated by high frequency modulations.

We also found that the AM and FM sensitivity of individual children, whether dyslexic or not, predicted their ability to read non-words, which is regarded as a task that particularly tests their phonological skills (Snowling et al., 1986). Auditory sensitivity to frequency and amplitude modulations accounted for nearly 50% of individual differences in phonological skill (Witton et al., 2002).

Paula Tallal was the first to suggest that developmental dysphasics may be poor at the auditory temporal processing that is required for the discrimination of speech sounds (Tallal & Piercy, 1973). In the last 5 years there have been over 100 studies testing basic auditory processing capabilities in dyslexics. Almost all have confirmed our finding that at least some dyslexics have auditory temporal processing deficits that could help to explain their phonological weaknesses (Banai et al., 2005; Boets et al., 2006; Stoodley et al., 2006).

Again, however, there are wide discrepancies in the prevalences claimed, ranging from 10–70%. Current psychophysical tests may not be sensitive enough to reveal the mild deficits that may cause reading problems. So it is still argued that there can be higher-level phonological problems without any evidence of lower-level auditory temporal processing impairments. However, using a mismatch negativity paradigm, we showed that even in the absence of a psychophysiologically demonstrable deficit, one can usually show some degree of low-level auditory processing impairment that correlates with the subjects' phonological problems (Stoodley et al., 2006).

In general, ERP studies of auditory processing in dyslexics have proved more sensitive than psychophysical ones, and most people would now accept that dyslexics with phonological problems have some degree of underlying impaired low-level auditory processing of transient stimuli to explain their phonological deficit.

Auditory magnocellular system?

This low-level auditory processing deficit may be associated with impaired development of the large M-like neurons in the brainstem that mediate auditory transient processing for tracking frequency and amplitude modulations. Like visual magno cells, they are recognized by M-specific antibodies, such as CAT 301 (Lurie et al., 1997), so that they form part of the extended M system described earlier.

It is significant that in dyslexics poor visual magnocellular function is often accompanied by poor auditory temporal processing suggesting that both visual and auditory M systems are impaired in dyslexia (Talcott et al., 2000b). This has been confirmed pathologically.

Galaburda et al. (1994) found in the dyslexic brains they studied, like those in the dyslexic LGN the magnocellular division of the thalamic auditory medial geniculate nucleus (MGN) contained fewer large cells on the left. Impaired development of large M-like cells in the auditory system might therefore underlie dyslexics' problems with acquiring good phonological skills.

Since not all dyslexics who show phonological problems can be shown to have either auditory or visual weaknesses, these are neither necessary nor sufficient to cause dyslexia. Some have argued from this that they cannot be considered causal at all (Ramus et al., 2003). But this is like saying that because smoking is neither necessary nor sufficient to cause lung cancer it can never cause it—patently false. The probability is that impaired auditory and visual temporal processing are important, but not the only, causes of impaired phonological processing.

The cerebellum

The cerebellum is the brain's autopilot responsible for automaticizing motor skills by building up internal models to represent their execution. Since accurate timing of sensory feedback and motor outflow is an essential requirement for this function, the cerebellum receives a rich input from visual, auditory, proprioceptive, and motor magnocellular systems (Stein, 1986; Eckert et al., 2005). Furthermore many precerebellar nuclear cells and cerebellar Purkinje cells stain for the magnocellular specific antigen CAT 301; hence the cerebellum can be considered part of the extended M system described earlier. Accordingly there is now a great deal of evidence that cerebellar function is mildly impaired in dyslexics and related neurodevelopmental conditions such as developmental coordination disorder (dyspraxia) (Nicolson, 2001a; Rae et al., 2002; Stoodley & Stein, 2011). This provides yet further indirect evidence for magnocellular involvement in dyslexic problems (Nicolson, 2001b).

Cutaneous sensation

The dorsal column somatosensory system is in many ways analogous to the dorsal visuomotor route, since it consists of large axons carrying rapidly adapting skin and muscle receptor signals. We therefore tested the vibration sensitivity of adult dyslexics compared with good readers. The dyslexics turned out to be significantly less sensitive to vibration at 3 Hz (P <0. 01) but no different at 100 Hz (Stoodley et al., 2000). Cutaneous sensory fibres can follow frequencies of 3 Hz in real time, but not at 100 Hz. This result is compatible with the hypothesis that a generalized, multisensory deficit of M-like cell temporal processing functions underlies dyslexia.

Functional imaging

Although there are no functional imaging studies directly examining the role of the peripheral visual M system in dyslexia (which would be very hard to carry out and still subject to the criticism that they are not pure M), there have been many studies whose findings are consistent with the M hypothesis. Thus in dyslexics the visual motion area MT/V5 has been shown to be less activated than in good readers in response to moving stimuli and it is one of the areas consistently less activated in dyslexics during reading (Eden et al., 1996; Demb et al., 1998b). Furthermore, in individuals the degree of activation of V5/MT during a visual motion task correlates with that person's reading skills, implying a significant association between dorsal stream function and reading (Demb et al., 1997).

Recently a new technique (diffusion tensor imaging) has been developed for tracing connections between areas in the intact human brain. This has shown that in dyslexics the connections linking the elements of the language network in the left hemisphere are weaker than in good readers (Odegard et al., 2009; Démonet & Reilhac, Chapter 1, this volume). This is consistent with their being thinner (i.e. the axons of smaller M cells). Importantly if a dyslexic's reading is successfully improved by training, these connections appear to strengthen (Gabrieli, 2009) and there are also morphological improvements (Krafnick et al., 2011). This is probably not associated with increased myelination of the fibres, but rather by reorientation of microtubules within the fibres. This may occur after they have been experiencing heavier electrical traffic, as would occur during successfully learning associations between visually identified letters, eye movements, letter sounds and word meanings.

There is a general consensus that there are three main left-sided language areas that are less activated in dyslexics than in good readers when reading. The first is on the dorsal where pathway in the left occipital-parietal-temporal junction around the supramarginal and angular gyri (Shaywitz et al., 1998; Pugh et al., 2005). The visual input to the these areas is known to be dominated by the magnocellular system, so that the relative underactivity there is consistent with depleted M input in dyslexics.

The second area implicated is the VWFA which lies in the ventral 'what' processing stream in the anterior part of the left fusiform gyrus on the undersurface of the occipito-temporal junction (Cohen & Dehaene, 2004). Even though it is on the ventral 'what' identification pathway, it receives about half its input from M cells that probably mediate the direction of its attention to visual word features. And almost all studies agree that VWFA is underactivated when dyslexics are reading compared with controls, again consistent with reduced M input.

The third area which is underactivated in dyslexics is in the anterior part of the left inferior frontal gyrus (Démonet & Reilhac, Chapter 1, this volume). In addition to receiving letter sound information from the anterior part of the temporal lobe via the uncinate fasciculus, this area is a major recipient of the visual dorsal pathway projection from the PPC via the arcuate fasciculus. So again its underactivity is consistent with an underactive M system.

Extended M-theory

Therefore one can speculate that perhaps all the visual, auditory, memory, and motor temporal processing impairments that are seen in dyslexics may be due to underlying weak development of this central nervous system-wide, pansensory, transient processing, magnocellular system (Stein & Walsh, 1997; Hari & Renvall, 2001; Stein, 2001). This impairment might idiosyncratically affect different individuals more in one system than another, so that one dyslexic might suffer mainly visual problems, whereas another may have mainly auditory difficulties, and yet a third mainly motor symptoms; he would then be termed 'dyspraxic'.

One can take this idea a stage further. Ramus showed in a small group of well-compensated undergraduate dyslexics that only a few of them had demonstrable auditory, visual, or motor problems, whereas despite their compensation most could still be shown to have residual phonological difficulties (Ramus et al., 2003). So he attributed the latter to a higher-level developmental abnormality, perhaps in the angular gyrus (Ramus, 2004). Since the angular gyrus is an important node in the M-cell dominated dorsal visuomotor stream, clearly this impairment might also involve impaired higher-level magnocellular connections.

There has been little opposition to or comment on the extension of the magnocellular theory to all kinds of temporal processing that is proposed here. CAT 301-staining magno cells have been shown to permeate the whole central nervous system. They have been shown to be specialized for processing transients in real time ('temporal processing') in both the visual and auditory systems, and they certainly contribute to it in the cerebellum. There is evidence that their development is impaired in the visual and auditory systems in at least some dyslexics and in other neurodevelopmental conditions as well. Furthermore there is a gradually emerging consensus that dyslexia is indeed associated with general temporal processing deficits. Final confirmation or refutation of the extended magnocellular theory will only come when the genetic mechanisms controlling the development and specialization of magno cells are fully understood. In the meantime the evidence will remain tentative and circumstantial. But in complex systems like this there is rarely one piece of evidence that is conclusive; rather, observations pile on each other until finally everyone is convinced one way or the other, and then they say it's obvious!

Causes of M-cell impairment

Of course the really interesting question is why dyslexics have impaired development of these magnocellular systems. There are three interacting factors that we consider here: genetic, immunological, and nutritional.

Dyslexia genetics

In his book *Hereditary Genius* (1869), Galton proposed that a system of arranged marriages between men of distinction and women of wealth would eventually produce a superior race. He coined the term 'eugenics' in 1883 to describe these eutopian arrangements and continued to expound their benefits until his death in 1911. Henry Maudsley, who rebuilt the Bedlam (now Maudsley) Hospital in London using his own money, initially supported these ideas. But later his psychiatric experience taught him to oppose them strongly. As the foremost psychiatrist of his day he observed that most of the great creative and successful families in Victorian England sheltered relatives who had 'mental' problems. He judged it dangerously simplistic to believe that mental disease was entirely hereditary and he feared that eliminating the genes that influence mental health might also eliminate creativity and imagination. He had worked out intuitively that the genes that help to cause conditions like dyslexia, depression, and schizophrenia would not be as common as they were unless they also contributed to the talents that made other members of these families so successful. But not until the 1930s did eugenic theories come under serious attack after the Nazis began to exploit them to support their extermination of Jews, gypsies, and homosexuals.

I begin this section on this note of caution to urge us to ponder why we should study the genetic basis of dyslexia at all. We certainly should not be trying to 'root out dyslexia genes' because thereby we might eliminate our chances of benefiting from future highly talented dyslexics, the likes of Da Vinci, Einstein, or Churchill. If pure curiosity to unravel the genetic basis of dyslexia were to have that effect, then we should vigorously oppose it.

Instead the main purpose of gaining understanding of how genes influence reading ability is to be able to make use of the incredibly powerful techniques of modern molecular genetics in order to work out the biochemical and developmental processes which cause the brain differences that underlie dyslexic reading problems—certainly not in order to diagnose it *in utero* for possible abortion.

Perhaps the most important gain that has already accrued from the uncontested demonstration that dyslexia has a strong genetic component is that this proves absolutely that dyslexia is a real neurological condition, and not a euphemism to hide middle-class children's laziness or stupidity. Demonstrating that dyslexia has a strong genetic basis has made it impossible to maintain that it is a myth or 'purely psychological'; rather it has a clear neurobiological reality. Knowing that his dyslexia is a respectable neurological diagnosis, and not another word for laziness or stupidity can transform a child's self-image. From losing all self-confidence because he could not keep up with his peers, giving a child the diagnosis of dyslexia can return to him, self-respect and hope. Then this often gives him the confidence to exploit the talents that many dyslexics undoubtedly possess but have lain hidden behind their desperate struggles to learn to read.

Writing was only invented *c*.4000 years ago, so literacy itself is a cultural development, and not likely to be under direct genetic control. Instead reading and writing must have piggy-backed on more fundamental sensory and motor processing functions that originally evolved for other purposes. These develop under the combined influence of genes and the environment. Modern genetic techniques are already helping us to elucidate the mechanisms by which certain alleles lead to vulnerability in the development of the nervous system that contribute to reading problems.

One great advantage of studying in particular the development of reading is that reading is much easier to measure precisely than many other higher functions, such as emotion, motivation, or delusional thinking. As a result, unlike the 600 or so genes of small effect that have been implicated in schizophrenia (Porteous, 2008), less than a dozen genes with much larger effects have now been associated with dyslexia and their role in reading is steadily being unravelled (Williams & O'Donovan, 2006).

We have taken advantage of the large number of families with children with reading problems that we have seen around Oxford to carry out whole genome quantitative trait linkage studies. We collected nearly 400 Oxford families and replicated many of our findings in 200 Colorado families provided by Dick Olsen. I shall just discuss one new gene that these analyses revealed.

KIAA0319

This is a gene situated on the short arm of chromosome 6 in amongst the MHC complex, a gene named *KIAA0319* (Paracchini et al., 2006). This is quite close to another gene, *DCDC2*, which has also been implicated in dyslexia. *KIAA0319* appears to be underexpressed in many dyslexics, and the protein it encodes is now known to be a partly extracellular, cell surface signalling molecule, perhaps controlling the expression of surface signature molecules such as those recognized by the M-selective antibody CAT 301. In the normal course of the early development of the cerebral cortex, neurons born in the ventricular zone migrate up the radial glia to their correct positions on the cortical surface to form the six layers of the cerebral cortex. But if *KIAA0319* is completely switched off by local electroporation of a specific inhibitory RNAi in the rat embryo brain, the cells fail to migrate at all and remain clustered around the ventricle (Paracchini et al., 2006).

Of course, in dyslexia *KIAA0319* is not completely knocked out, but it is thought to be 30% less expressed. Reduced production of such a vital cell–cell signalling molecule could explain the mismigration of M cells that is found in brains of dyslexics postmortem (Galaburda et al., 1985). As described earlier, these anomalies have been seen in the magnocellular layers of the visual LGN, the magnocellular portion of the left auditory MGN, and in the form of outgrowths of neurons (ectopias) in the cerebral cortex.

At least two other genes have also been associated with dyslexia that are involved in the control of neural migration early in the development of the brain (Galaburda et al., 2006). Unravelling the precise function of these promises to revolutionize our understanding of neurodevelopmental disorders, and with it, hopefully our ability to treat them successfully. This applies not only to dyslexia, but to the whole gamut of neurodevelopmental conditions that overlap with it, both genetically and phenotypically, such as developmental dysphasia (specific language impairment), dyscalculia, developmental dyspraxia, ADHD, and autistic spectrum disorders.

Autoimmunity

Because their development is under the control of the MHC gene complex with the gene *KIAA0319* in their midst, one way of identifying magno cells throughout the nervous system is to stain them for their characteristic surface antigen with antibodies such as CAT 301. Unfortunately magno cells, so vulnerable in other ways, also seem to be particularly vulnerable to antibody attack. Antineuronal antibodies are found in the blood in many general autoimmune conditions such as systemic lupus erythematosus (Lahita, 1988). The BSXB 'autoimmune' mouse has been bred as an animal model of lupus. This mouse develops ectopias similar to those seen in dyslexic brains. So it is not surprising to find a very high incidence of dyslexia and other neurodevelopmental conditions in the children of mothers with lupus.

Interestingly also, dyslexic children and their families consistently report a higher prevalence of immunological problems—not only lupus which is rare, but also much commoner conditions such as eczema, asthma, and allergies (Hugdahl et al., 1990). Although most antibodies circulating in a mother's blood are prevented from crossing the placenta to affect her fetus, some can cross over and even reach the fetal brain. We decided therefore to see whether mothers with dyslexic or autistic children showed any signs of circulating antimagnocellular antibodies in their blood. We took serum from mothers who had had two or more dyslexic or autistic children and injected it into pregnant mice. We then tested the offspring for behavioural abnormalities and looked for anomalies in cerebellar metabolism by magnetic resonance spectroscopy (MRS) and in cerebellar antibody binding. We found that indeed these young mice showed deficits in motor coordination. These abnormalities were associated with antibodies binding to the pup's cerebellar Purkinje cells and their severity correlated with MRS indices of impaired cerebellar metabolism (Vincent et al., 2002).

Taken together therefore, these findings about the association between autoimmunity, magnocellular development, and dyslexia provide further support for the hypothesis that a specific magnocellular impairment may underlie the manifold symptomatology of dyslexia and that this can be the result of immunological attack.

Nutrition—omega-3 fish oils

Another of the chromosomal sites that showed very strong linkage to reading difficulties in our Oxford and Colorado samples of dyslexic families was on chromosome 18 (18p11.2) very close to the melanocortin receptor 5 gene (*MCR5*). This receptor is not strongly expressed in the brain and so far we do not have any direct evidence that the gene is involved in dyslexia. But we do know that it is involved in appetite control, in particular affecting the metabolism of omega-3 essential fatty acids. The same site (18p11.2) has been implicated in bipolar depression susceptibility (Berrettini et al., 1994).

We are particularly interested in the possible role of this gene in the metabolism of omega-3 long-chain polyunsaturated fatty acids (LCPUFAs) derived from fish oils, because M cells seem to be particularly vulnerable to omega-3 LCPUFA deficiency. A single omega-3 LCPUFA, docosahexaenoic acid (DHA), constitutes 20% of neuronal membranes. Each of our brains contains 100 g of DHA because it has just the right properties to contribute flexibility and the correct electrostatic profile to the nerve membrane. As such, it has been conserved in eukaryotic membranes throughout evolution since the Cambrian explosion 600 million years ago. There are cogent reasons for believing that, evolving near water, our ready access to this molecule from eating fish, explains how our brains came to be so much larger in relation to our body size than is the case in other animals. It seems to be particularly important for proper magnocellular neuronal function because it is kinky and thus prevents lipid molecules from packing together too tightly. This confers sufficient flexibility in the membrane to allow M-ionic channels to open and close very fast.

But DHA is continuously leeched out of the membrane by phospholipases because it also forms the basis of many prostaglandin, leukotriene and interleukin signalling molecules. So it has to be replaced from dietary sources. Likewise another omega-3 LCPUFA, eicosapentaenoic acid (EPA), is the substrate for other eicosanoid prostaglandins, leukotrienes, and resolvins, which all tend to be anti-inflammatory, and also need to be replaced.

However, nowadays we eat far too little oily fish to replace them. The modern Western diet is dreadful; three-quarters of current teenagers eat no fish at all, so that they tend to be deficient not only in LCPUFAs but also fat-soluble vitamins, such as vitamins A and D and essential minerals. Hence a high proportion of the population, particularly from deprived households, is dangerously deficient in these essential nutrients. In contrast they are dangerously oversupplied with salt, sugar, saturated fat, and omega-6 fatty acids, the '4 Ss'; this imbalance goes a long way to explain our modern epidemic of heart disease, cancers, and psychiatric problems.

Because of the vulnerability of M cells to lack of omega-3 LCPUFAs we decided to see whether giving children supplement capsules containing EPA and DHA from oily fish could improve their focus of attention and their reading. In a double-blind randomized controlled trial Richardson & Montgomery (2005) were able to show that simply giving deprived 10-year-old children these supplements for 3 months improved their reading age by 9 months in the 3 months, compared with the group who received placebo capsules containing olive oil, whose reading advanced by only the 3 months you would expect of an average child.

We also observed that the children we were studying appeared calmer and less aggressive in the playground. So we began experimenting with giving young offenders in prison, many of whom are dyslexic, supplement capsules of fish oils, minerals, and vitamins. In a pilot double-blind randomized controlled trial we compared active supplements with placebo in nearly 300 male youths in a tough young offenders institute. The active supplements reduced these prisoners' rate of offending by a remarkable 33%—'peace on a plate' (Gesch et al., 2002). We are now completing a much larger study, hopefully to prove conclusively that simply improving these young lads' diets can help them to control themselves better and therefore to behave less antisocially. If such a simple and cheap solution really is that powerful, it will have profound implications.

Conclusion

Genetic, developmental, nutritional, neuroanatomical, physiological, and psychophysiological evidence all support the view that fundamentally the visual and/phonological reading problems that dyslexics suffer may be due to pervasive impaired development of magnocellular neurons throughout the brain.

References

Banai, K., Nicol, T., Zecker, S.G., & Kraus, N. (2005). Brainstem timing: Implications for cortical processing and literacy. *Journal of Neuroscience, 25*(43), 9850–7.

Bednarek, D.B., & Grabowska, A. (2002). Luminance and chromatic contrast sensitivity in dyslexia: the magnocellular deficit hypothesis revisited. *NeuroReport*, 13(18), 2521–5.

Ben-Yehudah, G., Sackett, E., Malchi-Ginzberg, L., & Ahissar, M. (2001). Impaired temporal contrast sensitivity in dyslexics is specific to retain-and-compare paradigms. *Brain*, 124, 1381–95.

Berrettini, W.H., Ferraro, T.N., Goldin, L.R., Weeks, D.E., Detera-Wadleigh, S., Nurnberger, J.I., *et al.* (1994). Chromosome 18 DNA markers and manic-depressive illness: evidence for a susceptibility gene. *Proceedings of the National Academy of Sciences of the United States of America*, 91(13), 5918–21.

Boets, B., Wouters, J., van Wieringen, A., & Ghesquiere, P. (2006). Auditory temporal information processing in preschool children at family risk for dyslexia: Relations with phonological abilities and developing literacy skills. *Brain and Language*, 97(1), 64–79.

Boets, B., Vandermosten, M., Cornelissen, P., Wouters, J., & Ghesquière, P. (2011). Coherent motion sensitivity and reading development in the transition from prereading to reading stage. *Child Development*, 82(3), 854–69.

Cestnick, L., & M., C. (1999). The relationship between language-processing and visual-processing deficits in developmental dyslexia. *Cognition*, 71, 231–55.

Chase, C.H., & Jenner, A. (1993). Magnocellular processing deficits affect temporal processing of dyslexics. *Annals of the New York Academy of Sciences*, 682, 326–30.

Cheng, A., Eysel, U., & Vidyasagar, T. (2004). The role of the magnocellular pathway in serial deployment of visual attention. *European Journal of Neuroscience*, 20, 2188–92.

Cohen, L., & Dehaene, S. (2004). Specialization within the ventral stream: the case for the visual word form area. *Neuroimage*, 22(1), 466–76.

Cornelissen, P., Richardson, A., Mason, A., Fowler, S., & Stein, J. (1995). Contrast sensitivity and coherent motion detection measured at photopic luminance levels in dyslexics and controls. *Vision Research*, 35(10), 1483–94.

Corriveau, R., Huh, G., & Shatz, C. (1998). Regulation of Class 1 MHC gene expression in the developing and mature CNS by neural activity. *Neuron*, 21, 505–20.

Crawford, T., & Higham, S. (2001). Dyslexia and centre of gravity effect. *Experimental Brain Research*, 137, 122–6.

Demb, J.B., Boynton, G.M., & Heeger, D.J. (1997). Brain activity in visual cortex predicts individual differences in reading performance. *Proceedings of the National Academy of Sciences of the United States of America*, 94(24), 13363–6.

Demb, J.B., Boynton, G.M., Best, M., & Heeger, D.J. (1998a). Psychophysical evidence for a magnocellular pathway deficit in dyslexia. *Vision Research*, 38(11), 1555–9.

Demb, J.B., Boynton, G.M., & Heeger, D.J. (1998b). Functional magnetic resonance imaging of early visual pathways in dyslexia. *Journal of Neuroscience*, 18(17), 6939–51.

Downie, A.L., Jakobson, L.S., Frisk, V., & Ushycky, I. (2003). Periventricular brain injury, visual motion processing, and reading and spelling abilities in children who were extremely low birthweight. *Journal of the International Neuropsychological Society*, 9(3), 440–9.

Eckert, M.A., Leonard, C.M., Wilke, M., Eckert, M., Richards, T., Richards, A., *et al.* (2005). Anatomical signatures of dyslexia in children: unique information from manual and voxel based morphometry brain measures. *Cortex*, 41(3), 304–15.

Eden, G.F., VanMeter, J.W., Rumsey, J.M., Maisog, J.M., Woods, R.P., & Zeffiro, T.A. (1996). Abnormal processing of visual motion in dyslexia revealed by functional brain imaging. *Nature*, 382(6586), 66–9.

Edwards, V.T., Giaschi, D.E., Dougherty, R.F., Edgell, D., Bjornson, B.H., Lyons, C., *et al.* (2004). Psychophysical indexes of temporal processing abnormalities in children with developmental dyslexia. *Developmental Neuropsychology*, 25, 321–54.

Elliot, J. (2006). Dyslexia: Diagnoses, debates and diatribes. *Education Canada*, 46(2), 14–17.

Facoetti, A., Paganoni, P., & Lorusso, M.L. (2000). The spatial distribution of visual attention in developmental dyslexia. *Experimental Brain Research, 132*(4), 531–8.

Facoetti, A., Turatto, M., Lorusso, M.L., & Mascetti, G.G. (2001). Orienting visual attention in dyslexia. *Experimental Brain Research, 138,* 46–53.

Felmingham, K.L., & Jakobson, L.S. (1995). Visual and visuomotor performance in dyslexic children. *Experimental Brain Research, 106*(3), 467–74.

Fischer, B., & Hartnegg, K. (2000). Stability of gaze control in dyslexia. *Strabismus, 8*(2), 119–22.

Fowler, M.S., Mason, A.J., Richardson, A., & Stein, J.F. (1991). Yellow spectacles to improve vision in children with binocular amblyopia. *Lancet, 338*(8775), 1109–10.

Fukushima, J., Tanaka, S., Williams, J., & Fukushima, K. (2005). Voluntary control of saccadic and smooth-pursuit eye movements in children with learning disorders. *Brain and Development, 27*(8), 579–88.

Gabrieli, J.D.E. (2009). Dyslexia: A new synergy between education and cognitive neuroscience. *Science, 325*(5938), 280–3.

Galaburda, A.M., LoTurco, J., Ramus, F., Fitch, R.H., & Rosen, G.D. (2006). From genes to behavior in developmental dyslexia. *Nature Neuroscience, 9*(10), 1213–17.

Galaburda, A.M., Menard, M.T., & Rosen, G.D. (1994). Evidence for aberrant auditory anatomy in developmental dyslexia. *Proceedings of the National Academy of Sciences of the United States of America, 91*(17), 8010–13.

Galaburda, A.M., Sherman, G.F., Rosen, G.D., Aboitiz, F., & Geschwind, N. (1985). Developmental dyslexia: four consecutive patients with cortical anomalies. *Annals of Neurology, 18*(2), 222–33.

Galton, F. (1869). *Hereditary Genius: An Inquiry into its Laws and Consequences.* London.

Geiger, G., & Lettvin, J.Y. (1987). Peripheral vision in persons with dyslexia. *New England Journal of Medicine, 316*(20), 1238–40.

Gesch, C.B., Hammond, S.M., Hampson, S.E., Eves, A., & Crowder, M.J. (2002). Influence of supplementary vitamins, minerals and essential fatty acids on the antisocial behaviour of young adult prisoners. Randomised, placebo-controlled trial. *British Journal of Psychiatry, 181,* 22–8.

Goodale, M.A., & Milner. A.D. (1992). Separate visual pathways for perception and action. *Trends in Neurosciences, 15,* 20.

Gross-Glen, K., Skottun, B.C., Glenn, W., Kushch, A., Lingua, R., Dunbar, M., *et al.* (1995). Contrast sensitivity in dyslexia. *Visual Neuroscience, 12*(1), 153–63.

Hankins, M.W., Peirson, S.N., & Foster, R.G. (2008). Melanopsin: an exciting photopigment. *Trends in Neurosciences, 31*(1), 27–36.

Hansen, P.C., Stein, J.F., Orde, S.R., Winter, J.L., & Talcott, J.B. (2001). Are dyslexics' visual deficits limited to measures of dorsal stream function? *NeuroReport, 12*(7), 1527–30.

Hari, R., & Renvall, H. (2001). Impaired processing of rapid stimulus sequences in dyslexia. *Trends in Cognitive Sciences, 5,* 525–32.

Hawelka, S., & Wimmer, H. (2005). Impaired visual processing of multi-element arrays is associated with increased number of eye movements in dyslexic reading. *Vision Research, 45*(7), 855–63.

Hill, G.T., & Raymond, J.E. (2002). Deficits of motion transparency perception in adult developmental dyslexics with normal unidirectional motion sensitivity. *Vision Research, 42*(9), 1195–203.

Hockfield, S., & Sur, M. (1990). Monoclonal Cat-301 identifies Y cells in cat LGN. *Journal of Comparative Neurology, 300,* 320–30.

Hugdahl, K., Synnevag, B., & Satz, P. (1990). Immune and autoimmune diseases in dyslexic children [published erratum appears in *Neuropsychologia,* 1991, 29(2), 211]. *Neuropsychologia, 28*(7), 673–9.

Iles, J., Walsh, V., & Richardson, A. (2000). Visual search performance in dyslexia. *Dyslexia, 6*(3), 163–77.

Kinsey, K., Rose, M., Hansen, P., Richardson, A., & Stein, J. (2004). Magnocellular mediated visual-spatial attention and reading ability. *NeuroReport, 15,* 2215–18.

Krafnick, A.J., Flowers, D.L., Napoliello, E.M., & Eden, G.F. (2011). Gray matter volume changes following reading intervention in dyslexic children. *Neuroimage*, 57(3), 733–41.

Kuba, M., Szanyi, J., Gayer, D., Kremlacek, J., & Kubova, Z. (2001). Electrophysiological testing of dyslexia. *Acta Medica (Hradec Kralove)*, 44(4), 131–4.

Lahita, R.G. (1988). Systemic lupus erythematosus: learning disability in the male offspring of female patients and relationship to laterality. *Psychoneuroendocrinology*, 13, 385–96.

Livingstone, M.S., Rosen, G.D., Drislane, F.W., & Galaburda, A.M. (1991). Physiological and anatomical evidence for a magnocellular deficit in developmental dyslexia. *Proceedings of the National Academy of Sciences of the United States of America*, 88, 7943–47.

Lovegrove, W., & Badcock, D. (1981). The effect of spatial frequency on colour selectivity in the tilt illusion. *Vision Research*, 21, 1235–7.

Lovegrove, W.J., Bowling, A., Badcock, D., & Blackwood, M. (1980). Specific reading disability: Differences in contrast sensitivity as a function of spatial frequency. *Science*, 210(4468), 439–40.

Lurie, D.I., Pasic, T.R., Hockfield, S.J., & Rubel, E.W. (1997). Development of Cat-301 immunoreactivity in auditory brainstem nuclei of the gerbil. *Journal of Comparative Neurology*, 380(3), 319–34.

Maddess, T., Goldberg, I., Dobinson, J., Wine, S., Welsh, A.-H., & James, A.-C. (1999). Testing for glaucoma with the spatial frequency doubling illusion. *Vision Research*, 39(25), 4258–73.

Manis, F., McBride-Chang, C., Seidenberg, M., Doi, L., & Petersen, A. (1997). On the bases of two subtypes of developmental dyslexia. *Cognition*, 58, 157–95.

Martin, F., & Lovegrove, W. (1984). The effects of field size and luminance on contrast sensitivity differences between specifically reading disabled and normal children. *Neuropsychologia*, 22, 73–7.

Martin, F., & Lovegrove, W. (1987). Flicker contrast sensitivity in normal and specifically disabled readers. *Perception*, 16, 215–21.

Mason, A., Cornelissen, P., Fowler, M.S., & Stein, J.F. (1993) Contrast sensitivity, ocular dominance and reading disability. *Clinical Visual Science*, 8, 345–53.

Maunsell, J.H. (1992). Functional visual streams. *Current Opinion in Neurobiology*, 2(4), 506–10.

McAnally, K.I., & Stein, J.F. (1996). Auditory temporal coding in dyslexia. *Proceedings of the Royal Society of London Series B Biological Sciences*, 263, 961–5.

Merigan, W.H., & Maunsell, J.H. (1990). Macaque vision after magnocellular lateral geniculate lesions. *Visual Neuroscience*, 5(4), 347–52.

Murakami, I., & Cavanagh, P. (1998). A jitter after-effect reveals motion-based stabilization of vision. *Nature*, 395, 798–801.

Nicolson, R.I. (2001a). Developmental dyslexia: the cerebellar deficit hypothesis. *Trends in Neurosciences*, 24(9), 508.

Nicolson, R.I. (2001b). Dyslexia, development and the cerebellum. *Trends in Neurosciences*, 24(9), 515.

Odegard, T.N., Farris, E.A., Ring, J., McColl, R., & Black, J. (2009). Brain connectivity in non-reading impaired children and children diagnosed with developmental dyslexia. *Neuropsychologia*, 47(8–9), 1972–7.

Pammer, K., & Wheatley, C. (2001). Isolating the M(y)-cell response in dyslexia using the spatial frequency doubling illusion. *Vision Research*, 41, 2139–48.

Paracchini, S., Thomas, A., Castro, S., Lai, C., Paramasivam, M., Wang, Y., *et al.* (2006). The chromosome 6p22 haplotype associated with dyslexia reduces the expression of KIAA0319, a novel gene involved in neuronal migration. *Human Molecular Genetics*, 15(10), 1659–66.

Porteous, D. (2008). Genetic causality in schizophrenia and bipolar disorder: out with the old and in with the new. *Current Opinion in Genetics & Development*, 18(3), 229–34.

Pugh, K.R., Sandak, R., Frost, S.J., Moore, D., & Mencl, W.E. (2005). Examing reading development and reading disability in English language learners: Potential contributions form functional neuroimaging. *Learning Disabilities Research & Practice*, 20(1), 24–30.

Rae, C., Harasty, J.A., Dzendrowskyj, T.E., Talcott, J.B., Simpson, J.M., Blamire, A.M., *et al.* (2002). Cerebellar morphology in developmental dyslexia. *Neuropsychologia,* 40(8), 1285–92.

Ramus, F. (2004). Neurobiology of dyslexia: a reinterpretation of the data. *Trends in Neurosciences,* 27(12), 720.

Ramus, F., Rosen, S., Dakin, S.C., Day, B.L., Castellote, J.M., White, S., *et al.* (2003). Theories of developmental dyslexia: insights from a multiple case study of dyslexic adults. *Brain,* 126, 841–65.

Rauschecker, J.P., & Tian, B. (2000). Mechanisms and streams for processing of 'what' and 'where' in auditory cortex. *Proceedings of the National Academy of Sciences of the United States of America,* 97(22), 11800–6.

Ray, N.J., Fowler, S., & Stein, J.F. (2005). Yellow filters can improve magnocellular function: motion sensitivity, convergence, accommodation, and reading. *Annals of the New York Academy of Science,* 1039, 283–93.

Richardson, A. J., & Montgomery, P. (2005). The Oxford-Durham study: a randomized, controlled trial of dietary supplementation with fatty acids in children with developmental coordination disorder. *Pediatrics,* 115(5), 1360–6.

Robichon, F., Besson, M., & Habib, M. (2002). An electrophysiological study of dyslexic and control adults in a sentence reading task. *Biological Psychology,* 59, 29–53.

Samar, V. J., & Parasnis, I. (2005). Dorsal stream deficits suggest hidden dyslexia among deaf poor readers: Correlated evidence from reduced perceptual speed and elevated coherent motion detection thresholds. *Brain and Cognition,* 58(3), 300–11.

Shaywitz, S., Shaywitz, B., Pugh, K., Fulbright, R., Constable, R., Mencl, W., *et al.* (1998). Functional disruption in the organization of the brain for reading in dyslexia. *Proceedings of the National Academy of Sciences of the United States of America,* 3(5), 2636–41.

Singleton, C., & Henderson, L. M. (2007). Computerized screening for visual stress in children with dyslexia. *Dyslexia,* 13(2), 130–51.

Skottun, B.C. (1997). The magnocellular deficit theory of dyslexia. *Trends in Neurosciences,* 20, 397–8.

Skottun, B.C. (2010). Rats, dyslexia, and the magnocellular system. *Cortex,* 46(6), 799.

Skottun, B.C., & Skoyles, J.R. (2011). On identifying magnocellular and parvocellular responses on the basis of contrast-response functions. *Schizophrenia Bulletin,* 37(1), 23–6.

Skoyles, J., & Skottun, B.C. (2004). On the prevalence of magnocellular deficits in the visual system of non-dyslexic individuals. *Brain and Language,* 88(1), 79–82.

Snowling, M. (2000). *Dyslexia.* Oxford: Blackwell Press.

Snowling, M., Goulandris, N., Bowlby, M., & Howell, P. (1986). Segmentation and speech perception in relation to reading skill: a developmental analysis. *Journal of Experimental Child Psychology,* 41(3), 489–507.

Sperling, A.J., Lu, Z.-L., Manis, F.R., & Seidenberg, M.S. (2005). Deficits in perceptual noise exclusion in developmental dyslexia. *Nature Neuroscience,* 8(7), 862–3.

Stanovich, K.E. (1996). Toward a more inclusive definition of dyslexia. *Dyslexia,* 2(3), 154–66.

Stein, J.F. (1986). Role of the cerebellum in the visual guidance of movement. *Nature,* 323(6085), 217–21.

Stein, J. (1992). The representation of egocentric space in the posterior parietal cortex. *Behavioral and Brain Sciences,* 15(4), 691–700.

Stein, J. (2001). The magnocellular theory of developmental dyslexia. *Dyslexia,* 7, 12–36.

Stein, J., & Fowler, S. (1985). Effect of monocular occlusion on visuomotor perception and reading in dyslexic children. *Lancet,* 2(8446), 69–73.

Stein, J., & Walsh, V. (1997). To see but not to read; the magnocellular theory of dyslexia. *Trends-Neurosci,* 20(4), 147–52.

Stein, J., & Fowler, S. (2005). Treatment of visual problems in children with reading difficulties. *PATOSS (Professional association of teachers in special situations) Bulletin*, 15–22.

Stein, J.F., & Fowler, S. (1982). Ocular motor dyslexia. *Dyslexia Review*, 5, 25–8.

Stein, J.F., Richardson, A.J., & Fowler, M.S. (2000). Monocular occlusion can improve binocular control and reading in dyslexics. *Brain*, 123(Pt 1), 164–70.

Stoodley, C., & Stein, J. (2011). The cerebellum and dyslexia. *Cortex*, 47, 101–16.

Stoodley, C., Talcott, J. B., Carter, E. L., Witton, C., & Stein, J. F. (2000). Selective deficits of vibrotactile sensitivity in dyslexic readers. *Neuroscience Letters*, 295(1–2), 13–16.

Stoodley, C.J., Hill, P.R., Stein, J.F., & Bishop, D.V. (2006). Auditory event-related potentials differ in dyslexics even when auditory psychophysical performance is normal. *Brain Research*, 1121(1), 190–9.

Talcott, J.B. (2003). Sensory and cognitive constraints on information processing during reading: Do the eyes have it? *Contemporary Psychology*, 48, 62–5.

Talcott, J.B., Hansen, P.C., Assoku, E.L., & Stein, J.F. (2000a). Visual motion sensitivity in dyslexia: evidence for temporal and motion energy integration deficits. *Neuropsychologia*, 38, 935–43.

Talcott, J.B., Witton, C., McLean, M.F., Hansen, P.C., Rees, A., Green, G.G., *et al.* (2000b). Dynamic sensory sensitivity and children's word decoding skills. *Proceedings of the National Academy of Sciences of the United States of America*, 97(6), 2952–7.

Tallal, P., & Piercy, M. (1973). Defects of non-verbal auditory perception in children with developmental aphasia. *Nature*, 241(5390), 468–9.

Ungerleider, L.G., & Mishkin, M. (1982). Two cortical visual systems. In: D.J. Ingle, M.A. Goodale, & R.J.W. Mansfield (Eds.) *The Analysis of Visual Behavior*, pp. 549–86. Cambridge, MA: MIT Press.

Vidyasagar, T.R. (2004). Neural underpinnings of dyslexia as a disorder of visuo-spatial attention. *Clinical and Experimental Optometry*, 87(1), 4–10.

Vincent, A., Deacon, R., Dalton, P., Salmond, C., Blamire, A.M., Pendlebury, S., *et al.* (2002). Maternal antibody mediated dyslexia? Evidence for a pathogenic serum factor in a mother of 2 dyslexic children shown by transfer to pregnant mice shown by behavioural and MRS studies. *Journal of Neuroimmunology*, 45, 87–9.

Wilkins, A.J., Evans, B.J., Brown, J.A., Busby, A.E., Wingfield, A.E., Jeanes, R.J., *et al.* (1994). Double-masked placebo-controlled trial of precision spectral filters in children who use coloured overlays. *Ophthalmic and Physiological Optics*, 14(4), 365–370.

Williams, J., & O'Donovan, M. (2006). The genetics of developmental dyslexia. *European Journal of Human Genetics*, 14(6), 681–9.

Williams, M.J., Stuart, G.W., Castles, A., & McAnally, K.I. (2003). Contrast sensitivity in subgroups of developmental dyslexia. *Vision Research*, 43(4), 467–77.

Witton, C., Stein, J.F., Stoodley, C.J., Rosner, B.S., & Talcott, J.B. (2002). Separate influences of acoustic AM and FM sensitivity on the phonological decoding skills of impaired and normal readers. *Journal of Cognitive Neuroscience*, 14, 866–74.

Yarbus, A.-L. (1965). *Role of eye movements in the visual process*. Moscow: Nauka.

Index